# NATURE'S CURES

## HELPS YOU FIND RELIEF THE NATURAL WAY

**ASTHMA**—On the verge of an asthma attack? Help may be just a cup of coffee away. Research shows that drinking a cup or two of coffee can actually ward off an asthma attack or treat one in an emergency. You may also breathe easier after a session of yoga, biofeedback or visualization.

**DIABETES**—Watching your diet? That's good, but don't deny yourself a healthy helping of beans. The soluble fiber in beans helps keep blood sugar under control and helps prevent heart disease. You may also find your condition responds to acupuncture, biofeedback, strength training and even pet therapy.

**PREVENTION OF HEART ATTACK**—A prescription for a healthy heart should include lots of carrots (packed with beta-carotene), black tea (rich in polyphenols), and a few good friends. Scientists say the more social connections you have the less likely you are to die from heart disease—or any other cause.

**PMS**—Feeling frazzled and out of sorts? Nothing spells relief like aromatherapy: just add a few drops of bergamot, chamomile, clary-sage, jonquil, and nutmeg oils to a bath and relax. Or try a session of therapeutic touch to rebalance your energy and leave you feeling unruffled.

S0-BED-043

# NATURE'S CURES

## MICHAEL CASTLEMAN

*Medical Reviewer:* Henry Edward Altenberg, M.D.,
Attending Geriatric Psychiatrist at Frisbee Memorial Hospital
in Rochester, New Hampshire, and Co-director of the
Spruce Creek Holistic Center in Kittery, Maine

**BANTAM BOOKS**
New York • Toronto • London • Sydney • Auckland

**Notice**
This book is intended as a reference volume only, not as a medical manual. The information given here is designed to help you make informed decisions about your health. It is not intended as a substitute for any treatment that may have been prescribed by your doctor. If you suspect that you have a medical problem, we urge you to seek competent medical help.

NATURE'S CURES

A Bantam Book/published by arrangement with Rodale Press, Inc.

Publishing History
Rodale Press edition published 1996
Bantam edition / June 1997

ISBN 0-553-57696-8

*Published simultaneously in the United States and Canada*

PRINTED IN THE UNITED STATES OF AMERICA

OPM   10   9   8   7   6   5   4   3   2

Pearl Rubin
(1903–1996)
A lifelong advocate of Nature's cures


*The healer of disease is Nature.*
—Hippocrates

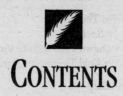

# CONTENTS

**Chapter 28: Visualization, Guided Imagery**
**and Self-Hypnosis** . . . . . . . . . . . . . . . .443
*Tapping into the Healing Power of Your Mind*
From Mesmerism to Visualization • The Healing Power of
Images • The Body Listens • Opening a Window to Better
Health • Beginning Deep Relaxation • Beginning Visualization:
The Beach • Visualizations for Specific Health Concerns

**Chapter 29: Vitamins and Minerals** . . . . . . . . . . .459
*The New Science of Sensible Supplementation*
Sweet Vindication • Antioxidants to the Rescue • RDAs,
Megadoses and Supplement Safety • Taking Supplements without
Getting Taken • Prevention and Treatment with Supplements

**Chapter 30: Walking** . . . . . . . . . . . . . . .481
*Terrific Exercise, One Step at a Time*
Walk It Off • Shoring Up Brittle Bones • Walking Away from
Illness • Getting Started • The Sole of Walking Shoes

**Chapter 31: Water** . . . . . . . . . . . . . . . .492
*The Elixir of Life*
Sip, Sip, Hooray! • Thirst Is Worst • Troubled Waters •
Let the Buyer Beware • Finding a Safe Supply

**Chapter 32: Weight Training** . . . . . . . . . . . .507
*Putting Muscle to Work for Health*
How Strength Benefits the Body • Getting Started

**Chapter 33: Yoga** . . . . . . . . . . . . . . . .513
*Stretch the Body, Mind and Spirit*
Doctors Take a Stand • Science Documents Yoga's Benefits •
Yoga, American-Style • How to Learn the Moves •
For Best Results

# ACKNOWLEDGMENTS

The love and companionship of Anne Simons and Jeffrey and Maya Castleman are my first-choice natural therapies for all of life's challenges.

Alice Feinstein, my editor at Rodale Press, deserves high praise for her vision, judgment and charm. Thanks also to Rodale research editor Bernadette Sukley and Debora Yost, vice-president and editorial director of Rodale Health and Fitness Books, for their support of *Nature's Cures*.

Thanks to Henry Edward Altenberg, M.D., for his thorough and careful medical review of this work.

Thanks also to Katinka Matson and John Brockman, my agents at Brockman, Inc., who have provided outstanding representation for 19 years.

I would also like to thank the many friends and editors who, over the years, have contributed to my understanding of Nature's cures or provided opportunities to learn more about them: Anne Alexander, Mark Bricklin, Deke Castleman, Mildred and Louis Castleman, Richard Day, M.D., Nancy Evens, Donna Farhi, David Fenton, Neshama Franklin, Wayne Kalyn, Jim Keough, Jeffrey Klein, Jon King, Carolyn Latteier, Paul Libassi, Jean Maguire, James Petersen, Carole Pisarczyk, Mark Powelson, Ted Rand, Tom Rawls, Amy Rennert, Robert Rodale, Emma Segal, Matt Segal, Linda Sparrowe, Jim Spaulding, Annie Stine, Barbara Tannenbaum, Bill Thomson, Trisha Thompson and Wallace Turner.

Finally, I would like to thank the researchers and practitioners whose generosity, expertise and insights helped shape *Nature's Cures*:

- William C. Adams, Ph.D., professor of physical education at the University of California at Davis.
- David Alper, D.P.M., podiatrist in Belmont, Massachusetts.
- Paul Amato, Ph.D., professor of sociology at the University of Nebraska at Lincoln.
- Phillip Ament, D.D.S., Ph.D., dentist and psychologist in Buffalo, New York.
- Linda Anderson, spokesperson for the National Cancer Institute.
- Jean Antonello, R.N., nurse in New Brighton, Minnesota.
- Dorothy Barbo, M.D., director of the Center for Women's Health at the University of New Mexico in Albuquerque.
- Neil Barnard, M.D., president of the Physicians Committee for Responsible Medicine in Washington, D.C.
- Robert Baron, Ph.D., professor in the School of Management at Rensselaer Polytechnic Institute in Troy, New York.
- Harriet Beinfield, L.Ac., San Francisco acupuncturist and practitioner of traditional Chinese medicine.
- Herbert Benson, M.D., associate professor of medicine at Harvard Medical School and president of the Mind/Body Medical Institute at New England Deaconess Hospital in Boston.
- Steven Blair, P.E.D., director of epidemiology at the Cooper Institute for Aerobics Research in Dallas.
- Gladys Block, Ph.D., professor of epidemology and nutrition at the University of California at Berkeley School of Public Health.
- Mark Blumenthal, executive director of the American Botanical Council in Austin, Texas.
- Helen Bonny, Ph.D., music therapist and president of the Bonny Foundation in Salina, Kansas.
- Joan Borysenko, Ph.D., president of Mind/Body Health Sciences in Boulder, Colorado.
- Ray Breitenbach, M.D., associate clinical professor of family medicine at Wayne State University School of Medicine in Detroit.

- Arline Bronzaft, Ph.D., professor of psychology at Lehman College of the City University of New York.
- Kelly Brownell, Ph.D., professor of psychology at Yale University.
- Al Bumanis, spokesperson for the National Association for Music Therapy in Silver Spring, Maryland.
- David Burns, M.D., professor of psychiatry and research clinical psychiatrist at the University of Pennsylvania Medical Center in Philadelphia.
- Francine Butler, Ph.D., executive director of the Association for Applied Psychophysiology and Biofeedback in Wheat Ridge, Colorado.
- Patricia Carrington, Ph.D., clinical associate professor of psychiatry at the University of Medicine and Dentistry of New Jersey/Robert Wood Johnson Medical School in Piscataway.
- Dennis Chernin, M.D., physician in Ann Arbor, Michigan.
- Nancy Clark, R.D., director of nutrition services at SportsMedicine in Brookline, Massachusetts.
- William E. Connor, M.D., professor of medicine and clinical nutrition at Oregon Health Sciences University in Portland.
- Robert K. Cooper, Ph.D., president of the Center for Health and Fitness Excellence in Bemidji, Minnesota.
- Edward Coyle, Ph.D., director of the Human Performance Laboratory at the University of Texas in Austin.
- Alison Crane, R.N., psychiatric nurse in Skokie, Illinois, and founder of the American Association of Therapeutic Humor.
- William Dement, M.D., Ph.D., professor of psychiatry and behavioral science at Stanford University and director of the Stanford Sleep Disorders Clinic.
- Elliot Dick, Ph.D., chief of the Respiratory Viruses Laboratory at the University of Wisconsin at Madison.
- Larry Dossey, M.D., co-chair of the Panel on Mind-Body Interventions of the Office of Alternative Medicine at the National Institutes of Health in Bethesda, Maryland.
- James Duke, Ph.D., botanist at the U.S. Department of Agriculture Research Station in Beltsville, Maryland.
- John Duncan, Ph.D., associate director of the Cooper Institute for Aerobics Research in Dallas.

- George Eby, president of Eby Research in Austin, Texas.
- Alan Elkin, Ph.D., psychotherapist and director of the Stress Management Counseling Center in New York City.
- Frank Falck, M.D., Ph.D., assistant clinical professor of surgery at the University of Connecticut School of Medicine in Farmington.
- Mark Fenton, of Cohasset, Massachusetts, five-time member of the U.S. National Racewalking Team and technical editor at *Walking* magazine.
- Tom Ferguson, M.D., self-care pioneer from Austin, Texas.
- Kenneth Ferraro, Ph.D., professor of sociology at Purdue University in West Lafayette, Indiana.
- William Fezler, Ph.D., psychotherapist in Beverly Hills.
- Maria Fiatarone, M.D., professor of medicine at Harvard Medical School.
- Tiffany Field, Ph.D., professor of psychology, pediatrics and psychiatry at the University of Miami Medical School and director of the Touch Research Institute there.
- Helen Flapan, co-founder (with Mark Flapan, Ph.D.) of the New York Scleroderma Society and the Scleroderma Federation.
- Carol Franz, Ph.D., visiting professor of psychology at Boston University.
- Dale Freeberg, O.D., behavioral optometrist in Hawthorne, California.
- Michael Freeman, M.D., psychiatrist in San Francisco.
- Meyer Friedman, M.D., cardiologist and director of the Meyer Friedman Research Institute at Mount Zion Medical Center in San Francisco.
- Michael Reed Gach, founder of the American Acupressure Institute in Berkeley, California.
- Cedric Garland, Ph.D., associate professor of epidemiology at the University of California at San Diego.
- Donald Getz, O.D., behavioral optometrist in Van Nuys, California.
- Leslie Gibson, R.N., founder of the Comedy Carts program at Morton Plant Hospital in Clearwater, Florida.
- Joel Goodman, Ed.D., executive director of The Humor Project in Saratoga Springs, New York.

- Ron Goor, M.D., and Nancy Goor, authorities on low-fat eating and weight control in Bethesda, Maryland.
- Arthur Grayzel, M.D., Philadelphia rheumatologist and consultant to the Arthritis Foundation.
- Joe Graedon and Teresa Graedon, Ph.D., pharmacists, authors, syndicated columnists and radio hosts.
- Shirley Grazsi, executive director of the New Jersey Coalition against Aircraft Noise in Cranford.
- Elmer Green, Ph.D., director emeritus of the Center for Applied Psychophysiology at the Menninger Clinic in Topeka, Kansas.
- Ronald Griffiths, Ph.D., professor of psychiatry and neuroscience at Johns Hopkins University School of Medicine in Baltimore.
- Jack Gwaltney, M.D., professor of medicine at the University of Virginia in Charlottesville.
- William Halcomb, D.O., physician in Mesa, Arizona.
- Diane Hanson, R.N., Ph.D., psychologist at the Pritikin Longevity Center in Santa Monica, California.
- Scott Hasson, Ed.D., associate professor of physical therapy at Texas Women's University in Houston.
- Peter Hauri, Ph.D., director of the Mayo Clinic Insomnia Research and Treatment Program in Rochester, Minnesota.
- Suzanne Havala, R.D., dietitian in Charlotte, North Carolina.
- Sheldon Saul Hendler, M.D., Ph.D., assistant clinical professor of medicine at the University of California at San Diego.
- J. Owen Hendley, professor of medicine at the University of Virginia in Charlottesville.
- Charles Hennekens, M.D., professor of medicine, ambulatory care and prevention at Harvard Medical School.
- Alan Hirsch, M.D., neurologic director of the Smell and Taste Research Foundation in Chicago.
- J. Allan Hobson, M.D., professor of psychiatry at Harvard University.
- Cynthia Husted, R.N., Ph.D., tai chi researcher at the University of California at Santa Barbara.
- William Jarvis, Ph.D., hematologist in Mountain View, California, professor of preventive medicine at Loma Linda University

Medical School in California and president of the National Coalition against Health Fraud.

- Jon Kabat-Zinn, Ph.D., associate professor of medicine at the University of Massachusetts Medical Center in Worcester and director of the Stress Reduction Clinic there.
- Gary Kaplan, M.D., physician and acupuncturist in Arlington, Virginia.
- Avi Karni, M.D., Ph.D., staff researcher at the National Institute of Mental Health Laboratory of Neurophysiology.
- Allen Klein, San Francisco "jollytologist" and authority on healing humor.
- Lawrence Klein, vice president of Thought Technology in Montreal, Quebec.
- Ronette Kolotkin, Ph.D., director of behavioral programs at the Duke University Diet and Fitness Center in Durham, North Carolina.
- Harvey Komet, M.D., San Antonio otolaryngologist.
- Stephen LaBerge, Ph.D., Stanford University dream researcher and director of the Lucidity Institute in Portola Valley, California.
- Marcel Lavabre, co-founder of the American Aromatherapy Association.
- Harold Leitenberg, Ph.D., professor of psychology at the University of Vermont in Burlington.
- Michael Lerner, Ph.D., director of the Commonweal Cancer Help Program in Bolinas, California.
- Arnold Levick, D.D.S., dentist in Albuquerque.
- Shari Lieberman, Ph.D., clinical nutritionist in New York City.
- Bonnie Liebman, director of nutrition at the Center for Science in the Public Interest in Washington, D.C.
- Allan Luks, director of Big Brothers/Big Sisters of New York.
- Edward Madara, director of the American Self-Help Clearinghouse in Denville, New Jersey.
- JoAnn Manson, M.D., associate professor of medicine at Harvard Medical School and director of women's health at Brigham and Women's Hospital in Boston.
- Mary Jane Massie, M.D., attending psychiatrist at Memorial Sloan-Kettering Cancer Center and professor of clinical

psychiatry at Cornell University Medical Center, both in
New York City.

- Alexander Mauskop, Ph.D., director of the New York
Headache Center in New York City.
- Emmett Miller, M.D., psychiatrist in Stanford, California.
- Stephen Miller, O.D., director of clinical care for the American
Optometric Association in St. Louis.
- George Milowe, M.D., Saratoga Springs, New York, psychiatrist.
- Edwin Morris, aromatherapist in Pelham, New York.
- Daniel Mowrey, Ph.D., director of the American Phytotherapy
Research Laboratory in Salt Lake City.
- Suki Munsell, Ph.D., director of the Dynamic Walking Institute
in Corte Madera, California.
- Alfred Munzer, M.D., former president of the American Lung
Association.
- David Nieman, D.H.Sc., professor of health promotions in the
Department of Health, Leisure and Exercise Science at Appala-
chian State University in Boone, North Carolina.
- Christiane Northrup, M.D., gynecologist in Yarmouth, Maine.
- Karen Olness, M.D., professor of pediatrics at Case Western
Reserve Medical Center in Cleveland.
- Susan Olson, Ph.D., psychologist and weight-loss consultant in
Portland, Oregon.
- Dean Ornish, M.D., president of the Preventive Medicine
Research Institute in Sausalito, California.
- Neal Owens, founder of the The SunBox Company in
Gaithersburg, Maryland.
- Bruce Paton, M.D., professor of surgery at the University of
Colorado School of Medicine in Denver.
- David Perlmutter, M.D., neurologist and preventive medical
specialist in Naples, Florida.
- David Phillips, Ph.D., professor of sociology at the University
of California at San Diego.
- Susan Potter, Ph.D., assistant professor of food sciences and
nutrition at the University of Illinois in Urbana-Champaign.
- Joan Price, a Sebastopol, California, aerobics instructor and
weight-control authority.

- Mary Pullig Schatz, M.D., Nashville pathologist on the staff of the Centennial Medical Center and a member of the American College of Sports Medicine.
- Trish Ratto, R.D., coordinator of Health Matters, the employee wellness program at the University of California at Berkeley.
- Stephen Rennard, M.D., chief of pulmonary and critical care medicine at the University of Nebraska in Omaha.
- Stella Resnick, Ph.D., Los Angeles clinical psychologist.
- James Rippe, M.D., director of the Exercise Physiology and Nutrition Laboratory at the University of Massachusetts Medical Center in Worcester.
- Sheah Rorback, R.D., Miami dietitian.
- Martin Rossman, M.D., clinical associate professor of medicine at the University of California's San Francisco Medical Center.
- Thomas Roth, Ph.D., director of the Henry Ford Hospital Sleep Disorders Center in Detroit.
- Julia Rowland, Ph.D., assistant professor of psychiatry at Georgetown University Medical Center in Washington, D.C., and director of psycho-oncology at the Vincent T. Lombardi Cancer Center there.
- Kenneth Sancier, Ph.D., staff member of the Chi Gong Institute in San Francisco.
- Susan Schiffman, Ph.D., professor of psychology at Duke University in Durham, North Carolina.
- Jay Schindler, Ph.D., professor of health education at the University of Wisconsin in LaCrosse.
- Nancy Schwartz, biofeedback therapist in Orange, Florida.
- George Schwartz, M.D., specialist in emergency medicine and toxicology in Santa Fe, New Mexico.
- Dean Shapiro, Ph.D., associate professor of psychiatry and human behavior at the University of California at Irvine.
- Anne Simons, M.D., assistant clinical professor of family and community medicine at the University of California's San Francisco Medical Center.
- Maria Simonson, Ph.D., Sc.D., director of the Health, Weight and Stress Clinic at Johns Hopkins University in Baltimore.

- Mark Sisti, Ph.D., associate director of the Center for Cognitive Therapy in New York City.
- David Sobel, M.D., regional director of patient education and director of the regional education department at Kaiser Permanente Medical Care Program of Northern California.
- William Sonis, M.D., professor of psychiatry at the University of Pennsylvania in Philadelphia.
- Olive Soriero, M.D., gynecologic oncologist on the staff of St. Vincent's Hospital in Indianapolis.
- David Spiegel, M.D., professor of psychiatry at Stanford University and director of the Psychosocial Treatment Laboratory there.
- Waneen Spirduso, Ed.D., professor of kinesiology and health eduation at the University of Texas in Austin.
- Bryant Stamford, Ph.D., director of the Health Promotion Center at the University of Louisville School of Medicine in Kentucky.
- Steven Subotnick, D.P.M., podiatrist in Hayward, California.
- Rob Sweetgall, president of Creative Walking, Inc., in Clayton, Missouri.
- Leonard Syme, Ph.D., professor of epidemiology at the University of California at Berkeley School of Public Health.
- Michael Terman, Ph.D., director of the Light Therapy Unit at Columbia Presbyterian Medical Center in New York City.
- Varro Tyler, Ph.D., professor of pharmacognosy (natural product pharmacy) at Purdue University in West Lafayette, Indiana.
- George Ulett, M.D., Ph.D., director of the Department of Psychiatry at Deaconess Hospital in St. Louis and clinical professor of psychiatry at the University of Missouri School of Medicine.
- Dana Ullman, president of Homeopathic Educational Services in Berkeley, California, and author of several books on homeopathy.
- Thomas Wadden, Ph.D., director of the Center for Health and Behavior at Syracuse University in New York.
- James Walsh, Ph.D., director of the Sleep Disorders Clinic at St. Luke's Medical Center in St. Louis, Missouri.

- Hope Warshaw, R.D., dietitian in Newton, Massachusetts.
- Andrew Weil, M.D., professor of preventive medicine, director of the Program in Integrative Medicine and associate director of the Division of Social Perspectives in Medicine at the University of Arizona College of Medicine in Tucson.
- James White, Ph.D., professor emeritus of physical education at the University of California at San Diego and director of the Human Performance Laboratory there.
- Laurens White, M.D., clinical professor of oncology at the University of California's San Francisco Medical Center.
- Walter Willett, M.D., Dr.P.H., chair of the Department of Nutrition at Harvard University.
- Eileen Marie Wright, M.D., physician in Maitland, Florida.
- Bruce Zahn, director of psychology and cognitive therapy at Presbyterian Medical Center in Philadelphia.
- Mitchell Zeller, special assistant for policy at the Food and Drug Administration in Rockville, Maryland.

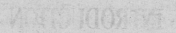

# INTRODUCTION

## Safe, Effective, Natural Self-Care

*Nature's Cures* explores 33 valuable and fascinating healing arts—some ancient, others recently discovered; some from folk healing traditions, others from scientific laboratories; some probably familiar, others possibly exotic. But despite their differences, they are all safe, effective, self-care-oriented and natural. These terms require a bit of explanation.

*Safe* means that when used appropriately, all the therapies in *Nature's Cures* can be used confidently, without fear that they might cause harm. Of course, when used inappropriately, some of Nature's cures *can* cause harm. Where appropriate, the book includes safety warnings, which readers should take seriously.

*Effective* means that rigorous scientific studies support the therapies' value. Those interested in the scientific references demonstrating the therapies' effectiveness may consult the Bibliography Note on page 525.

*Self-care–oriented* means that most of the therapies in *Nature's Cures* can be used without the help of professional practitioners. However, some require professional care. It's not prudent to perform acupuncture on oneself, so *Nature's Cures* focuses on acupressure, or massage of the same points, which in most cases can be self-administered. Where appropriate, the book also includes suggestions for finding professional practitioners: acupuncturists, biofeedback trainers, behavioral optometrists, yoga and tai chi teachers and so on.

*Natural* is a word whose meaning has been, unfortunately, warped by misuse and debased by often-questionable advertising claims. As used here, natural connotes a philosophy of healing distinct from that of conventional medicine. The table on the opposite page shows the differences.

No single school of healing has all the answers, but most schools offer reasonable approaches to at least some conditions. Despite the shortcomings of conventional medicine, it has achieved some astonishing therapeutic results no other healing system can match in the treatment of trauma, medical emergencies, serious infections and burns and premature birth, as well as in cosmetic and rehabilitative procedures such as orthodontics and reattachment of severed limbs.

But conventional medicine has been considerably less successful in dealing with chronic degenerative conditions, such as heart disease, cancer and stroke (the nation's three leading causes of death), and the myriad of conditions that are stress-related—everything from asthma to chronic stomach distress. Nature's cures can often help treat these and other conditions.

## From "Alternative" to "Natural and Complementary"

Some of the therapies discussed in *Nature's Cures* are alternative, that is, they exist largely outside of conventional medicine. Examples are acupuncture, aromatherapy, herbal medicine and homeopathy. But in recent years, the term *alternative* has become increasingly problematic. Although these therapies are still outside the medical mainstream, growing numbers of physicians now include acupuncture, homeopathy and herbal medicine in their practices.

In addition, over the last decade, several natural therapies that were once considered alternative have become largely integrated into conventional medicine. Among them are exercise, low-fat diet, massage, meditation, dietary supplements and

# Conventional versus Natural

What's the difference between conventional and natural medicine? A whole world of philosophy and outlook.

| Conventional Medicine | Natural Medicine |
| --- | --- |
| Emphasizes diagnosis and treatment. | Emphasizes disease prevention. |
| Views the mind and body as separate, with little effect on each other. | Views the mind and body as one, the "bodymind." Anything that affects one affects the other. |
| Views the body as essentially a machine with disease resulting when parts break. | Views the body as a living microcosm of the universe, with disease resulting when forces that act on it become unbalanced. |
| Views medicine as a military campaign. Seeks better "weapons" to "combat" disease. | Views medicine as an effort to restore mind/body harmony. |
| Views the body as the passive recipient of treatments that "fix" it. | Views the body as capable of self-repair and administers treatments to support self-healing. |
| Patients obey doctors' orders. | Individuals take an active role in their healing. |
| Primary treatments include pharmaceuticals, surgery and radiation. | Primary treatments include diet, exercise, stress management, social support and herbal medicines. |
| Focuses on disease. | Focuses on illness, the human experience of disease. |
| Focuses on pain. | Focuses on suffering, the human experience of pain. |
| Goal is cure. | Goal is healing, the individual's experience of physical, mental and spiritual wholeness. |

yoga. Finally, some natural therapies that may appear alternative actually emerged from conventional medical research: biofeedback, bright light therapy, cognitive therapy, lucid dreaming and vision therapy.

*Alternative* implies an either/or situation: You either take drugs for your back pain or you try an alternative, such as yoga. But as Nature's cures become increasingly incorporated into conventional medicine, we see fewer either/or situations and more reliance on judicious combinations of mainstream procedures and natural therapies. Someone with severe back pain might be advised to take pain medication for a few days and then begin a walking program, enroll in a yoga class and lose weight by adopting a low-fat diet.

Finally, the very notion that, say, herbal medicine is "alternative" while antidepressant medications are "mainstream" is myopic. The large majority of the world's population has relied on herbal medicine for the vast majority of recorded history, while antidepressants have been used by only a tiny fraction of humanity for a very brief period of time. If healing arts were judged by worldwide numerical support or duration of use, many "alternative" therapies would be "mainstream," and vice versa.

Experts who chart medical trends no longer call Nature's cures alternative but complementary. These cures don't replace what's taught in medical schools but rather complete it. They fill in what's been missing—an appreciation for the body's innate self-healing abilities supported by diet, exercise, the mind, human touch, social connections, traditional healing arts and spiritual exploration.

Use the natural therapies described in *Nature's Cures* to enhance your well-being and prevent illness. When illness strikes, use them to complement your physician's treatment plan.

—Michael Castleman

# NATURE'S CURE-FINDER

## Selecting the Best Treatment

When you want to treat a disease or condition, how do you know which method is best? Simply look up the condition in this guide to find which methods hold the greatest promise.

### CHAPTER 1

# ACUPUNCTURE AND ACUPRESSURE

**W**hen something hurts, you rub it. Since the dawn of time, people around the world have rubbed, poked and massaged the body to heal dozens of ailments.

The ancient Chinese were well aware of the healing power of touch, but thousands of years ago, they gave it their own unique spin. According to legend, on the eve of a battle, a Chinese soldier had an illness his physicians could not cure. During the fighting, he was hit by an arrow and received a superficial wound. The wound healed, and oddly, so did his illness.

Over time, other soldiers who received penetrating injuries from knives, spears or arrows also experienced unexpected relief from health problems elsewhere in their bodies. Intrigued, ancient Chinese physicians began recording the places where stab wounds produced improbable healing. Eventually their observations became the foundation for acupuncture and its offshoots, acupressure, shiatsu and reflexology.

Acupuncture involves the insertion of fine needles into the skin at specific points around the body. Acupressure and its

17

Japanese counterpart, shiatsu, dispense with needles and use deep fingertip massage of the same points. (*Shiatsu* is a combination of two Japanese words, *shi*, meaning "finger" and *atsu*, meaning "pressure.") Reflexology uses finger pressure on just the feet, hands and ears.

Needle acupuncture is better known and more popular than its fingertip cousins, and experts consider it more effective. Acupressure puts some people off because they doubt their ability to find the therapeutic points for self-treatment. In fact, it's easy to find useful points. For some detailed instructions on how to treat several common ailments with acupressure, see "Press Your Way to Better Health" on page 32.

Unless otherwise noted, this chapter uses the term *acupuncture* to mean both the needle and finger-pressure therapies.

## Acupuncture Comes to the West

More than 2,000 years ago, acupuncture became a major adjunct to Chinese herbal medicine. It spread to Korea around A.D. 300 and to Japan in the seventeenth century. During the late nineteenth century, a few Western physicians—notably Sir William Osler, M.D., a Canadian physician whose medical textbooks earned him knighthood in England and a distinguished professorship at Johns Hopkins University School of Medicine in Baltimore—became fascinated by it.

In the 1912 edition of his book, *Principles and Practices of Medicine,* Dr. Osler wrote, "For lumbago, acupuncture is, in acute cases, the most efficient treatment." (Lumbago is muscle pain in the lower back.) This endorsement was deleted from subsequent editions, and outside of America's Asian communities, acupuncture remained largely unknown until 1971, when Richard Nixon became the first president to visit the People's Republic of China.

During Nixon's visit, television news programs broadcast astonishing footage of Chinese patients undergoing major surgery while fully conscious—their only anesthesia provided by a few acupuncture needles in their ears and feet. *New York Times* columnist James Reston accompanied Nixon and witnessed acupuncture anesthesia firsthand. While in China, he had to have an emergency appendectomy and decided to try acupuncture instead of narcotics to control his postsurgical pain. In his column, Reston wrote, "I've seen the past, and it works." Such praise in the nation's leading newspaper spurred tremendous interest in acupuncture—and a great deal of controversy.

Health-care consumers who felt alienated from mainstream medicine eagerly embraced acupuncture and Chinese medicine. Today acupuncturists practice in all 50 states, and experts estimate that several million Americans have been "needled."

Organized medicine, however, still tends to scoff at this age-old healing art. The American Medical Association's (AMA) Council on Scientific Affairs—its official arbiter of medical controversies—was suspicious from the moment James Reston first put pen to paper. The council viewed acupuncture as a foreign, folk-medical superstition that rode into the United States on a wave of breathless media reports without laboratory evidence of effectiveness and without any explanation of how it worked that made sense in Western scientific terms. In 1981, the AMA dismissed acupuncture as an "unproven therapy." Today more than 5,000 M.D.'s include acupuncture in their practices or refer patients to acupuncturists.

## Assessing the Evidence

When TV newscasts first showed acupuncture anesthesia in China, the American physicians who rolled their eyes included both dyed-in-the-wool medical conservatives and many advocates of mind/body medicine, who suggested that acupuncture anesthesia might actually be a form of hypnosis and that its other purported benefits might result from placebo effects.

Hypnosis can indeed be used for anesthesia. And typically, 30 percent of people who take medically worthless pills for their ills report benefit, thanks to what's known as the placebo effect—healing that takes place due to the conviction that the therapy has the power to heal.

(continued on page 22)

# A Venerable Tradition:
# A Brief Introduction to Chinese Medicine

Western medicine values the latest scientific discoveries. Chinese medicine values a tradition dating back more than 2,000 years. It's not surprising that the approach is a little different.

Chinese medicine is based on the *Nei Ching, The Yellow Emperor's Classic of Internal Medicine,* a book reportedly written long before the birth of Hippocrates, the father of Western medicine. The *Nei Ching* is a dialogue between the legendary ruler Huang-Ti and his court physician, Chi Po. Since the *Nei Ching,* thousands of books have been written about Chinese medicine, but practitioners continue to study and revere *The Yellow Emperor's Classic.*

Western medicine has been heavily influenced by Darwin's concept of the survival of the fittest, which says that all life is in constant struggle and that only the most successful competitors survive and reproduce. As the theory is applied to medicine, humans live under continual attack by the thousands of microorganisms that, in the Western view, cause most disease. We defend ourselves and counterattack with treatments that combat and ideally vanquish the microscopic enemy. Western medicine is a military campaign, a fight literally to the death, pitting "us" against "them."

## ACHIEVING THE GREAT BALANCE

Chinese medicine, in contrast, is based on the idea of balance. Life energy (*chi, qi* or *ki*) constantly flows throughout the body. In health, it is properly balanced, but if it becomes unbalanced, the result is illness. The traditional Chinese physician's job is to restore the balance using diet, acupuncture and herbal medicine.

Chi comes in two opposite but complementary forms, yin and yang, often likened to the shady and sunny sides of a hill. Neither is better than the other; they simply have different qualities. Yin phenomena include the earth, moon, night, fall and winter, cold, wetness, darkness, the feet, the left side, the female sex, tissue growth and a passive, following temperament. Yang counterparts are the heavens, the sun, day, spring and summer, heat, dryness, light, the head, the right side, the male sex, tissue breakdown and aggressive, leading temperaments. All individuals—both male and female—consist of unique combinations of yin and yang, requiring Chinese physicians to tailor treatments to individual qualities.

In Chinese medicine, all change and all healing occur in five stages that unite the outer world around us with the inner world of the body. Each stage is associated with one of the five seasons: fall, winter, spring, summer and late summer (from mid-July to mid-September). Intimately linked to the five seasons are the five elements: fire, earth, wood, metal and water. These "elements" have nothing to do with the Periodic Table of chemistry (hydrogen, oxygen, carbon and so forth). Rather, they are aspects of yin and yang chi—changeable forms of energy.

Each Chinese element relates to one season, one color and two organ systems, and they all interact in subtle, complicated ways.

Like Western doctors, Chinese physicians talk to their patients and take a medical history. But after that things get very different. A Chinese medical exam is short on Western lab tests and long on pulse-taking. Chinese physicians may spend 20 minutes feeling the pulse, inferring a good deal about the person's condition from 28 different pulse qualities: quick, taut, thready, weak and so forth. They also pay great attention to the state of the tongue and to the sound of one's breathing.

## THE DIFFERENCE IN PRACTICE

To illustrate the differences between Western and Chinese medicine, let's take the case of Maria of San Francisco, who developed red welts. Her M.D. diagnosed hives, which, according to Western medicine, are an allergic reaction caused by the body's release of excess histamine. He gave her the standard Western medication, an antihistamine, to suppress the offending chemical's activity. The an-

*(continued)*

# A Venerable Tradition: A Brief Introduction to Chinese Medicine—*Continued*

tihistamine helped, but it did not cure Maria's hives. It also made her sleepy. Her doctor switched her to a nonsedating antihistamine, but it too provided only partial relief. Frustrated, Maria decided to try Chinese medicine.

She consulted Harriet Beinfield, a licensed acupuncturist who practices Chinese medicine in San Francisco and is co-author of *Between Heaven and Earth: A Guide to Chinese Medicine*. Beinfield also diagnosed hives, but she treated the condition from a completely different perspective.

In response to Beinfield's questions, Maria mentioned that she often felt warm, dry and thirsty and that she'd been plagued for years by frequent bladder infections and canker sores. During the physical exam, Beinfield noticed that Maria had a soft, weak, rapid pulse and a red tongue.

"In Chinese medical terms," Beinfield explains, "Maria had a fire-element imbalance. Her heart, a fire organ, was overactive, and its heat was trying to escape through her skin, causing her hives. Her red tongue, canker sores, thirst and feeling of warmth provided additional

---

Studies by acupuncture researcher George A. Ulett, M.D., Ph.D., director of the Department of Psychiatry at Deaconess Hospital in St. Louis and clinical professor of psychiatry at the University of Missouri School of Medicine, suggest that acupuncture is neither hypnosis nor a placebo.

In one study, Dr. Ulett treated people who were in pain first with hypnosis and then with acupuncture. The two treatments elicited different physiological responses, and significantly, those who responded poorly to hypnosis responded well to acupuncture. "Acupuncture is not a form of hypnosis," Dr. Ulett insists.

It's also not a placebo response. Placebos (nontherapeutic "dummy" treatments) produce benefits in about one-third of those who take them, but studies sponsored by the National In-evidence that her fire chi was out of balance—too much heat (yang), and not enough moisture (yin)." Beinfield says a fire imbalance also explained Maria's history of bladder infections: "Fire from the heart typically descends to the lower body, notably the kidney, and an excess of heat in the kidney can cause bladder infections."

Beinfield inserted several acupuncture needles along Maria's pericardium meridian to "cool her heart fire" and more needles along the large intestine meridian to relieve her itching and "redirect her heart fire out through the digestive tract." She also prescribed Chinese medicinal herbs and a diet rich in cooling foods: juicy fruits and vegetables, legumes and root vegetables with a minimum of hot spices.

After six weeks of twice-weekly acupuncture treatments, Maria's hives had largely cleared, and she reported a noticeable decrease in bladder infections. As the months passed, when either symptom flared up again, she returned to Beinfield for more herbs and an acupuncture "tune-up."

stitutes of Health show that acupuncture treatment of pain—including pain from migraines and arthritis—is effective in about 60 percent of cases.

"Most good studies of acupuncture pain relief show effectiveness in the range of 55 to 85 percent," Dr. Ulett explains. "I've used it to treat several thousand people with many different painful conditions, including low back pain, arthritis, sciatica, headaches, sports injuries and carpal tunnel syndrome. They tried acupuncture after standard Western therapies gave them no relief. My results, on the whole, have been most gratifying."

In fact, a number of studies have shown acupuncture to be effective for a variety of conditions. Swiss researchers tested its effectiveness in treating fibromyalgia—a form of arthritis that often resists Western medical therapies. Over a period of three weeks, they gave 35 people with fibromyalgia six sessions of electro-acupuncture—a type of acupuncture that uses needles connected to a low-voltage electrical generator. The electrical stimulation reportedly enhances acupuncture's effects. Another group of 35 people with fibromyalgia had needles inserted into nonacupuncture points. The sham-treatment group gained no benefits, but 25 percent of those who received electro-acupuncture reported complete relief, and 50 percent experienced significant improvement.

Researchers at McMaster University Medical Center in Ontario measured stomach acid production after real or sham electro-acupuncture. The sham procedure had no effect, but electro-acupuncture significantly reduced acid output.

Acupuncture has also been used with some success in the West to treat depression, anxiety, tension, stress-related insomnia and narcotic addiction. According to the World Health Organization, it is widely used around the world to treat dozens of conditions, among them allergies, bronchitis, cerebral palsy, diabetes, hemorrhoids, hepatitis, herpes, infertility, menstrual and premenstrual symptoms, polio, stroke and ulcers.

"I've had good results using acupuncture to treat asthma," says Gary Kaplan, M.D., an Arlington, Virginia, physician who has included acupuncture in his practice since 1983. "Recently I treated an asthmatic man in his late forties. He was on several medications, and they weren't giving him much relief. I urged him to adopt a hypoallergenic diet—no milk, wheat or red meat—and I gave him acupuncture. Over several months, he gradually stopped taking all but one of his medications, and now he uses that one only occasionally."

But Dr. Kaplan cautions that acupuncture is not a cure-all. "No therapy is 100 percent effective all the time," he says. "Chinese physicians use it in combination with dietary recommendations and herbs. I use it in combination with mainstream medical therapies. It's one tool among several."

# How Acupuncture Works

Traditional Chinese medicine is based on the concept of a life energy that constantly circulates throughout the body. They call this life energy *chi* (*chee*). Sometimes it's spelled *ki* or even *qi*. Traditional Chinese healers hold that chi comes in two opposite and complementary forms, known as yin and yang. When these two types of chi are well-balanced, the result is good health, they believe. But when yin and yang become unbalanced, illness is sure to follow.

Chi is thought to circulate through the body along meandering pathways called meridians, each linked to a particular organ system. Meridians are not anatomical structures. They are invisible and cannot be found by dissection, a fact that Chinese medical texts have recognized since the writing of the oldest known work on acupuncture—*Systematic Classic of Acupuncture*—way back in A.D. 282.

The meridians' invisibility accounts for a good deal of the controversy surrounding acupuncture and Chinese medicine in general. Critics dismiss invisible meridians as mystical fantasy. But to traditional Chinese physicians, the meridians are as real as the heart or lungs. Their invisibility has never bothered Chinese physicians. They insist that acupuncture has been proven effective over thousands of years of use, therefore meridian theory must be correct.

In the Chinese view, each meridian passes close to the skin's surface at places called *hsueh*, meaning "cave" or "hollow" and translated as "point." Chinese physicians describe acupuncture points as slight depressions, tender spots or nodules under the skin. At these points, the insertion of needles or the use of firm finger pressure affects the flow of chi. A skilled acupuncturist who diagnoses chi weakness or excess along any meridian or in its related organs can strengthen or weaken the chi by manipulating specific acupuncture points.

There are 14 major meridians and, depending on the source cited, 360 to 365 classic points on the body, many with poetic names such as "The Elegant Mansion" or "The Sea of Tranquillity." But over time, practitioners added additional points, and some texts suggest as many as 2,000, though few acupuncturists use more than 150. Points are particularly plentiful where meridians converge—on the hands and feet and especially on the ears, which contain more than 100 classic points.

Traditional Chinese acupuncturists supplement needling with a heat treatment—moxibustion—which involves burning the medicinal herb moxa (mugwort). Powdered mugwort is shaped into small cones similar to incense. These may be burned directly over acupuncture points or on the end of the acupuncture needles themselves. Chinese physicians believe that moxibustion increases acupuncture's effectiveness. Modern acupuncturists have largely replaced moxibustion with low-voltage electrical stimulation.

## Looking for Answers

American acupuncturists—including many physicians who practice this ancient healing art—tend to believe in meridians and in traditional Chinese acupuncture theory in general. "Chinese medical theory has a great deal to offer the West, especially for the treatment of chronic illnesses," says George Milowe, M.D., a Saratoga Springs, New York, psychiatrist who also practices acupuncture and Chinese herbal medicine.

Meanwhile, the AMA—and Western medical science in general—continues to scoff at the very idea of meridians. This controversy has led to a classic medical stalemate that has largely stymied research into this fascinating healing art. Acupuncture believers say, "We know acupuncture works. Why should we waste time doing research to prove what we already know is true?" Meanwhile, skeptics unfamiliar with the modest but largely positive scientific literature on acupuncture retort, "We know acupuncture can't possibly work. Why waste time studying something we know is worthless?"

Fortunately, a handful of scientists around the world—among them Dr. Ulett; Bruce Pomeranz, M.D., Ph.D., professor of neurosurgery at the University of Toronto; Richard Chapman, M.D., Ph.D., professor of anesthesiology at the University of Washington in Seattle; and several researchers in China, France and Scandinavia—have quietly studied acupuncture for more than 20 years, looking for a scientific explanation of its effectiveness. Their conclusion: Acupuncture works, and you don't need meridians to explain it.

"The available evidence suggests that acupuncture works neuroelectrically," Dr. Ulett explains. "The meridians are not invisible. In fact, they are the motor nerves, the nerves connected to the major muscles. Stimulating acupuncture points changes the flow of bioelectrical energy along the nerves and triggers the release of specific neurotransmitters. These neurotransmitters produce acupuncture's effects." (Neurotransmitters are chemicals that allow nerve cells to communicate.)

As evidence, Dr. Ulett cites studies in his own laboratory and in several others around the world, particularly the work of Dr. Pomeranz and Dr. Ji-Sheng Han, a researcher at the Medical University of Beijing.

When Dr. Ulett demonstrated that acupuncture is not a form of hypnosis, he also examined acupuncture points with sensitive electrical instruments and noticed that the classic points and the tissue surrounding them carry different electrical charges. "I believe these electrical differences result from the underlying anatomy," he explains. "Points occur over places where the motor nerves penetrate the muscles."

Theorizing that bioelectrical energy plays a role in acupuncture's effects, Dr. Ulett tested its ability to relieve the pain of identical mild electrical shocks in volunteers treated in four different ways: (1) with needles alone placed randomly around the body at sham points, (2) with needles at false points with electrical stimulation, (3) with needles alone at true points and (4) with needles at true points with electrical stimulation. The needles at the sham points produced no significant pain relief. The needles at the true points did. But compared with needles alone at the true points, true-point needling with electrical stimulation produced twice as much relief.

(continued on page 30)

# Want Relief? You're Stepping on It

Many years ago, at an early—and enormous—holistic health convention, this author attended too many seminars, wolfed his lunch too quickly and ran around too much to too many booths.

By late afternoon, I had an upset stomach and a tense, sore neck. I craved a place to sit and rest, but my hotel, which was across the street, seemed light-years away. Then I spied a sign: Free Reflexology Foot Massage.

Back then, in the late 1970s, I had only a glancing acquaintance with reflexology. I knew its practitioners considered the foot to be a map of the body. Tender spots coincided with problems elsewhere, and massaging them supposedly healed many ailments. At the time, I was unaware of reflexology's roots in acupuncture, and I viewed it skeptically. But the booth had something I really wanted—a place to sit down. In fact, it had a big, inviting recliner with a pop-out footrest.

I'd always enjoyed foot massage. I figured I could put up with the reflexologist's spiel until I felt rested and then be on my way.

I eased into the recliner (ahhh . . . ) and removed my shoes and socks. The woman staffing the booth made no inquiries about my health, and I volunteered no information about my sore neck and upset stomach. She began with some whole-palm massage strokes to relax me and prepare my feet for her probing. Then she pressed here and there with her fingers. "Tell me if I hit anything tender," she said.

## READING THE BODY'S PAIN MAP

It didn't take her long to locate a tender spot at the base of my big toe. "Hmm," she ventured, "does your neck hurt?" I began paying more attention. She found another tender spot in the middle of my foot. "Is your stomach upset?" she asked.

She massaged my neck and stomach points for perhaps ten minutes, and by the time she finished, my neck felt relaxed and my stomach felt better. Was it a coincidence or did reflexology really work? I had no idea, but I left the booth impressed, and during the years since that experience, my respect for reflexology has grown.

Reflexology is an offshoot of acupuncture. According to Chinese medical theory, the meridians converge in the feet, hands and ears, and many acupuncture points are located on them. Massaging the feet and hands changes the flow of chi, which has an effect on the entire body.

Western acupuncture researchers offer a different yet similar explanation. The hands and feet are richly endowed with motor nerves, and the ear is the only place on the body where the vagus nerve comes close to the skin.

"Because of the importance of hearing, walking and manipulating objects, a significant portion of the brain is involved in processing bioelectrical nerve impulses from the ears, hands and feet," explains acupuncture researcher George A. Ulett, M.D., Ph.D., director of the Department of Psychiatry at Deaconess Hospital in St. Louis and clinical professor of psychiatry at the University of Missouri School of Medicine.

"Massaging them releases neurotransmitters along these nerve lines and in the brain, which could affect other parts of the body," says Dr. Ulett. (Neurotransmitters are chemicals that allow nerve cells to communicate.)

Reflexology is easy to learn and easy to practice on yourself. There's no need to consult manuals about the acupuncture points appropriate for a given condition. The hands, feet and ears are fairly small. Simply massage them, focusing on any tender spots you find, and you're bound to send chi or bioelectrical energy where you want it to go.

Self-reflexology can be enjoyed almost anywhere. Feel blah at a meeting? Just press here and there on your hands and ears. Want to invest in your health while watching TV? Pull off your shoes and massage your feet.

(continued)

# Want Relief?
## You're Stepping on It—*Continued*

Reflexology is also the perfect skeptic's introduction to acupuncture or massage. It's easy to learn and it's nonintrusive. Many people feel uncomfortable removing their clothing for massage or acupressure, and most acupuncture first-timers feel leery about its needles. But few people object to hand, foot or ear massage. Even if the recipient has no particular physical complaints, this type of massage is marvelously relaxing.

"Electro-acupuncture at the true points produced as much pain relief as injecting ten milligrams of morphine," Dr. Ulett says. "That's a major effect."

In his studies, Dr. Han gave volunteers electro-acupuncture and measured pain relief over time. Relief gradually increased, peaked and then declined, suggesting that the needle treatment triggered the release into the blood of some pain-fighting substance that had druglike action. But which pain-fighting chemicals?

The chemicals are neurotransmitters, particularly serotonin and endorphins, according to Dr. Pomeranz and other researchers. (Endorphins are the body's pain relievers and mood elevators. They are also released by exercise, which is why physical activity has pain-relieving and antidepressant effects.)

Swedish researchers have shown that endorphin levels in the brain double 30 minutes after acupuncture. When experimental animals are pretreated with chemicals that enhance the effects of serotonin and the endorphins, acupuncture pain relief increases. But when pretreated with chemicals that interfere with the effects of these neurotransmitters, acupuncture becomes less effective.

For centuries, traditional acupuncturists have known that needles placed at the same points can have different effects, depending on how they are manipulated. Several researchers have shown that changing the frequency of electrical stimulation at any acupuncture point changes the neurotransmitters produced. "Acupuncture's effects have more to do with the frequency of electrical stimulation than with the points themselves," Dr. Ulett says.

Pain specialists have shown that electro-acupuncture has pain-relieving effects similar to those of transcutaneous electrical nerve stimulation (TENS), which involves attaching electrodes to various points on the skin. Significantly, several studies that found acupuncture ineffective for pain relief—the ones critics cite to prove that it is merely a placebo—used needles alone, without electrical stimulation.

The neuro-electrical explanation for acupuncture also sheds light on why so many points are located on the hands and feet. The hands and feet are richly supplied with motor nerves.

Although electro-acupuncture produces the greatest effects, needling alone also produces significant health benefits, and so does acupressure. "With vigorous finger pressure," Dr. Ulett says, "you get some bioelectrical effects. If people want to start with self-treatment using acupressure, that's fine. It may produce sufficient relief. But if it doesn't, they shouldn't write off acupuncture as worthless. They should consult a professional, ideally one who practices electro-acupuncture, because that produces the greatest benefits."

Which explanation of acupuncture is correct: the traditional Chinese view with its meridians and chi flow or the Western view with its motor nerves and release of neurotransmitters? "They're both right," Dr. Kaplan says. "They're two different perspectives on the same phenomenon, two sides of the same coin. What's most important is that no matter how you explain this ancient healing art, it works."

## Safe and Painless Therapy

Does acupuncture hurt? Rarely. The needles are very fine, and insertion typically feels no worse than a little pinch followed by other possible sensations: numbness, warmth, tingling, heaviness or a dull ache. Many people also experience relaxation, mood elevation and a dreamy sense of well-being. Afterward, some people feel energized; others feel drowsy.

Some people report a temporary increase in the severity of symptoms following acupuncture treatment. This, Chinese physicians say, is a sign that the body is marshaling its energy to overcome the problem.

Is acupuncture safe? "Very, assuming that the practitioner uses sterile needles," insists Dr. Ulett. "There are fewer side effects with acupuncture than with painkilling drugs." However, dizziness and fainting are possible, especially in those experiencing acupuncture for the first time. Sometimes the needles cause minor bleeding, and on rare occasions, needles may become difficult to withdraw. Relaxation of the affected area by massage or insertion of additional needles at nearby points typically resolves the problem.

"I've treated several thousand patients," Dr. Ulett says, "and I've never had a case of needle-related infection."

## Press Your Way to Better Health

"Acupressure is not as powerful as acupuncture," says Dr. Milowe, "but it's easy to learn, convenient for self-care and, for many conditions, it provides real benefits. I often teach it to my patients."

If you'd like to try acupressure for yourself, the healing points for several common conditions are described below. And if you'd like to use acupressure on a regular basis, a good book that maps the points and provides details on how to treat specific diseases and conditions is essential. *Acupressure's Potent Points* by Michael Reed Gach, founder of the American Acupressure Institute in Berkeley, California, is probably the best available.

Here are a few acupressure basics from Gach: Once you think you've located the appropriate point, probe the area with a fingertip or the second joint of the index finger, boring into the skin in tight circles in the general location of the point. Points announce themselves with a feeling of tenderness, tingling, soreness or minor discomfort. Press each point firmly for one

# How to Find a Good Acupuncturist

We're talking needles here. While safe and effective in the right hands, acupuncture is one of the more invasive natural healing therapies. If you're going to try this ancient Chinese treatment, make sure you're working with an expert.

The best way to find a good acupuncturist—or any other health professional, for that matter—is to ask for recommendations from people you trust.

Beyond personal endorsements, there are a couple of other things you can look for. Good acupuncturists are certified by the National Commission for the Certification of Acupuncturists (NCCA), established in 1985. Certified acupuncturists have passed an exam administered by the NCCA that includes a section devoted to clean-needle techniques, which are crucial in the age of AIDS and other serious bloodborne infections.

To take the exam, candidates must have completed three years of full-time training, apprenticed with a certified acupuncturist for three years or practiced acupuncture for four years. (The last category is for immigrant acupuncturists trained abroad.) Of the 25 states (plus the District of Columbia) that currently license acupuncturists, almost all use NCCA certification as the basis for licensure.

If you opt for an acupuncturist who is not certified by the NCCA, ask about the person's training and needle hygiene. Needles must be sterilized. The safest needles are disposable.

An estimated 5,000 American doctors now include acupuncture in their practices. Most are family physicians, anesthesiologists, orthopedists and pain specialists. Few M.D.'s are NCCA-certified, but most are certified by the American Academy of Medical Acupuncture instead.

minute, then stop for a few seconds before pressing again. Work each point for 5 to 20 minutes. While pressing, breathe deeply. You need not use all of the points recommended for each condition. Experiment for yourself and find the one or more that work best for you.

*Allergies. Point number one:* Hold out your open hand, palm down. You'll find the point on the back of your hand in the center of the fleshy webbing between the thumb and index finger. (Pregnant women should not stimulate this point; it may encourage uterine contractions.) *Point number two:* This one is on top of the foot in the valley between the big toe and second toe. *Point number three:* Hold your arm out, palm down. The point is located on top of the forearm 2½ finger-widths above the wrist crease between the two arm bones. *Point number four:* Hold your arm out, palm down. Find the point on the outer elbow crease. *Point number five:* This point is on both sides of the spine, one finger-width below the base of the back of the skull on the muscles one finger-width from the spine. *Point number six:* Find this point high on the chest in the hollow below the collarbone and next to the breastbone. *Point number seven:* This one is two finger-widths directly below the navel.

*Arthritis. Point number one:* Hold out your open hand, palm down. You'll find the first point in the center of the fleshy webbing between the thumb and index finger. (Pregnant women should not stimulate this point; it may encourage uterine contractions.) *Point number two:* Hold your arm out, palm down. You'll find this point on top of the forearm 2½ finger-widths above the wrist crease between the two arm bones. *Point number three:* This point is four finger-widths below the kneecap and one finger-width to the outside of the shinbone. *Point number four:* Hold your arm out, palm down, and find this point on the outer elbow crease. *Point number five:* This point is at the base of the back of the skull in the hollow above the two large vertical neck muscles.

*Constipation. Point number one:* Open your hand, palm down, and find this point in the center of the fleshy webbing between the thumb and index finger. (Pregnant women should not stimulate this point; it may encourage uterine contractions.) *Point number two:* This point is four finger-widths below the kneecap and one finger-width to the outside of the shinbone. *Point number three:* Hold your arm out, palm down, and find this point on the outer elbow crease. *Point number four:* This point is two finger-widths directly below the navel.

*Headache. Point number one:* Hold your hand open, palm down, and find this point in the center of the fleshy webbing between the thumb and index finger. (Pregnant women should not stimulate this point; it may stimulate uterine contractions.) *Point number two:* Find this point on top of the foot in the valley between the big toe and second toe. *Point number three:* This point is at the base of the back of the skull in the hollow above the two large vertical neck muscles. *Point number four:* This point is in the back of the head in the center of the hollow at the base of the skull. *Point number five:* Find this point in the hollow above the inner eyes, where the bridge of the nose meets the ridge of the eyebrows. *Point number six:* This point lies between the eyebrows in the indentation where the bridge of the nose meets the forehead. *Point number seven:* You'll find this point on top of the foot, two finger-widths above the webbing of the fourth and fifth toes in the groove between the bones.

*Hiccups. Point number one:* This point lies in the indentation behind each earlobe. *Point number two:* This point is located at the base of the throat in the center of the collarbone. *Point number three:* You'll find this point on the center of the breastbone three thumb-widths up from the base of the bone. *Point number four:* This point is located in the pit of the abdomen on the midline three finger-widths below the base of the breastbone. (Press this point only on an empty stomach. If you are healthy, do not press this point for more than two minutes. If you are ill, do not press this point at all.)

*Insomnia. Point number one:* The first point is found on the back between the shoulder blades and the spine at heart level. *Point number two:* You can find this point in the middle of the inner forearm 2½ finger-widths from the wrist crease. *Point number three:* This point is on the inside of the wrist crease in line with the little finger. *Point number four:* Find this one just one finger-width below the base of the back of the skull on the muscles one finger-width out on both sides of the spine. *Point number five:* This point is located on the back of the head in the center of the hollow at the base of the skull. *Point number six:* You can find this one between the eyebrows in the indentation where the bridge of the nose meets the forehead. *Point number seven:* This point is on the center of the breastbone three thumb-widths up from the base of the bone.

*Nausea (morning sickness, motion sickness). Point number one:* You can find this point in the indentation between the ear-lobe and the jawbone. *Point number two:* Look for this point four finger-widths above the center of the inner wrist crease be-tween the tendons. *Point number three:* This point is located in the middle of the inner side of the forearm 2½ finger-widths above the wrist crease. *Point number four:* Look for this one four finger-widths below the kneecap and one finger-width out-side the shinbone, where the muscle flexes as the foot moves up and down. *Point number five:* This one is on top of the foot in the valley between the big toe and second toe. *Point number six:* You'll find this one on the outside of the base of the nail of the second toe.

CHAPTER 2

# AROMATHERAPY

## When Healing Makes "Scents"

Seventy-five years ago, French fragrance chemist René-Maurice Gattefossé was in his lab hard at work on a new perfume. He was lost in thought while blending essential oils—the super-concentrated aromatic essences of fragrant plants—and a sudden explosion burned his arm. Frantic with pain, he plunged his arm into the nearest cold liquid, which happened to be a bowl of lavender oil.

Immediately he noticed surprising pain relief, and instead of requiring the extended healing process he had experienced during recovery from previous burns—which caused redness, heat, inflammation, blisters and scarring—this burn healed remarkably quickly, with minimal discomfort and no scarring. Perhaps, he thought, a powerful healer was hiding right under our noses. Perhaps the fragrant oils that people had used for thousands of years as perfumes to attract mates and manipulate mood could also be used to improve physical health.

Gattefossé went on to devote his life to studying essential oils' influence on health and healing. In 1928 he published *Aromatherapie,* coining the term now used to describe the art of inhaling aromatic plant oils or massaging them into the skin for physical or emotional benefits.

At the time, scientists generally ignored Gattefossé's work, but slowly a few of his colleagues began nosing around aromatherapy. In the 1930s, one reported success using lavender oil to treat black widow spider bites. During World War II, French army surgeon Jean Valnet, M.D., used essential oils successfully to treat battlefield wounds and infections when penicillin ran low. After the war, Dr. Valnet experimented with aromatherapy for anxiety and other emotional problems. In 1964, he borrowed Gattefossé's title for his own book, *Aromatherapie*, which stands today as the field's basic medical text.

## The New Science of Smell

Inside your nose are some five million smell-sensing cells that sit atop your nasal passages. Each cell has 6 to 12 hairlike receptors that hang down into the stream of air that rushes into your nose as you inhale. These receptors form a tiny comblike structure that catches all sorts of molecules floating in inhaled air. When a fragrance molecule lands on the comb, your smell-sensing cells send a message to the olfactory center in your brain and you smell its aroma.

Unlike vision and hearing, the sense of smell is fully functional at birth. Soon after their first attempt at breastfeeding, newborns can recognize their mothers by smell. We know this because they turn toward cotton pads that have been swabbed against their mothers' necks and away from pads swabbed against strangers' necks. Olfaction, it seems, is at the root of parent/child love and bonding.

It may also play a role in adult relationships. When people fall in love, the popular phrase is that they have "good chemistry." That saying may be literally true. Research suggests that the subtle brain chemistry of olfaction plays a key role in sexual attraction.

Without a functioning sense of smell, the sense of taste largely disappears. That's the reason food loses flavor when you have a cold—you can't smell it as well with a stuffed nose. As you age, your sight and hearing become less acute. Your sense of smell slowly declines as well, taking along with it some of your ability to taste.

But if your nose doesn't know as much as it used to, aging may have nothing to do with it. Olfactory impairment can be a sign of zinc deficiency. To get enough of this essential nutrient, eat plenty of whole grains, cereals, breads, beans, low-fat dairy products, shellfish, fish, poultry and lean meats.

Olfactory impairment may also be a sign of several illnesses, among them allergies, epilepsy, Parkinsonism, Alzheimer's disease, nasal polyps, thyroid problems, multiple sclerosis and certain brain tumors.

In fact, researchers at Duke University in Durham, North Carolina, showed that a smell test might be used to diagnose Alzheimer's before it becomes apparent using standard cognitive tests. A research team studied 22 pairs of individuals matched for age, gender, race and education. One member of each pair had a family history that suggested considerable risk of Alzheimer's. The pairs were given mental and sensory tests. For the most part there were no differences in the pairs—except that those at risk for Alzheimer's scored lower on ability to recall odors. The researchers speculate that olfactory deterioration may be the earliest sign of this tragic, mind-robbing condition.

Loss of the sense of smell may also signal an emotional problem. The nose's olfactory nerve is wired directly into the limbic system of the brain—a primitive, poorly understood area that plays a key role in emotions, memory, hormone secretion and such mind/body functions as appetite and sexuality.

Alan R. Hirsch, M.D., neurological director of the Smell and Taste Treatment and Research Foundation in Chicago, first became interested in the link between scent and emotion during his psychiatric residency, when he noticed that many people with mental health disorders—particularly depression and anxiety—also had problems with their sense of smell.

"There's a whole world out there at the tip of our noses," Dr. Hirsch says. "We've found that the sense of smell can evoke powerful memories and change people's perceptions and behavior. But until recently, olfaction has been largely ignored by the scientific community."

## From Cleopatra's Nose to Olfactory Muzak

Scientists may have discovered the power of fragrance only recently, but cultures around the world have recognized it for thousands of years. The perfume industry is one of the world's oldest. The Bible records brisk trade in such aromatic herbs as frankincense, myrrh and cinnamon. As Cleopatra awaited the arrival of Marc Antony, she had her servants fill the entryway ankle-deep with rose petals, hoping that the fragrance would open him to her seductive charms. From all accounts, it did.

Cleopatra's aromatic greeting was no accident. Ancient Egyptian physicians routinely used aromatic plant oils to affect the emotions and treat mental health problems, among them the disorder now known as depression. The ancient Chinese and Ayurvedic physicians in early India also used aromatic oils therapeutically. In the fourth century B.C., Hippocrates, the father of Western medicine, reportedly said, "The way to health is to have an aromatic bath and scented massage every day." Around the same time, another Greek physician, Theophrastus, wrote the first aromatherapy treatise, *Concerning Odors*.

In Europe after the fall of Rome, perfumes became rare, and the medical use of aromatic oils virtually died out. But aromatherapy survived in the Middle East. The tenth-century Arab physician Avicenna wrote an entire book on the healing benefits of rosewater. The Arabs' Muslim religion may have been blasphemy to Christian Crusaders, but the Europeans who traveled to the Holy Land became quick converts to their enemy's perfumes and aromatic medical preparations. Perfumes captivated European royalty, especially in France, which became the world capital of perfumery.

Today perfumes are a $6-billion-a-year industry worldwide. But aromatic oils' medicinal uses were largely lost—until Gattefossé burned his arm in the 1920s.

Modern research has demonstrated that Gattefossé and the

ancient aromatherapists were clearly on to something. Brain wave studies by Dr. Hirsch have shown that some scents, such as lavender, increase alpha brain waves associated with relaxation, while others, like jasmine, boost beta waves linked to alertness.

"When we first presented our findings at scientific meetings," Dr. Hirsch recalls, "people generally thumbed their noses. Their attitude was: So what?"

Dr. Hirsch went on to show that his findings might open a whole new field, "aroma-marketing," which would allow merchants to manipulate unsuspecting consumers into liking products more and spending more on them. "Basically," Dr. Hirsch says, "smell sells, and people are surprisingly willing to pay through the nose—literally."

Studies going back decades have shown that light music increases consumers' willingness to spend, which is why Muzak is ubiquitous in malls. And one of the oldest marketing tricks in real estate is to bake bread or cookies during open houses.

"Those smells bring back pleasant memories of childhood and grandma's house," says Paul Selinger, a real estate investor in Inverness, California. "They help people feel at home—and often push them over the edge to make an offer."

One day soon, you may waltz into your favorite supermarket or department store and find yourself engulfed not only by Muzak but also by sweet floral aromas.

In one experiment, Dr. Hirsch ushered volunteers into one of two rooms containing an identical pair of Nike athletic shoes and asked them to fill out a questionnaire about them. One room was unscented, while the other was infused with a pleasant floral fragrance. Compared with those who considered the shoes in the unscented room, those in the perfumed room liked the shoes more and said they would be willing to pay an average of $10.33 more for them.

Both men and women liked the shoes more in the scented room, but women reacted more positively to the fragrance than men. (The only group that liked the Nikes less in the scented room were cigarette smokers. It is well-known that smoking impairs the sense of smell.)

(continued on page 44)

# How Good Is Your Sense of Smell? ━━━━

A good deal of the healing potential of aromatherapy relies on your sense of smell. If your sense of smell is impaired, this might not be the best kind of therapy for you. To find out how well your nose is doing its job, take this simple test, created by Alan R. Hirsch, M.D., neurological director of the Smell and Taste Treatment and Research Foundation in Chicago.

## PART I

For every yes answer, give yourself 1 point. For every no, score 0.

1. Have you ever been told (or gotten the feeling) that you're wearing too much perfume?
2. In general, do you think foods taste blander than they used to?
3. Lately, have you been adding more salt, spices and sugar to your food?
4. Has coffee been tasting especially bitter lately? (Coffee's bitter taste is offset by its sweet smell. But as olfactory acuity declines, coffee tastes increasingly bitter.)
5. Do other people notice scents that you don't?
6. When you're cooking, has the smoke alarm ever gone off before you noticed that something was burning?
7. When you're at a service station, do you not notice the smell of gasoline?
8. When shining your shoes, do you fail to smell the polish?
9. At the movies, do you never notice the aroma of popcorn?
10. When you first turn on a gas stove, do you fail to smell the gas?

## PART II

You'll need a partner for these questions so you can take the smell-and-taste tests blind. For every yes, score 0. For every no, give yourself 1 point.

11. Cut sliver-thin slices of apple and onion. Close your eyes and have your partner place one or the other on your tongue. Can you identify it? (Apples and onions taste the same to people with an impaired sense of smell.)

12. Place a scoop of vanilla ice cream in one bowl and a scoop of chocolate in another. Close your eyes and have your partner feed you a spoonful of one or the other. Can you identify it?

13. Close your eyes and have your partner spray one tissue with a scented deodorant and another with an unscented deodorant. Open your eyes and smell the tissues. Can you tell which is which?

14. Cut some bubble gum and a stick of fruit-flavored gum (not mint-flavored) into similar-size pieces. Close your eyes and have your partner give you one. Can you identify the flavor?

15. Place an eraser in one cup and a piece of Swiss cheese in another. Close your eyes and have your partner wave one or the other under your nose. Can you tell which is which?

## SCORING

0–1 point. Congratulations. Your sense of smell is fine. To keep it that way, don't smoke, and be sure to wear a seat belt in cars and a helmet whenever you ride a bike. Smoking impairs olfaction, and head injuries are a leading cause of olfactory impairment. Also get enough smell-supporting zinc by eating whole grains, fruits, beans and leafy green vegetables.

2–15 points. Your sense of smell may not be up to snuff. Consult a physician to rule out illness and a zinc deficiency. If your doctor says you're healthy and you have no nutritional deficiencies, don't smoke, and prevent head injuries.

In another study, when Dr. Hirsch infused a pleasant aroma into a Las Vegas casino, gamblers happily plunked down 45 to 53 percent more money. "The more intense the fragrance, the more they spent," says Dr. Hirsch.

But keeping a tight rein on your credit cards whenever you sense aroma-marketing may not save you from its effects. Even vanishingly faint scents can boost spending. Dr. Hirsch asked participants in another study about what they thought various consumer items were worth. He conducted some of the interviews in an unscented room and others in a room infused with a minute amount of fragrance undetectable to the average nose. Conscious awareness of the aroma didn't matter. Those interviewed in the undetectably scented room still said they'd pay more for the merchandise.

The effects of fragrance go beyond spending. People in a pleasant-smelling environment are also more productive. Robert Baron, Ph.D., professor in the School of Management at Rensselaer Polytechnic Institute in Troy, New York, gave 120 students two mental tasks—proofreading and unscrambling letters to form words. Half of the students worked in an unscented room, while half worked in a room containing floral and fruit/herbal fragrances such as apple-cinnamon. Those in the scented room performed 25 percent better. "The fragrance itself doesn't matter," Dr. Baron says, "as long as people find it pleasant."

A similar experiment in Japan showed that when the aroma of lemon—which aromatherapists consider uplifting—was added to an office building's ventilation system, clerical errors declined 53 percent. These studies give new meaning to the old phrase "nose to the grindstone."

## The Sweet Smell of Healing

Other researchers have focused on aromatherapy's use in healing. At Memorial Sloan-Kettering Cancer Center in New York City, physicians became concerned about the anxiety attacks many patients experience during magnetic resonance imaging (MRI)—a high-tech procedure that involves claustrophobic full-body enclosure in a large, noisy machine. Before their MRIs, some patients were given heliotropin, a close relative of vanilla oil, whose scent aromatherapists often recommend for relaxation. Compared with those who received no aromatherapy, the heliotropin group reported significantly less anxiety.

Researchers at Duke University explored how fragrant aromas might sweeten the interpersonal atmosphere on New York City subways. They had a subtle scent piped into one car and then compared riders' behavior with that of riders in an adjacent, unscented car. In the scented car, pushing, shoving and other aggressive acts dropped by as much as 40 percent.

"When you ask people why they find walks in the woods or by the seashore relaxing," Dr. Hirsch says, "they typically reply that they like the beautiful vistas or the pounding surf or the wind whistling through the trees. But there's something else going on as well. Forests, beaches, golf courses, baseball stadiums—anything people find stress-reducing or invigorating—also have an important olfactory dimension that leads us by our noses."

## Oils with Special Powers

What are these aromas with such powerful potential to affect people's mood and health?

Although they're called essential oils, the term oil is somewhat misleading. The oils used in aromatherapy do not feel oily—nowhere near as oily as, say, olive oil. But chemically they are oils. They do not mix with water but mix well with vegetable oils.

Essential oils are also known as volatile oils, from the Latin word for flying. Open a vial of essential oil and some of the molecules fly off as a gas, which is how they get into your nose and smell aromatic.

Plant oils are incredibly concentrated. For a chamomile bath, it might take several handfuls of fresh or dried flowers but only a few drops of chamomile oil. One drop of an essential oil is the medical equivalent of one ounce of its parent plant material, ac-

# Safety Alert: Essential Oils Are Strong Medicine

Medicines should only be taken in the prescribed manner at the recommended dosage, and essential oils are no exception. They should not be taken by mouth. When ingested, surprisingly modest amounts can be fatal. Professional aromatherapists may occasionally recommend ingestion of dilute solutions of certain oils for specific ailments, but amateur aromatherapists should never ingest these oils. Whiff them or mix them with vegetable oil for use in massage.

In addition, British aromatherapist Valerie Ann Worwood, author of *The Complete Book of Essential Oils and Aromatherapy*, cautions against using the following oils at all because of possible adverse effects: bitter almond, boldo leaf, calamus, yellow camphor, horseradish, jaborandi leaf, mugwort, mustard, pennyroyal, rue, sassafras, savin, southernwood, tansy, thuja, wintergreen, wormseed and wormwood. Leave these oils to the professionals.

A few oils—among them clove and bergamot—are phototoxic and can cause severe sunburn and rash.

Finally, any essential oil massaged into the skin may cause allergic irritation in some people. Be careful if you have sensitive skin. In fact, if you have allergies, you should also be cautious about inhaling essential oil aromas. If you experience a rash or any kind of discomfort from using any essential oil, discontinue use.

cording to Marcel Lavabre, co-founder of the American Aromatherapy Association, owner of Aroma Vera, an essential oil company in Culver City, California, and author of *The Aromatherapy Workbook*.

Essential oils can be extracted from their parent plants in several ways, but the typical process used is distillation, which scientific historians believe was developed in ancient Egypt to produce aromatic embalming fluids.

Depending on the plant, its oil comes from specialized oil or resin cells, glandular tissue, pockets within scales or intercellular spaces. There isn't much of it in each plant, and the harder it is to obtain, the more expensive it becomes.

Lavender contains a good deal of oil. It takes "only" two pounds of lavender to produce one ounce of this relatively inexpensive oil (approximately $15 to $25 per ounce). Rose oil is considerably rarer (one ounce requires 60,000 rose blossoms) and more costly (about $400 per ounce). Jasmine oil is one of the rarest and most expensive. To produce one ounce, it takes 250,000 blossoms picked on the first day they open; cost is approximately $200 to $400 an ounce.

No matter which part of the plant they come from, essential oils have the same purposes—to keep the plant from becoming dehydrated and to protect it from predators, particularly microorganisms. Because they have an antimicrobial mission, all essential oils are antibacterial, antiviral and antifungal—attributes that make them quite useful to us humans as antiseptics.

Thyme oil was once widely used as a disinfectant in hospitals, and it's still the active ingredient in Listerine. Today the chemical phenol is the most widely used household antiseptic— it's the active ingredient in Lysol. Phenol is considerably less expensive than essential plant oils, but it's also less effective. Drop for drop, lavender oil is more than 4 times the more potent germ-killer; rosemary, 5 times; rose, 7 times; clove, 9 times and thyme, 12 times.

Many insects are also put off by essential oils. Pennyroyal oil is the standard active ingredient in natural flea collars for dogs and cats.

Essential oils are chemically extremely complex. They contain hundreds of different chemicals, all of which, aromatherapists say, are critical to their effectiveness. Some scientific researchers claim that synthetic approximations have indistinguishable effects at much lower cost. The vanilla-like scent that relaxed the MRI patients, for example, was synthetic, so it's clear that synthetics can have considerable value as well.

Professional aromatherapists use up to 300 oils, but most people can meet their needs with less than two dozen. Valerie Anne Worwood, British aromatherapist and author of The

*Complete Book of Essential Oils and Aromatherapy,* maintains that most people can fulfill the majority of their needs with just 10: chamomile, clove, eucalyptus, geranium, lavender, lemon, peppermint, rosemary, tea tree and thyme.

Aromatherapist Edwin T. Morris, of Pelham, New York, who teaches aromatherapy at the New York Botanical Gardens and is the author of *Fragrance: The Story of Perfume from Cleopatra to Chanel,* says that French lavender oil is his favorite. "It's the most versatile oil I've ever encountered," he says. "It can be used undiluted on the skin. A drop is wonderful in a bath. And I've never found anyone to be allergic to it. It's uplifting, bright, bracing and antiseptic."

Essential oils must be stored carefully in brown or dark vials away from heat, light and dampness. When not in use, keep them tightly closed. Aromatherapists differ on the shelf life of essential oils, but most say they last for at least two years.

## Healing with Aromatherapy

Aromatherapy is an offshoot of herbal medicine. Frequently, aromatherapists' use of aromatic oils parallels herbalists' use of the flowers, stems, leaves and roots of the same plants. Valerian root, for example, is a well-known herbal sedative that's also recommended for stress management. At least one study shows that valerian oil reduces blood pressure and relieves stress. Aromatherapists often recommend it to relieve anxiety. And although many of aromatherapy's benefits come through the sense of smell, aromatherapists also advise topical applications of many essential oils because of the oils' healing benefits. (Remember Gattefossé's experience using lavender on his burns.)

Research demonstrating aromatherapy's effectiveness is not as plentiful as studies of medicinal herb preparations given as teas or in capsules. But several studies—and a great deal of clinical experience by aromatherapists—suggest that essential oils can be effective for a variety of ailments, especially those that involve mind/body interactions.

*Compulsive eating.* For several years, Susan Schiffman, Ph.D., professor of psychology at Duke University, has been using apricot oil to help patients at Duke's weight-loss clinic control their eating. Weight management researchers have shown that many obese people often eat not because they're hungry but because they feel anxious.

Dr. Schiffman teaches relaxation techniques to participants in the Duke weight-loss program and at the same time has them inhale whiffs of apricot oil, so they associate the aroma with feeling calm. Then they carry a vial of the oil with them and inhale it whenever they feel anxious, in effect substituting apricot's relaxing effect for their former stress reliever, eating. Dr. Schiffman claims her aromatherapy technique has helped control compulsive eating in more than half of those who have adopted the technique.

*Menopausal problems.* Dr. Schiffman has also discovered that pleasant floral scents help women cope with the emotional symptoms of menopause: tension, anxiety, depression, fatigue and confusion. Pleasant aromas appear to suppress negative emotions and allow more positive emotions to express themselves.

The following recommendations come from the books by Worwood and Lavabre and *The Aromatherapy Book* by San Francisco herbalist Jeanne Rose.

*Abrasions, cuts, burns and scrapes.* After washing with soap and water, apply one to three drops of lavender oil or tea tree oil to the wound or to a bandage. Reapply the oil twice a day until the area is substantially healed.

*Athlete's foot.* Mix two drops of lavender oil and one drop of tea tree oil. Using a cotton swab, apply it between the toes. Then dilute five drops of tea tree oil and one drop of lemon oil in one teaspoon of vegetable oil. Use this to massage the entire foot.

*Bee stings.* Apply one drop of chamomile oil three times a day for two days.

*Blisters.* Never open a blister. Apply one drop of lavender oil and one drop of chamomile oil.

*Chapped lips.* Add two drops of chamomile oil and two drops of geranium oil to two teaspoons of aloe vera gel. Apply to the lips.

*The common cold.* Add three drops of lemon oil, two drops of thyme oil, two drops of tea tree oil and one drop of eucalyptus oil to a hot bath. Lie back and inhale deeply.

*Cough.* Add three drops of eucalyptus oil and two drops of thyme oil to two teaspoons of vegetable oil. Massage this mixture into the neck and chest. The old standby, Vicks Vaporub, is essentially an aromatherapy product. Its decongestant vapors come from eucalyptus oil.

*Depression.* To a bath, add 15 drops of geranium oil, 10 drops of bergamot and 5 drops of lavender.

*Dry skin.* Add ten drops of geranium oil, ten drops of chamomile oil, five drops of lemon oil and five drops of lavender oil to two teaspoons of vegetable oil. Massage into the affected area.

*Fear of flying.* Place one drop of lavender oil and one drop of geranium oil in a plastic sandwich bag. Keep the bag in your pocket or purse. Whenever you feel anxious, open it for a moment and inhale.

*Hay fever.* Begin by placing one drop of chamomile oil and one drop of lemon oil into a tissue, then inhale. If this does not provide sufficient relief, experiment with combinations of these two oils plus the oils of peppermint, clove, rosemary, lavender and geranium.

*Headache.* Massage around the temples, the base of the skull and along the hairline with three drops of lavender oil and one drop of peppermint oil blended with one drop of vegetable oil. Or substitute one drop of chamomile, rosemary or clove oil for the peppermint.

*Hiccups.* Place one drop of chamomile oil in a small brown paper bag. Hold it over your nose and mouth and breathe deeply through your nose. You can also try lemon oil.

*Insomnia.* To a bath, add a mixture of two tablespoons of vegetable oil and 30 drops of any combination of the following oils: chamomile, clary-sage, lemon, marjoram, sandalwood and valerian.

*Menstrual cramps.* Mix ten drops of peppermint oil, ten drops of nutmeg, five drops of lavender and five drops of cypress with two tablespoons of vegetable oil. Massage the abdomen, lower back and shoulders.

*Premenstrual irritability.* Add to a bath seven to nine drops of the following oils in the combination that works best for you: bergamot, chamomile, clary-sage, geranium, jonquil and nutmeg.

*Sinus infection.* Place the following mixture on a tissue and inhale: two drops of rosemary oil, one drop of geranium and one drop of eucalyptus.

*Stress.* Mix five drops of grapefruit oil, four drops of cypress and two drops of geranium with one teaspoon of vegetable oil. Inhale the aroma or massage the face, neck, shoulders, chest and back.

## CHAPTER 3
# BIOFEEDBACK

### Mind over Body

Nancy Schwartz had always believed the old saying, "cold hands, warm heart." Her hands usually felt cold, but in 1985, the then-30-year-old psychology student at the University of North Florida (UNF) had no time to worry about chilly fingers. In the midst of a divorce, she had no idea how she could support her two children with just a B.A. in psychology, a degree that was virtually useless in the job market. She also had terrible migraine headaches that sent her to bed several days a month. She'd taken several drugs, but even the most effective provided only minimal relief.

One day Schwartz mentioned her job anxieties to a friend, who suggested she look into biofeedback: "You can get a job with little more than a B.A., and UNF has a biofeedback training program."

Schwartz had never heard of biofeedback, but the course would count toward her degree, and the job possibilities intrigued her.

In the class, the professor explained that people receive feedback from their bodies all the time. After a few hours of not eating, we feel hungry. When running leaves us winded, we rest to catch our breath. And when stress piles up, certain muscles become tense.

These forms of biological feedback—or biofeedback—are easy to sense and require no amplification. Other types of body feedback are more difficult to discern. The techniques learned in biofeedback training amplify these subtle physiological signals, allowing people to gain control over them. Biofeedback can be used to treat all sorts of medical conditions, from anxiety to chronic high blood pressure.

After explaining all this, the professor produced a biofeedback device, a tiny thermometer connected to a small electronic box with a display meter and a loudspeaker. He taped the thermometer, or thermistor, to his finger. The meter read 78° and the loudspeaker emitted a high-pitched tone.

Then he announced that he was going to warm his hands. He closed his eyes and took a few deep breaths, and moments later, the temperature meter started to rise and the tone's pitch began to drop. Soon the professor's finger temperature was 92°, and the tone was low.

"To earn an A in this class," he announced, "you'll all have to raise your finger temperature to 92°, first with a biofeedback device and then without one."

Schwartz was skeptical. Her finger temperature was 72°. She doubted she could raise it 20°. Perhaps, she thought grimly, that old saying should be revised from "cold hands, warm heart" to "cold hands, low grade."

For two weeks, Schwartz struggled to raise her finger temperature and lower the machine's tone. First she willed her finger temperature up, with no luck. The thermometer stayed low and the tone stayed high. Then she tried a visualization, imagining herself at the beach. It raised her finger temperature a few degrees and the tone dropped, but only slightly. Finally, she focused on an image of warm blood rushing into her fingertips. The tone dropped. The thermometer rose to 92°. Within a few weeks, she could warm her hands whenever she wanted, with and without the biofeedback device. Schwartz earned her A.

She also reaped an unexpected reward. Once she could warm

her hands with biofeedback, her migraines all but disappeared. The experience had a profound impact on her. She became a certified biofeedback therapist in 1986 and now practices in Orange Park, Florida.

"Biofeedback helps people take more responsibility for their health," she says. "I don't 'fix' them. I'm an educator, a coach. I explain how they can resolve their health problem by learning greater physiological control, and then I help them learn it. One great thing about biofeedback is that it doesn't take long. Very quickly, even people who come in more skeptical than I was say, 'Wow, I can do this.' "

## Asian Mysteries, Western Science

Starting in the 1950s, reports of amazing, seemingly impossible physiological feats reached American researchers. Asian scientists were documenting the claims of Indian yoga masters and Japanese Zen masters who claimed they could voluntarily control body functions that physiologists had long considered completely involuntary.

Japanese Zen monks could take a few deep breaths and almost immediately slow their metabolic rate and decrease their oxygen consumption by 20 percent. The only other examples of these kinds of changes that Western science has found are in animals during hibernation and in humans during their deepest stages of sleep. Even more amazing was film from India showing a yoga master being locked into a sealed metal chamber. Researchers then evacuated most of the chamber's air, enough to suffocate anyone who was breathing normally. Long after the average person would have died, the researchers opened the door. The yogi got up and walked out, none the worse for his experience. "How did you survive?" the researchers asked. "Simple," he replied. "I stopped breathing."

Many Western scientists assumed these supposed feats were frauds. But not Neal Miller, Ph.D., then head of the Laboratory of Physiological Psychology at Rockefeller University in New

York. Dr. Miller became fascinated by the similarities between the Asian reports and the work of B. F. Skinner, the Harvard psychologist who developed operant conditioning—a system of simple rewards and punishments used to train animals to perform complex tasks. If Skinner's conditioning could teach pigeons to do things long thought beyond them—such as pecking at a target only when a certain combination of lights was illuminated—then perhaps "involuntary" human body functions were not entirely beyond conscious control. Perhaps the yogis and Zen masters used a kind of internal Skinnerian conditioning to alter their physiology.

In a classic series of experiments, Dr. Miller used Skinnerian rewards and punishments to teach rats to raise and lower their heart rate, blood pressure, ear temperature, kidney function and intestinal muscle contractions. Publication of his results in 1969 in *Science*, the nation's top research journal, changed forever how Western science viewed learning. It was clear that with the right feedback, biological processes could be modified, hence "biofeedback."

Other researchers soon picked up where Dr. Miller left off. One was cardiologist Herbert Benson, M.D., associate professor of medicine at Harvard Medical School and president of the Mind/Body Medical Institute at New England Deaconess Hospital in Boston, whose biofeedback experiments with blood pressure control in monkeys led to his discovery of the relaxation response. Others repeated Dr. Miller's experiments in humans and discovered that people could affect many "involuntary" body functions when trained to use simple, inexpensive biofeedback devices that measured breathing, finger temperature, pulse rate, muscle tension or minute changes in perspiration.

The biofeedback industry was born. Today several thousand certified biofeedback therapists teach the technique to tens of thousands of people with dozens of ailments. Thousands more people learn biofeedback themselves using small home devices and the instruction books that come with them.

## Healing with Biofeedback

"Biofeedback is not a cure-all," says Francine Butler, Ph.D., executive director of the Association for Applied Psychophysiology and Biofeedback in Wheat Ridge, Colorado, "but it helps treat all the stress-related health problems."

Here's a look a some of the conditions that biofeedback can help.

*Anxiety.* Biofeedback teaches people to relax deeply. In that regard, it's similar to meditation and visualization and is often used in conjunction with visualization exercises.

"It's certainly possible to learn to relax without biofeedback," Schwartz explains, "but many people are so stressed and so out of touch with their bodies that they truly don't know how to relax, and when they do, they can't recognize it. With biofeedback, you simply look at the monitor and you can see yourself relax. Clients often say, 'Oh, so that's what deep relaxation feels like.' "

*Asthma.* In a 1992 study, Erik Peper, Ph.D., associate director of the Institute for Holistic Healing Studies at San Francisco State University, used biofeedback to teach 21 people with asthma to breathe slowly and deeply from their diaphragms. He hoped the training would help prevent the rapid, shallow gasping and wheezing of asthma attacks. After 15 months, 17 of the participants (80 percent) reported fewer attacks and emergency room visits and less use of asthma medication.

*Bruxism.* Bruxism is the dental term for clenching or grinding the teeth. That was how David Kahle of Cleveland dealt with his stress. He clenched his teeth so tightly that his jaw was chronically sore and he developed frequent tension headaches.

He knew he should relax his jaw, but he couldn't do it. As fate would have it, his boss at the time was using biofeedback to control his high blood pressure. He mentioned his success to Kahle, who thought it might help his bruxism. With muscle-tension sensors attached to his jaw, Kahle quickly learned to relax his facial muscles. In 12 sessions, his jaw soreness cleared up and his headaches vanished. That was ten years ago, and Kahle has had no problems with bruxism since.

*Chronic pain.* Chronic pain and anxiety form a vicious cycle. The pain causes anxiety, which lowers the pain threshold. Biofeedback relieves anxiety, which raises the pain threshold and helps control chronic pain. In addition, a good deal of back pain results from muscle tension up and down the back. Biofeedback can teach people to relax all the muscles from the neck to the buttocks.

Biofeedback is also useful in treating shortness of breath due to congestive heart failure as well as vaginismus (vaginal muscle contraction that makes intercourse painful or impossible) and other conditions. It is also helpful during stroke rehabilitation and artificial limb training—situations that require people to relearn the use of certain muscles.

*Constipation.* In a 1993 study, researchers at the University of Amsterdam in the Netherlands recruited 29 children who had chronic constipation because of an inability to relax the anal sphincter. After an average of five biofeedback training sessions, 90 percent learned sphincter relaxation and considered their problem cured. Over time, some of the children relapsed, but one year after their biofeedback training, 55 percent were still free of the problem.

*Diabetes.* Many people with diabetes experience circulatory impairment in the feet and legs, which sometimes necessitates amputation of a toe, foot or limb. In a 1992 study, Jay Schindler, Ph.D., then a professor of health education at the University of Wisconsin at La Crosse, and Birgitta Rice, a registered pharmacist and a researcher there, recruited 40 people with diabetes, ages 17 to 73, and asked them to select a relaxation technique, such as deep breathing or meditation, that appealed to them.

During the relaxation exercise, their toe temperature increased 9 percent and blood volume in the toe rose 2 percent. Then they were taught to increase blood flow to their toes using biofeedback. Their toe temperature soared 31 percent and their blood volume jumped 22 percent.

Biofeedback can also apparently help with a key problem for people with diabetes—keeping their blood sugar (glucose) under control. Under stress we all pump glucose into the blood. Our muscles need it to react to whatever stress there is. People with diabetes, though, cannot produce enough insulin to get glucose to the cells that need it, so they have higher blood glucose levels under stressful conditions—not an ideal situation. Worse, the stress hormones released during a stressful event can make whatever insulin is present less efficient.

"People with diabetes who learn to relax with biofeedback, however, can reduce their blood glucose levels," says Angele McGrady, Ph.D., associate professor at the Medical College of Ohio in Toledo. In two of her small preliminary studies, people doing biofeedback experienced lower stress and glucose levels when compared with untrained people.

"Consistent stress levels as well as peak responses to stressful events can be lowered," says Dr. McGrady. "You're also able to shorten the length of your stress response."

**Headaches.** "Biofeedback is one of the most effective treatments for migraine and tension headaches," says Alexander Mauskop, M.D., director of the New York Headache Center in New York City. With sensors placed on the head and neck, people who regularly have tension headaches become more aware of their tense spots and are better able to relax them.

Migraines are believed to involve unnatural expansion and constriction of certain blood vessels in the brain. Biofeedback can teach people who often have migraines to correct this. And while biofeedback is not a cure for headaches, "about half of clients improve by 50 to 80 percent," Schwartz says. Dr. Mauskop adds that at least one study shows 80 percent improvement *five years* after biofeedback training.

**High blood pressure.** Some of the original biofeedback studies showed that the technique could teach laboratory animals to raise or lower their blood pressure. "Many people use biofeedback to help control mild to moderate high blood pressure," Dr. Butler says.

**Incontinence.** "Nursing homes have a big problem with incontinence," Dr. Butler explains. "The patients hate the loss of control, and the nursing staff winds up spending a great deal of time cleaning people up and changing their clothes and linens.

Using special muscle-tension sensors, biofeedback can re-establish urinary and anal sphincter control."

Biofeedback may also strengthen the pelvic muscles needed for proper urinary control. In one study, 123 incontinent women were split into three groups—some were placed in a biofeedback/pelvic exercise group, some in just a pelvic exercise group and some in a group that did not do exercise or biofeedback. Those who tried biofeedback (using a vaginal probe) in combination with pelvic muscle exercises known as Kegels significantly lowered the number of incontinence episodes.

Women with moderate to severe symptoms maintained improvement for six months. Those who were doing only Kegels had similar results, although the biofeedback-guided exercises showed better "pelvic muscle activity"—a sign of more improved control.

"Biofeedback helps improve the person's ability to do the pelvic muscle exercises," says Patricia Burns, Ph.D., associate professor at the School of Nursing at the State University of New York at Buffalo.

In some cases, women can actually be cured of incontinence. When they stop treatment, though, incontinence can return. "Those who continue the therapy are likely to get the most benefit," says Dr. Burns.

*Raynaud's disease.* This common condition involves constriction of blood vessels in the fingers (and sometimes toes), that leads to cold extremities and painful extremities in cold weather. Schwartz says that most people given biofeedback instruction that teaches them to control their circulation reduce their discomfort by at least two-thirds.

*TMJ syndrome.* The temporomandibular joint (TMJ) is near the ear and connects the jaw to the skull. Thousands of people experience TMJ pain, which has several possible causes, among them chronic tension in the jaw muscle. Studies by Leonard Hukzinski, Ph.D., director of biofeedback services in the Department of Psychiatry at the Ochsner Medical Foundation in New Orleans, have shown that in tension-related TMJ syndrome, biofeedback provides effective long-term relief.

# Branches on the Biofeedback Tree

Any body function that can be monitored can be used for biofeedback. But over the years, therapists and equipment manufacturers have favored feedback that's easy to monitor, easy to learn and relatively inexpensive. The following types of biofeedback are most popular.

***Brain waves.*** Brain waves are measured using an electroencephalogram (EEG). EEG biofeedback may help in treating addictions and attention deficit disorder in children.

***Breathing.*** Using sensors placed on the chest or over the mouth and nose, this form of biofeedback measures breath rate, volume and rhythm. The feedback is usually visual, on one or more meters. Users learn to breathe more deeply, slowly and regularly. Breathing biofeedback is used to treat asthma and the rapid breathing (hyperventilation) of anxiety and panic attacks.

***Galvanic Skin Response (GSR).*** People perspire all the time, even when they're unaware of it. Anxiety increases this hidden perspiration, and relaxation decreases it. As the amount of perspiration changes, the electrical conductivity of the skin, or GSR, also changes. GSR biofeedback is used to treat anxiety, insomnia, obesity, chemical dependencies and overactive sweat glands (hyperhidrosis).

## Finding a Biofeedback Therapist

If you'd like to be coached in biofeedback by a certified therapist, send a self-addressed, stamped envelope to the Biofeedback Certification Institute at 10200 West 44th Avenue, Suite 304, Wheat Ridge, CO 80033 for a list of certified therapists in your area. Your doctor might also be able to give you a referral.

Professional biofeedback training costs from $75 to $150 per hour and requires 1 to 20 sessions. Occasionally people need a refresher course, but not often. "It's like riding a bike," biofeedback therapist Nancy Schwartz says. "Once you learn, you don't forget." Some health insurers cover biofeedback; others do not. Check your policy.

*Muscle tension.* Also known as electromyographic (EMG) biofeedback, this form uses sensors attached to the skin to detect electrical activity related to muscle activity. The feedback, either visual or aural, reflects muscle tension. EMG biofeedback may be used to treat tension headaches, back pain, incontinence and chronic muscle pain. It's also used in rehabilitation programs for those who have had strokes or serious injuries in accidents.

*Pulse.* Pulse biofeedback measures heart rate with sensors typically attached to one or more fingers. Pulse biofeedback may be used to treat anxiety, high blood pressure and some heart rate irregularities (cardiac arrhythmias).

*Thermal.* This form of biofeedback uses special thermometers called thermistors to measure skin temperature. Sometimes thermistors are taped to the forehead or chest, but often they are attached to one or two fingers. Muscle tension in the fingers reflects tension elsewhere, and muscle tension constricts the blood vessels, reducing blood flow and skin temperature. As the muscles relax, blood flow increases and temperature rises. Thermal biofeedback is frequently used to treat migraines, high blood pressure and anxiety.

For many problems—including everyday stress, headaches or insomnia—professional therapy might not be necessary. For the cost of one or two professional sessions, you can buy a home biofeedback system and possibly heal yourself.

Most biofeedback therapists have nothing against home systems. In fact, many rent or lend them to clients for practice. But they say their coaching helps produce the best results, just as coaching in sports improves athletes' performance. "I'd hate to see someone not get relief from a home biofeedback system and give up on it," Dr. Butler says. "Professional biofeedback therapy might help them." Remember this caveat if you try a home system without professional guidance, but if you'd rather do it yourself, excellent home equipment is available.

## Do-It-Yourself Therapy

The first practical home biofeedback device was developed in 1974 by Hal Myers, Ph.D., then a graduate student in biomedical engineering in Montreal.

Dr. Myers was using biofeedback to help a woman overcome an elevator phobia. He hooked her up to a device that measured her galvanic skin response (GSR)—the electrical conductivity of her skin. GSR is a sensitive measure of anxiety. A tone generator translated her anxiety level into sound—the higher the pitch, the more anxiety.

Her assignment was to approach and then ride the elevator in Dr. Myers's building while keeping the tone low. The woman made steady progress, but the biofeedback equipment was a hassle. GSR electrodes had to be attached to her with wires, and the monitor and tone generator were so large and unwieldy that she had to roll them along beside her on a cart.

Dr. Myers built a smaller unit using a display meter and tone generator that could be held in one hand and a GSR sensor resembling a computer mouse with two grooves for the index and middle fingers that could be held in the other hand. The minisystem worked just as well as the big one.

Shortly after Dr. Myers developed his machine, he was visited by a childhood friend, Lawrence Klein, who was footloose back home in Canada after working in Europe as a ski instructor. Dr. Myers proudly showed his friend the midget biofeedback system and asked what he thought of it.

Klein was so impressed he suggested they go into business together selling the device. The following year, they founded Thought Technology, with Dr. Myers as president and Klein as vice president. Today, Thought Technology is the world's leading manufacturer of home biofeedback equipment. The company has sold more than 250,000 biofeedback devices to individuals and to more than 10,000 clinicians, who use them professionally in more than 3,000 hospitals and clinics in 85 countries.

Even after he went into the business of biofeedback, Klein remained passionate about skiing, and he wondered if his company's major product, the GSR-2, combined with a visualization program, might be able to improve athletic performance.

He recruited the Canadian military biathlon team for a test. Biathlon is a sporting version of alpine hunting that combines cross-country skiing and riflery. The cross-country ski component demands rigorous aerobic exercise, with the athletes' heart rates rising to more than 150 beats per minute. But the riflery component demands composure and steady hands, which are best achieved with a heart rate below 90 beats per minute. Klein theorized that using the GSR, biathletes might be able to bring their heart rates down more quickly and improve their shooting.

In the test, half of the biathlon team used the real GSR with a variable-pitch tone that fell as heart rate decreased, and half used a sham GSR with a constant-pitch tone that gave no feedback about heart rate. The sham GSR group showed no improvement in shooting, but marksmanship in the real GSR group improved significantly.

Unexpectedly, the real GSR also improved the group's ski times. "That surprised us," Klein recalls. "When we asked the athletes about it, they said the GSR training helped them concentrate so they could better visualize their skiing."

Klein went on to produce "Mind over Muscle: Athletic Concentration Training," a program that combines a GSR-2 with a two-cassette visualization tape and an instruction booklet. Many Olympians have used it, including the U.S. and Canadian ski teams and half of the Japanese athletes who won medals in Seoul.

But most people use home biofeedback systems therapeutically for health problems. Bruce Thomson, a Quebec businessman, experienced on-the-job stress so severe that he experienced migraines, heartburn, rashes and eventually tachycardia—a frighteningly rapid heart rate. His doctor advised him to slow down and relax, but he didn't know how.

At a trade show in 1982, he chanced to see a GSR-2. "I began using it almost every day. Instead of getting headaches twice a week, I now get one about once a year. The same is true for my heartburn. My heart disturbances ceased years ago. But the best of it isn't my better health. I have become a more rested, more confident person, and I enjoy a more peaceful life," Thomson says.

"Biofeedback is a really a bridge between Eastern meditative practice and Western science," Klein says. "It's deep relaxation without the spirituality. Personally, I have tremendous respect for yoga and Asian spiritual disciplines. But in the West, many people just want results. For them, biofeedback can be very effective."

## CHAPTER 4

# COGNITIVE THERAPY

*Thinking Yourself Better*

In 1976, Philadelphia psychiatrist David D. Burns, M.D., became the father of a son, David Erik. The birth was normal, but something was clearly wrong with the newborn. His skin looked blue. He had difficulty breathing and gasped for air. The obstetrician reassured Dr. Burns and his wife that David Erik's condition did not appear serious and explained that there was not enough oxygen in the infant's bloodstream. As a precaution, the obstetrician said he'd like to send David Erik to the intensive care nursery for extra oxygen.

Dr. Burns consented—then panicked. Intensive care meant something must be terribly wrong, he told himself. His thinking spiraled downward from there: His baby son wasn't getting enough oxygen. That meant that his brain wasn't getting enough. He could be brain-damaged. Dr. Burns flashed on his own future, ruled by the needs of a severely handicapped child. He wondered if he could love such a child and imagined guiltily that people would think less of him for having a handicapped son.

### Getting Real

Feeling himself becoming overwrought, Dr. Burns decided to try the disarmingly simple therapeutic technique his colleague,

Aaron Beck, M.D., had pioneered. It involved writing down negative thoughts and then seeing if they were really true or somehow illogical. But the moment the idea occurred to him, Dr. Burns dismissed it as absurd: That approach was fine for his patients. They were imagining their problems. His problem was *real*.

Of course, Dr. Burns's patients had often made the identical comment to him, so he told himself what he always told them: Just try it. What do you have to lose?

It didn't take the panicky psychiatrist long to identify his negative thoughts: Intensive care meant the worst. His son was brain-damaged. His life would be ruined caring for a handicapped child. And his child's problems would diminish him in others' eyes.

Next Dr. Burns looked for fact or fallacy in his stated feelings—and found major distortions. The obstetrician had said intensive care was a precaution, that David Erik's condition did not look serious. By assuming the worst, he'd "mentally filtered" the information available to him, seeing only the most dire possibility, when his son might well be fine. Thinking that his son was brain-damaged, he'd "jumped to a conclusion" that was unjustified. Even if his son were handicapped, he'd "magnified" the problem by assuming it would ruin his life. Plenty of people live full, rich, rewarding lives despite their children's— or their own—handicaps.

Finally, by assuming that others would think less of him because his son was handicapped, he'd engaged in "overgeneralization." On reflection, he realized that his friends would judge him for himself, just as he judged them, independent of their children.

This simple exercise immediately calmed Dr. Burns. Soon after, he learned that David Erik was breathing normally and that his skin had turned a healthy pink. Subsequently he learned that the boy's brain was fine.

In addition, Dr. Burns learned that the technique he'd used could benefit not just those with major psychiatric problems but anyone dealing with an emotional challenge. Dr. Burns, professor of psychiatry and research clinical psychiatrist at the University of Pennsylvania Medical Center in Philadelphia, went on to write *Feeling Good: The New Mood Therapy* and *The Feeling Good Handbook,* both pioneering popular guides to cognitive therapy.

*Cognitive* refers to thought processes. Cognitive therapy is a deceptively simple, powerful self-help technique for dealing with emotional negativity by consciously changing the way we think.

## What Causes Negative Feelings?

Are you depressed? Are you anxious or troubled by guilt, frustration, anger or other negative emotions?

The true cause of negative emotions is a matter of opinion. To Freudian psychoanalysts, they are the result of repressed feelings that typically date back to childhood relationships with one's parents. To biological psychiatrists, they stem from chemical imbalances in the brain. To cognitive therapists, they represent distorted thinking. This view may be comparatively new to the mental health profession, but it was first espoused more than 2,000 years ago by the Greek philosopher Epictetus, who said, "People are not disturbed by events themselves, but rather by the views they take of them."

Some emotional turmoil is clearly the result of problems early in life—for example, childhood abuse—and Freudian-style talk therapies can help. "But most people don't have to spend a great deal of time understanding the past to improve how they react to potentially upsetting situations in the present," says psychologist Mark Sisti, Ph.D., associate director of the Center for Cognitive Therapy in New York City.

Some mental health problems are caused by chemical imbalances in the brain, and in recent years new antidepressants have been hailed by some biological psychiatrists as the answer to all mood problems. "Antidepressants can help people with severe depression," Dr. Sisti says, "but in mild to moderate depression, cognitive therapy works as well or better. In addition, it costs less and has no side effects. For other mood problems—anxiety, stress, guilt or phobias—cognitive therapy is more helpful than medication."

Scientific research supports Dr. Sisti. In a study, researchers at the University of British Columbia in Vancouver analyzed 28 separate studies comparing how people fared after different types of mental health therapy. Those using cognitive therapy did better than 98 percent of those who had no other therapy, better than 70 percent of those who took antidepressant drugs, better than 70 percent of those who tried the various forms of talk psychotherapy and better than 67 percent of those who tried behavior therapy (such as changing routines to break bad habits).

## The Ten Forms of Distorted Thinking

Could cognitive therapy help you deal with negative emotions? Perhaps. Dr. Burns has documented ten types of distorted thinking that lead to problems with negative emotions. How many of these emotional traps have you fallen into?

*All-or-nothing thinking.* You see things as black or white. If you're not perfect, you think of yourself as a total failure. You make one mistake at work and decide you're going to be fired. You get a B on a test and it's the end of the world. Your husband reprimands you for not checking the oil when you got gas and you decide he doesn't love you.

Dr. Burns says he was guilty of this one himself. "Like many people, I was a perfectionist," he explains. "Either I was terrific or I was nothing. Either I pleased my boss, spouse, parents or friends or else I was good for nothing. It made me terribly anxious, and I spent a good deal of my life ashamed of myself because, of course, I wasn't perfect."

*Labeling.* This practice is an extension of all-or-nothing thinking. You make a mistake, but instead of thinking "I made a mistake," you label yourself: "I'm a jerk." Your girlfriend breaks up with you, but instead of thinking "She doesn't love me," you decide "I'm unlovable."

Dr. Sisti felt himself slipping into labeling during a six-hour professional licensing exam. When he came to a section he found difficult, his first thought was "This is really tough. I must be an idiot."

"But then I took a deep breath and realized that I'd completed other sections that weren't so hard and that everyone else in the room was probably having as tough a time as I was," he recalls.

*Overgeneralization.* The tip-offs to this kind of distorted thinking are the use of the words always or never. You drop something and think "I'm always so clumsy." You make a mistake and think "I'll never get it right."

*Mental filtering.* In complicated situations that involve both positive and negative elements, you dwell on the negative. Your mother clearly enjoys the dinner party you throw in her honor but comments that the cake was a bit dry. You filter out all her positive comments and whip yourself for being such a lousy baker.

"As a perfectionist," says Bruce Zahn, Ed.D., director of psychology and cognitive therapy at Presbyterian Medical Center in Philadelphia, "I sometimes slip into mental filtering. I usually get good feedback on my job and in my personal relationships, but when people give me minor criticism, I'm apt to think the worst: 'They're going to fire me. They don't love me.' Then I realize 'No, this is a minor criticism, and all I have to do is correct it.' "

*Discounting the positive.* The tip-offs to this kind of distorted thinking are the phrases "That doesn't count," "That wasn't good enough," or "Anyone could have done it." You do well on a test and think "It doesn't count." Your colleagues praise a presentation and you think "It wasn't good enough." You win a commendation and think "Anyone could have done it."

*Jumping to conclusions.* You assume the worst based on no evidence. There are two subcategories here—mind reading and fortune-telling. In mind reading, you decide that another person is reacting negatively to you. Two of your co-workers are chatting at the coffee machine at work, but as you approach, they fall silent. Chances are they'd simply finished their conversation, but you assume they've been criticizing you behind your back.

In fortune-telling, you predict the worst possible outcome. A test is difficult, so you decide you'll fail. The sky is cloudy before your lawn party, so you decide a thunderstorm must be imminent.

Dr. Sisti slipped into fortune-telling when he realized he'd lost his automatic teller machine bank card: "My blood pressure shot up as I imagined that I'd lose all my money. Then I thought, What's the worst thing that could happen? Someone might use my card. But no one could—not without my personal identification number. But what if I'd left it in the machine? Then someone could withdraw $250. That would have been a loss, but not a terrible one."

*Magnification.* In this kind of distorted thinking, you exaggerate the importance of problems, shortcomings and minor annoyances. Your toilet backs up and you believe you need your entire plumbing system replaced. You forget to close a window before it rains and imagine that you'll return to a flooded home. A neighbor's dog tramples a few flowers and you decide your garden is ruined.

*Emotional reasoning.* When you fall into emotional reasoning, you mistake your emotions for reality. "I feel nervous about flying, therefore it must be dangerous." "I feel guilty about forgetting my brother's birthday, therefore I'm a bad person." "I feel lonely, therefore I must not be good company."

*"Should" and "shouldn't" statements.* This kind of thinking involves blaming yourself. You play well in the company volleyball tournament but miss one shot and berate yourself: "I should have made that shot. I shouldn't have missed." You eat a doughnut and think "I shouldn't have done that. I should lose ten pounds." Other self-denigrating tip-offs include *must*, *ought to* and *have to*.

*Personalizing the blame.* Here you hold yourself personally responsible for things beyond your control. Your child misbehaves at school and you think "I'm a bad mother."

"Occasionally I've been late for an appointment because of

heavy traffic," Dr. Sisti says, "and I've felt tempted to personalize it, as in 'I must be irresponsible.' But then I've realized that I'd allowed what should have been enough time and that the traffic jam is beyond my control. People understand if you get stuck in traffic. It happens to everyone."

## Seven Ways to Untwist Your Thinking

"When you feel bad," Dr. Burns explains, "your thinking becomes negative. This is the ABC of emotion: 'A' stands for the Actual event, 'B' for your Beliefs about it and 'C' for the Consequences you experience because of your beliefs." If you can somehow prevent erroneous negative beliefs from forming around an actual event, you've gone a long way toward protecting yourself from the unnecessary negative emotions that are sure to follow from such distorted thinking.

Dr. Burns recommends seven techniques to protect yourself from negative, distorted thinking. These techniques work for many unpleasant experiences, but let's use as an example a particularly unpleasant divorce.

In the throes of a nasty divorce you might be tempted to believe many of the charges your ex levels against you: You're selfish, uncaring and vindictive, and not only that, you're lousy in bed. If you buy into this picture of yourself, the consequences might well be low self-esteem and guilt, not to mention severe depression. Cognitive therapy tries to change the Bs—your beliefs—so you don't experience the Cs—negative consequences. Here's how to cope.

**Talk to yourself as you would to a best friend.** Dr. Burns says, suppose a friend were getting divorced and felt like a selfish, uncaring, vindictive failure. What would you say? Probably something like: "You're not a failure simply because your relationship ended. Many marriages end in divorce, and many winning teams lose a game now and then. It's rough to endure a divorce, and break-ups never bring out the best in people, but I've known you for years, and you're a warm, kind, caring person."

(continued on page 74)

# The Burns Anxiety Inventory ━━━━━━━━

Nearly everyone suffers from anxiety and worry from time to time. This self-test lists 33 common symptoms of anxiety. When answering each question, think about your thoughts, feelings and health during the last week. Score each question numerically, then add up your score.

0 for "not at all"    2 for "moderately"
1 for "a little"      3 for "very much"

1. Have you felt nervous, worried or afraid? _____
2. Have you felt that things around you seem strange or unusual? _____
3. Have you felt detatched from all or part of your body? _____
4. Have you felt at all panicky? _____
5. Have you felt apprehensive or a sense of impending doom? _____
6. Have you felt tense, stressed, uptight or on edge? _____
7. Have you had difficulty concentrating? _____
8. Have your thoughts raced or jumped from one subject to another? _____
9. Have you had frightening fantasies or daydreams? _____
10. Have you felt on the verge of losing control? _____
11. Have you feared cracking up or going crazy? _____
12. Have you feared fainting or passing out? _____
13. Have you feared dying from a heart attack or other serious illness? _____
14. Have you felt concerned about appearing foolish or inadequate in front of other people? _____
15. Have you feared being isolated, abandoned or left alone? _____
16. Have you feared criticism or disapproval? _____
17. Have you been afraid that something terrible is about to happen? _____
18. Have you had heart palpitations (racing or skipping beats)? _____

19. Have you felt pain, pressure or tightness in your chest? _____
20. Have your fingers and/or toes tingled or felt numb? _____
21. Have you experienced stomach upset, distress or butterflies? _____
22. Have you had constipation or diarrhea? _____
23. Have you been restless or jumpy? _____
24. Have your muscles felt tight or tense? _____
25. Have you perspired noticeably in cool places? _____
26. Have you felt a lump in your throat? _____
27. Have you experienced trembling or shaking? _____
28. Have your legs felt weak or rubbery? _____
29. Have you felt dizzy, light-headed or off-balance? _____
30. Have you experienced choking or smothering sensations or had difficulty breathing? _____
31. Have you suffered headaches, backaches or neck pain? _____
32. Have you experienced hot flashes or cold chills unrelated to fever? _____
33. Have you felt weak, tired or easily exhausted? _____

## SCORING:

| | | | |
|---|---|---|---|
| 0–4 | Minimal anxiety | 21–30 | Moderate anxiety |
| 5–10 | Borderline anxiety | 31–50 | Severe anxiety |
| 11–20 | Mild anxiety | 51+ | Extreme anxiety, panic |

NOTE: This quiz is not intended to be a substitute for proper mental health care. Those with mild to moderate symptoms of anxiety can often benefit from self-help books such as *The Feeling Good Handbook* and *Nature's Cures*. However, anyone with an elevated score or persistent symptoms of anxiety that last more than two weeks should seek consultation with a mental health professional.

SOURCE: Reprinted with permission from *The Feeling Good Handbook* by David D. Burns, M.D. (New York: Plume/Penguin, 1989). Not to be reproduced without permission of the author.

**Examine the evidence.** Take in the big picture. Write it down if you have to. Your ex says you're lousy in bed, but are you really? Until you learned of your ex's unfaithfulness, the two of you had a great sexual relationship. Of course, after your heart was broken, you didn't have any energy for sex, especially with the person who'd rejected you. That's not being lousy in bed. That's a normal reaction to betrayal.

**Experiment.** See how this negative thinking about yourself in this one area stacks up against your behavior in other areas. Your ex called you selfish for wanting to keep the house, but are you really? If you were truly selfish, you wouldn't give to charity, wouldn't help friends in need and wouldn't share credit for your group's accomplishments at work. Test your reactions the next time a charitable solicitation arrives or a friend calls with a problem or your group's efforts are recognized. If you write a check, offer to lend a hand or praise a co-worker, you're not entirely selfish. You may not be as magnanimous as you'd like to be, but you're not the ogre your ex says you are.

**Look for partial successes.** Instead of thinking that your marriage was a complete failure, consider the many ways that it was successful: You took turns putting each other through school, and now you both have much more fulfilling careers than you had when you met. You have two great kids, and the problems that led to your breakup have given you valuable new insights into the kind of person you'll look for in your next relationship.

**Take a survey.** Your ex insists that your refusal to take the kids for an extra day after a holiday weekend proves you're vindictive. You maintain that you're open to rescheduling time with the children, but not when the real reason is to allow your ex to jet off to a luxurious resort with a new lover. You feel justified, but after a screaming argument on the phone, your confidence is shaken. Perhaps you are a vindictive creep. Now's the time to call a few friends and solicit their views. Chances are they'll say you're justified.

**Define your terms.** You had no idea your ex was having affairs. You were blind. Define *blind*. The dictionary says, "completely without sight." That wasn't you. You saw that your ex was withdrawn from you and was spending an enormous amount of time "working late." You weren't blind, just too trusting of someone you had every reason to believe was trustworthy.

**Solve the problem.** You blew up when you came home early and found your ex, who moved out months ago, unexpectedly in your house. Since that ugly scene, you've been thinking that your "terrible temper" has turned you into a "monster." Possibly, but the problem in this case is not your temper. The real problem is that your ex still has keys to your house. Maybe it's time to change the locks.

## Seven Steps to Feeling Better

What if negative thinking does creep in and you find yourself mired in unpleasant emotions. Then what?

Cognitive therapy calls for tackling the problem in seven easy steps. Seven steps may not sound like many, but "simplicity is one of cognitive therapy's major strengths," Dr. Sisti explains. "It's quick and easy, and once people understand the basic concepts, almost anyone can practice it."

Sometimes, though, cognitive therapy's very simplicity puts people off. They say, "It's so simple, it can't work." When that happens, Dr. Sisti points out that they're jumping to a conclusion—the "fortune-telling" kind—and urges them to try the steps anyway. Give it a try for any given problem and see what happens.

**Step 1: Write everything down.** "The act of writing automatically puts some distance between you and your negative thought," Dr. Sisti says. "Jotting things down provides perspective and helps people detect distorted thinking more easily." If you are in a situation where you just can't put pen to paper, Dr. Sisti recommends saying things out loud.

**Step 2: Identify the upsetting event.** What's really bothering you? Is it simply the fact that you got a flat tire? Or is it that you soiled your outfit while changing it? Or that you knew you

# The Burns Depression Checklist

Everyone gets "the blues" when disappointed. And everyone gets depressed over job layoffs, a divorce, the death of a loved one or other major loss. A certain amount of sadness is a normal part of life. But when sadness never returns to gladness, it becomes what many authorities call the nation's leading mental health problem—clinical depression.

This self-test can help identify the symptoms of depression. How have you felt during the last week? Score each question numerically, then add up your score.

0 for "not at all"   2 for "moderately"
1 for "a little"      3 for "very much"

1. Have you been feeling sad or down in the dumps? _____
2. Does the future look hopeless? _____
3. Do you feel worthless or a failure? _____
4. Do you feel inadequate or inferior to others? _____
5. When things go wrong, do you criticize and blame yourself? _____
6. Do you have trouble making up your mind? _____
7. Have you been feeling resentful and angry a lot lately? _____
8. Have you lost interest in your job, hobbies, family or friends? _____
9. Do you feel overwhelmed and find you have to push yourself hard to get things done? _____

needed a new tire but didn't replace it? Or that the flat made you late for your daughter's soccer game?

**Step 3: Identify your negative emotions.** You might feel annoyed about the flat, frustrated that replacing it soiled your outfit, angry at yourself for not replacing it in time and guilty for being late for the soccer game.

**Step 4: Identify the negative thoughts that accompany your negative emotions.** About failing to replace the tire: "I always

10. Do you think you look old or unattractive? _____
11. Have you lost your appetite or engaged in binge eating? _____
12. Do you have trouble sleeping or sleep too much? _____
13. Have you lost interest in sex? _____
14. Do you worry a great deal about your health? _____
15. Do you ever think life isn't worth living or that you might be better off dead? ___

## SCORING:

| | | | |
|---|---|---|---|
| 0–4 | Normal ups and downs | 21–30 | Moderate depression |
| 5–10 | Borderline depression | 31–45 | Severe depression |
| 11–20 | Mild depression | | |

NOTE: This quiz is not intended as a substitute for proper mental health care. Those with mild to moderate symptoms of depression can often benefit from self-help books such as *The Feeling Good Handbook* and *Nature's Cures*. However, anyone with an elevated score, persistent symptoms of depression that last more than two weeks or suicidal impulses should seek consultation with a mental health professional.

procrastinate. I never take care of things in time." About soiling the outfit: "I'm a slob. I can't go anywhere and look okay." About being late for the game: "My daughter will make a scene. She'll think I don't love her. And the other adults there will think I'm a bad parent."

**Step 5: Identify distortions and substitute rational responses.** About the tire: "I don't always procrastinate. I juggle my job and family and accomplish just about everything that has to get done. I would have replaced that tire in time, but I had to deal with an emergency at work, and the tire just got by me." About the stained outfit: "I'm not a slob. I'm usually very careful about my appearance, more so than most people, which is why things like this upset me." About the tardiness: "My daughter knows I love her. She knows that if I'm late, whatever detained me was beyond my control. She's unlikely to make a scene, but if she does, the other adults there will comfort her. I've done the same for their kids and never thought them to be bad parents. No one will think the worst of me."

**Step 6: Reconsider your upset.** Are you still heading for an emotional tailspin? Probably not. But you still feel annoyed about getting the flat.

**Step 7: Plan corrective action.** "As soon as the game is over, we're getting that tire. That will take the time I'd planned to spend cooking dinner, so I'll pick up some take-out instead."

## Count Your Blessings

"A major task of adulthood is to balance striving to do well and accepting one's limits," Dr. Burns says. "Cognitive therapy has helped me accept my limits without feeling ashamed."

"Cognitive therapy is simply a more organized way to implement traditional psychological self-care advice," says psychotherapist Alan Elkin, Ph.D., director of the Stress Management Counseling Center in New York City. "It boils down to counting your blessings. Most stressful, depressing or anxiety-producing events are not inherently awful. What makes them feel awful is the way we react to them. Counting your blessings forces you to step back, get some perspective and see challenges in a larger context.

"The problem with 'count your blessings' is that it's vague. Cognitive therapy is a step-by-step program, and when negative thoughts are spinning out of control, an organized program helps," says Dr. Elkin.

CHAPTER 5

# COLD AND FLU THERAPY

## Natural Ways to Fight Back

What do Americans do when they feel the scratchy throat that signals a cold coming on? They typically respond in one of three ways: with fatalism, with pharmaceuticals or with natural therapies.

The fatalists believe the old saying that if you ignore a cold, it lasts a week, but if you treat it aggressively, you can get rid of it in just seven days. They are mistaken. There's a great deal you can do to prevent and treat the common cold.

Those who favor pharmaceuticals reach for drugstore cold formulas, believing that these products provide fast, fast, *fast* relief. The drug-takers are sadly misinformed. They spend more than $1 billion a year on products that neither prevent nor treat colds. All those dozens of cold formulas do is suppress cold symptoms, cost you money, cause annoying side effects and possibly even increase your cancer risk. (See "Cold Remedies: The Downside" on page 92.)

Those who gravitate toward natural medicine are on the right track, but few people who take the nation's most popular natural cold remedy—vitamin C—understand how to gain maximum benefit from it. And fewer still appreciate the fact that vitamin C is just one of many natural approaches to preventing

79

and treating humanity's number one infectious illness. As a result, they too often suffer needlessly from the sore throat, nasal congestion, runny nose, hacking cough and general misery of the all-too-common cold.

## Boost Your Immunity

Colds can be caused by any of about 200 viruses. Viruses are baffling bundles of genetic material. They're so tiny that if a human throat cell were the size of a typical house, a cold virus would be about the size of a window. Using the common definition of *life*, viruses are barely even alive. They don't breathe, digest food or eliminate wastes. Their only lifelike attribute is reproduction, which they do with a vengeance whenever they infect cells at the junction of the nose and the throat (the nasopharynx) and start creating more viruses.

Technically, each cold virus causes a "different" cold, but because all colds produce similar symptoms, we consider the common cold a single illness.

Americans get an estimated one billion colds a year, but contrary to what the fatalists believe, colds are not inevitable. There are two ways to beat them—fortify your immune system so the viruses you encounter don't cause infection and avoid viral encounters whenever possible so they can't infect you.

To boost your immunity, try these strategies.

**Manage your stress.** Ever catch a cold while studying for final exams or rushing to meet a deadline? Blame emotional stress. In one study, Sheldon Cohen, Ph.D., professor of psychology at Carnegie-Mellon University in Pittsburgh, used a battery of psychological tests to determine stress levels in 400 volunteers. Then he squirted live cold virus up their noses. Compared with the lowest-stress group, those with the highest stress levels were twice as likely to catch the cold. Why does stress increase susceptibility? Because it impairs the immune system's ability to fight off colds.

Final exams and major deadlines loom large in our emotional lives, but even minor daily ups and downs, the kind most people hardly notice, can affect cold susceptibility. In a study at the State University of New York Medical School in Stony Brook, 100 healthy adults were asked to keep detailed diaries for three months, recording all their ups and downs. Ups consisted of things such as compliments from co-workers and hugs from loved ones and downs were things like getting stuck in traffic.

Participants in the study donated daily saliva samples that were analyzed for secretory IgA. IgA is an immune system protein that's secreted in the mouth and upper respiratory tract; it acts as the body's first line of defense against cold viruses. The higher the IgA level, the better the chance of fending off colds. All the daily "downers," particularly those at work, significantly depressed IgA levels on the day they occurred. But life's little joys boosted IgA levels for up to two days.

Other studies have shown that relaxation exercises, such as meditation, raise IgA levels. The spontaneous relaxation produced by laughter has the same effect. In a study by Kathleen Dillon, Ph.D., professor of psychology at Western New England College in Springfield, Massachusetts, volunteers were shown one of two videos—either a serious educational program about anxiety or the comedy *Richard Pryor Live*. Those who watched the educational video experienced no change in IgA levels, but after watching the Richard Pryor tape, viewers' IgA levels jumped significantly.

Ditto for massage. Boston researchers divided 32 elderly volunteers into two groups. Members of one group lay on massage tables for ten minutes but did not receive massages. The other group enjoyed a ten-minute back rub. Both groups provided saliva samples before and after. Those in the group that were not massaged showed no change in IgA levels. But in the massaged group, IgA levels increased significantly.

The ability to inspire immune-enhancing relaxation may even explain some of the successes claimed by faith healers. Harvard researchers assembled a group of volunteers who were developing colds and took them to a Boston faith healer. Half the group had only brief, impersonal contact with the healer. The rest spent a long time with him. He gave them a great deal of personal attention, told them they were wonderful and laid his hands on them to help them relax and experience the calm of a meditative state. In the "impersonal" group, 11 of the 13 developed full-blown colds, but in the "healed" group only 2 did.

**Get regular exercise—but don't overdo it.** Researchers at Loma Linda University in California divided 50 sedentary women into two groups. Half continued their inactive lifestyle. The other half took brisk, 45-minute walks five days a week for 15 weeks. Compared with the stay-at-homes, the exercisers boosted their immune function and experienced only half as many days with cold symptoms, says David Nieman, D.H.Sc., professor of health promotions in the Department of Health, Leisure and Exercise Science at Appalachian State University in Boone, North Carolina, who headed the study. However, ultra-strenuous exercise depresses the immune system and increases risk of colds, according to another study of 2,300 runners training for the Los Angeles Marathon. During the two months before the race, runners who logged 60 miles a week were twice as likely to get colds as those who ran only 20 miles a week.

**Reduce your sweets.** Sugars (sucrose, fructose, glucose, honey) are apparently as bad for your immune system as they are for your teeth. Sweets impair the activity of infection-fighting white blood cells called neutrophils, according to Joseph Pizzorno, Jr., N.D., president of Bastyr College, the naturopathic medical school in Seattle. As cold-infected cells die, they release chemicals that draw neutrophils into the area to engulf and digest the invading microorganisms. But neutrophils become lethargic if you've been eating sweets. In one study, researchers gave people 100 grams of sugar (about the amount in two cans of soda or a few cups of yogurt with fruit) and then watched as neutrophil activity plummeted 50 percent. Five hours later, it was still substantially below normal.

**Eat less fat and more fresh fruits and vegetables.** Many studies have shown that a high-fat diet increases the risk of heart disease and several cancers, notably breast, colon and prostate cancer. But long before you develop diagnosable heart disease or cancer, the immune system must work overtime to prevent these

# The Flu Finder

You know you're sick, but do you know whether you have a bad cold or mild flu? Usually when a cold is mild or a flu is really mean, you know which one you have. But there's a whole gray area where it's hard to tell a bad cold from a mild case of flu. Here's a chart to help you sort them out. (And if any of these symptoms persist, see your doctor.)

| Symptom | Cold | Flu |
| --- | --- | --- |
| Fever | Rare in adults | Typical, high (102°–104°); lasts 3 to 4 days |
| Headache | Rare, except with sinus congestion | Typical |
| Aches, pains | Mild | Typical, often severe |
| Fatigue, weakness | Mild | Severe; can last up to 2 weeks |
| Exhaustion | Rare | Typical, suddenly you feel you must go to bed |
| Stuffiness | Typical | Sometimes |
| Sneezing | Typical | Sometimes |
| Cough | Typical, mild to moderate | Typical, can become severe |

diseases, and it may become less able to fight off colds. A 1992 review of 156 studies on diet and cancer risk showed persuasively that as fruit and vegetable consumption increases, risk of every major cancer decreases.

A plant-based diet supports the immune system's fight against not only cancer but all illnesses, because plant foods are high in vitamins and minerals. So do your immune system a favor: Eat less fat and enjoy more fruits and vegetables. The main sources of fat in the American diet are meats, dairy foods and fried foods, which include most junk snacks like potato chips and corn chips. The National Cancer Institute now recommends that Americans "strive for five," that is, five servings of fruits and vegetables a day.

**Drink water, tea and juices.** The nasopharynx is lined with protective mucus that acts almost like flypaper, trapping cold viruses and then carrying them to the stomach, where powerful digestive acids kill them. Grandma always advised drinking fluids as a cold treatment, and she may have been onto something. Research shows that fluids also help prevent colds.

"Adequate fluid intake helps maintain the integrity of the mucous membranes that line the throat," says Robert K. Cooper, Ph.D., health educator, president of the Center for Health and Fitness Excellence in Bemidji, Minnesota, and author of *Health and Fitness Excellence: The Scientific Action Plan.* When that mucus is moist, it's in top form for trapping cold viruses. But if even minor dehydration reduces the mucus layer's moisture content, cold viruses may penetrate it and infect throat cells. This is particularly true for office workers, as the air in today's climate-controlled buildings is usually quite dry.

"Keep a cup of water on your desk and sip it frequently during the day," advises Dr. Cooper, who advocates drinking six to eight cups of water a day.

**Watch the alcohol.** An occasional beer or glass of wine probably won't increase your risk of catching a cold (and many studies show that modest consumption of alcohol reduces heart disease risk). But research shows that daily drinking impairs neutrophil activity, increasing your risk of infection.

**Use immune-strengthening herbs.** When someone in your family or a co-worker has a cold, your risk of catching it goes way up. That's the time to give your immune system an extra tweak with any of several immune-boosting herbs, including echinacea, goldenseal, chamomile and ginger.

Echinacea and goldenseal are the most powerful immune enhancers. Echinacea appears to act like the body's own antiviral creation, interferon. Before cold-infected cells die, they release a tiny amount of interferon, which increases the ability of the surrounding cells to resist the infection. Researchers bathed cells in echinacea, then exposed them to two powerful viruses (influenza and herpes). Compared with untreated cells, those exposed to echinacea resisted infection significantly more effectively. Goldenseal contains the powerful natural antibiotic berberine, which is also an immune stimulant.

The most convenient way to take echinacea and goldenseal is to buy commercially prepared tinctures and add the recommended amount to a beverage tea, ideally chamomile or ginger tea, which also have immune-boosting benefits. Dr. Pizzorno cautions against taking echinacea or goldenseal daily, however. For daily immune enhancement, use the other approaches discussed in this section and reserve these herbs for times when you are actually threatened with a cold or other illness. Echinacea causes temporary tingling or numbing of the tongue, which is harmless. (For more on using medicinal herbs safely, see Herbal Healing on page 239.)

**Take vitamin C.** Many people take vitamin C as a cold preventive. The vitamin is an effective cold treatment, but a Finnish review of 21 scientific studies of vitamin C showed that even high doses have no cold-preventive value. What about the people who swear that since they've begun taking vitamin C, they've caught fewer colds? Perhaps they haven't documented their experience rigorously. Or maybe they're experiencing a placebo effect.

Placebos are dummy treatments that have no pharmacological value. But study after study shows that placebos consistently benefit about one-third of people who use them. (That's why good studies test new treatments against a placebo. The new treatment must perform significantly better to be considered effective.)

Scientists who take a mechanistic view of the human body consider placebo effects proof of people's gullibility: Give these turkeys anything and they'll say they feel better. But more thoughtful researchers understand that placebos are actually beautiful examples of mind/body healing. When you take something you believe to be beneficial, your emotions rev up your immune system and bingo, the treatment works. If you really believe that vitamin C helps prevent your colds, ignore the studies that show no benefit and keep taking it. In doses of a few thousand milligrams a day, vitamin C is safe for the vast majority of people. (If you have kidney disease, consult your physician before taking vitamin C supplements.)

**Try a homeopathic remedy.** Homeopathic physicians recommend a remedy known as *Oscillococcinum (AH-sill-oh-cock-SINE-um)* to prevent flu.

Like the common cold, flu is an upper respiratory viral infection, but the similarity ends there. Colds are minor illnesses that rarely cause fever in otherwise healthy adults. But one of the three flu viruses, influenza A, causes high fever, severe body aches and that awful death-warmed-over feeling that sends many otherwise healthy adults to their beds for several days. Type-A flu may also lead to pneumonia, and the combination kills thousands of Americans every year, mostly the elderly and those with chronic diseases. That's why public health officials urge annual vaccination every fall to prevent this flu.

The homeopathic medicine *Oscillococcinum* can also help. "For flu prevention," says Dennis Chernin, M.D., a physician in private practice in Ann Arbor, Michigan, "I recommend one dose a week. I recommend taking it throughout the fall and winter flu season."

A British study showed that this homeopathic medicine, available over the counter at many health food stores, provided significant relief of flu symptoms (fever, body aches and loss of appetite and energy). *Oscillococcinum* comes in tiny beads packaged in a capped vial; one dose is a capful of beads.

## Outwit Cold and Flu Viruses

A robust immune system certainly helps defeat any cold viruses you encounter. But why tempt fate? With a little information on cold transmission, you can often avoid cold viruses altogether.

Colds spread in two ways: through the air and by hand-to-nose contact. Ever since the nineteenth century, when Louis Pas-

# Cold Symptoms?
## Blame the Immune System, Not the Virus

Cold viruses don't cause cold symptoms. The sore throat, congestion, runny nose and cough result from the immune system's battle against the infection.

Before cold-infected throat cells die, they release special chemicals that rally the body's self-defense forces to arms. As the immune system swings into action, the tiny blood vessels in the throat expand. This allows extra blood to flow into the nose and throat, bringing with it infection-fighting white blood cells and other immune warriors. Eventually the swollen blood vessels activate local pain nerves and you feel "a sore throat coming on." The phrase is ironic, because by the time the sore throat develops, the infection has already been present for 24 to 48 hours.

As the days pass, the extra fluid drawn to the throat to fight the infection clogs the sinus cavities around the nose, causing nasal congestion. Some of it leaks out as a runny nose or triggers sneezing. Eventually the immune system's fight against the infection irritates the throat and bronchial tubes, causing a dry, hacking cough. People feel fine as they become infected with colds. They start to feel ill when the body starts making them well.

teur popularized the idea that microorganisms cause infectious diseases, people have believed that colds spread through the air when people with colds cough or sneeze. But this commonsense explanation remained unproven until the 1980s, when Elliot Dick, Ph.D., chief of the Respiratory Viruses Laboratory at the University of Wisconsin at Madison, began organizing unusual poker games.

Dr. Dick promised healthy college students a week of free room and board plus a nonstop poker marathon if they would move into a sealed suite of rooms and risk catching a cold. After locking his healthy volunteers into the suite, Dr. Dick added a few people with colds to the poker game and watched what hap-

## Flu-Related Pneumonia: Beware!

In the elderly and those with chronic illnesses, one type of flu, influenza A, can lead to a deadly form of pneumonia. Flu-related pneumonia is the nation's sixth leading cause of death, claiming thousands of American lives every winter.

The high death rate from flu-related pneumonia is the reason those at risk should get flu shots every year. The danger signs include shortness of breath, difficulty breathing and/or a second fever a few days to three weeks after the initial flu fever subsides.

If you or anyone you know—especially anyone over age 60—develops these symptoms, call a doctor immediately.

pened. In one experiment, all the healthy volunteers caught the cold—and so did more than half of the researchers who visited the room. Clearly, the cold had spread through the air.

But after many poker experiments, Dr. Dick came to an astonishing conclusion: Contrary to popular opinion, under natural conditions, colds are not that easy to transmit. In one test, when the experimental room was unsealed and ventilated as a typical home would be, only 20 percent of the uninfected volunteers caught the cold.

Enter J. Owen Hendley, M.D., and Jack Gwaltney, M.D., professors of medicine at the University of Virginia in Charlottesville, who discovered that when people with colds touch their noses, their fingers pick up live virus. When those contaminated fingers touch hard, nonporous objects—such as doorknobs, telephones and countertops—they deposit some virus, which can survive until it dries out. When the fingers of the uninfected touch cold-contaminated objects, they literally pick up the virus and can inoculate themselves by touching their own noses or rubbing their eyes. (The tear ducts in the inner corners of the eyes are connected to the nasopharynx by a tiny tube.) Most people unconsciously touch their noses several times an hour, allowing ample opportunity for people with colds to leave a trail of virus and for others to risk self-inoculation.

The discovery of the hand-to-nose route cast doubt on Dr. Dick's earlier findings: Perhaps his poker players had caught their colds by touch. So Dr. Dick organized another poker marathon, only this time his healthy subjects wore restraints that prevented them from touching their noses and eyes. Many still caught the cold. Now scientists generally agree that colds can be spread through the air and by finger contamination.

You can use the findings on cold transmission to keep those wily viruses out of your throat.

**Increase ventilation.** This disperses cold viruses in the air, and the fewer that get into your throat, the better off you are. You may not want to open the windows in winter, but do what you can to keep the air moving. Invest in some small fans. If you have forced-air heat, check the filters and the cold air return to make sure the air flows freely.

**Wash your hands often.** This minimizes hand-to-nose transmission.

**Don't touch your nose or rub your eyes.** This is not as easy as it sounds, but with some effort you can train yourself to keep your hands away from your face. If you must rub your nose or eyes, don't use a possibly contaminated fingertip. Use a knuckle, which is less likely to be tainted with virus.

**Retire your cloth handkerchiefs.** Live virus can survive for several hours in cloth hankies, and every time you pull them out, you recontaminate your fingers. Switch to disposables. They're used once, then discarded, thus limiting finger contact with the virus. Washing your hands removes any lingering virus from your fingers.

**Disinfect everyday surfaces.** Disinfectants remove cold viruses from doorknobs, telephones and other surfaces. In one study, Dr. Gwaltney contaminated a countertop with cold virus, then sprayed it with Lysol disinfectant. Lysol treatment greatly reduced the amount of cold virus. But Lysol is not the only antiseptic disinfectant. Most kitchen herbs—such as rosemary, sage, the mints, thyme, cinnamon and ginger—have antiseptic properties. Natural disinfectants made with these spices should have a similar effect.

**Don't worry too much about kissing.** To test the widely held belief that kissing spreads colds, Dr. Dick infected one member of each of 16 couples with a cold virus and had them plant an extended kiss on their spouses' mouths. Only one partner (6 percent) caught the cold. During colds, the virus generally stays in the nose and throat. The mouth remains remarkably virus-free.

Then Dr. Dick infected one member of each of 24 married couples and tracked them as they lived their daily lives together for more than a week. Only nine of the spouses (38 percent) caught the cold, and the risk was unrelated to their kissing or lovemaking. The only risk factor was the total amount of time they spent together. There's no reason to refrain from kissing someone with a cold, especially if the kiss is merely a peck on the cheek. "Just don't rub noses with them," Dr. Dick advises, "or you risk passing the cold by nose-to-nose transmission."

**When you cough or sneeze, cover your mouth.** People with colds expel millions of virus particles when they cough and sneeze. Covering the mouth helps trap particles before they spread through the air.

**Avoid anyone with the flu as much as possible.** Flu viruses also spread through the air, but compared with the common cold, flu spreads much more easily. In one case, a passenger with the flu boarded a commercial airliner. After being exposed to this person's exhalations for just three hours, an astonishing 72 percent of the other passengers developed the illness.

How can you tell if a friend or loved one has the flu and not just a bad cold? Colds almost never cause physical collapse, but people with the flu typically spend several days in bed, barely able to move. Colds rarely cause fever, headache and body aches, but these symptoms are typical of flu.

## Parents, Kids and Colds

Even if you exercise regularly, become a vegan, take echinacea, meditate like Buddha and wash your hands like Lady Macbeth, you'll still probably catch an occasional cold—especially if you spend a great deal of time with children under five. There's probably nothing wrong with your immune system. Young children catch the most colds by far—six to nine a year—and proximity to all that virus raises cold risk. (Because most adults who care for kids are women, women catch more colds than men.)

Children catch the most colds for three reasons: First, their immune systems are not fully developed, so compared with adults, they can't fight off colds as well. Second, each cold confers a three- to ten-year (and possibly longer) immunity to that specific virus and a few of its close relatives. Young children haven't lived long enough and endured enough colds to have acquired much of this virus-specific immunity, so compared with older children and adults, they're vulnerable to more viruses. Finally, few kids relish hand washing, and it's unrealistic to expect them to keep their fingers away from their noses (or other people's).

If you spend time with children, follow the preventive suggestions above and try not to get too stressed about your cold risk. Remember, stress increases susceptibility.

But before fear of colds makes you reject parenthood or a career in day care, consider this: Parents and those who work with children catch more colds, but only for the first few years. Because each cold confers fairly long-standing immunity to that virus, over time the defenses of those in close contact with children improve and they catch fewer colds.

The same thing happens to children in day care. In one study, toddlers enrolled in day care programs had 60 percent more colds than children cared for at home. But those extra colds equipped them with extra immunity. Later, from age three to five, the day care kids caught only half as many colds as the children cared for at home.

Finally, contrary to what moms have said since time immemorial, being cold has nothing to do with catching a cold. Extended exposure to low temperatures can cause life-threatening hypothermia, but ordinary, everyday chills don't increase susceptibility to colds. British researchers had subjects take hot baths and then spend a half-hour in a drafty hallway wearing

# Cold Remedies: The Downside

Hundreds of over-the-counter (OTC) cold formulas claim to relieve every major cold symptom. Do they work? The actors in the commercials gain instant relief, but scientific investigations have produced decidedly mixed results. Antihistamines in particular have often been declared useless—and possibly hazardous.

Two Canadian pediatricians, Michael Smith, M.D., of Nova Scotia, and William Feldman, M.D., of Toronto, reviewed 51 studies of OTC cold formulas published from 1950 to 1991. Their findings: Cold remedies do nothing to attack cold viruses or boost the immune system's fight against them, so they have *no effect* on the duration of colds. All they do is suppress symptoms, providing modest relief from nasal congestion, runny nose and cough—but only for those over age five. In preschoolers, the researchers found that OTC cold formulas have no benefit at all.

Of the five antihistamines commonly used to treat colds, Dr. Smith and Dr. Feldman concluded that only one, chlorpheniramine (*klor-fen-EAR-uh-mean*) maleate, actually helps dry a runny nose. But before you reach for an OTC containing it, you should be aware that a study published in the *Journal of the National Cancer Institute* suggested that antihistamines might spur tumor growth.

Antihistamines have chemical structures similar to DPPE, a chemical used in cancer research to produce tumors in experimental animals. Canadian researchers wondered if antihistamines might do the

only wet bathing suits and wet socks until they became thoroughly chilled. But chilling alone never produced any colds. You need viral exposure to catch a cold. So the researchers then squirted live cold virus up the noses of another group of people, half of whom endured the same chilling treatment; the other half spent their time ensconced in warm, cozy rooms watching TV. The chilled group did not catch any more colds or worse colds than the warm people.

same. They injected mice with two types of tumor cells and then divided them into six groups. One group received no antihistamines; the other five received one of five antihistamines in daily doses equivalent to what humans take for colds. After three weeks, the researchers examined the tumors.

The largest tumors developed in the mice given three of the five antihistamines. This study does not prove that antihistamines are hazardous. But most antihistamines have no effect on cold symptoms, they're expensive, and they might stimulate tumor growth. Why use them?

Much of the more than $1 billion a year consumers spend on cold remedies goes for all-in-one cold formulas, but most doctors discourage taking them. Cold formulas do indeed contain ingredients to relieve every major cold symptom, but cold symptoms develop serially, not all at once. Why pay for a cough suppressant when what's bothering you is a stuffed nose? And why risk side effects from medicines you may not need—drowsiness from antihistamines and jitters and insomnia from decongestants?

Nature's cures for the common cold don't just suppress symptoms. Most boost the immune system's effectiveness against it, and some have antiviral action. Natural approaches also have fewer side effects than pharmaceuticals, and most are considerably cheaper.

## Cold Treatment: Grandma Was Right

For colds, Grandma always said to rest, drink plenty of hot fluids and have some chicken soup. There's wisdom in these recommendations—and in many other natural remedies as well.

**Get plenty of rest.** Most colds aren't serious enough to send people to bed, but if possible, take it easy for a few days. It's hard work for your immune system to vanquish those viruses.

That's why anyone with a cold feels tired. Support your immune system by resting.

If possible, take a day off from work. Educate your boss that a brief self-quarantine for colds protects co-workers from your virus, and in the long run can increase group productivity.

**Drink hot fluids.** Cold viruses reproduce best at temperatures slightly below normal body temperature. Hot liquids warm the throat and help impair viral replication. They also soothe a sore throat and cough. And hot liquids have a mild decongestant effect that helps relieve nasal congestion.

**Take enough vitamin C.** Ever since 1970, when the late Linus Pauling, Ph.D., published *Vitamin C and the Common Cold,* vitamin C has been the nation's most controversial cold remedy. Some studies have shown clear benefit from using vitamin C as a treatment; others have not.

Wisconsin's Dr. Dick was one of those who scoffed at the vitamin's value. Then Dr. Pauling himself buttonholed Dr. Dick at a scientific meeting and challenged him to test vitamin C in one of his poker-game experiments. In three studies, Dr. Dick had some of his volunteers take four 500-milligram tablets (2,000 milligrams) of vitamin C daily for several weeks before they moved into his experimental room along with volunteers who had not taken the vitamin. Then he brought in people with colds. The vitamin users caught as many colds as the untreated people. These results lined up with almost two dozen other studies showing that vitamin C has no cold-*preventive* value. But in every test, the vitamin C group had significantly milder symptoms, showing a clear *treatment* benefit. Dr. Dick, the former skeptic, was won over: "At the first sign of a cold," he says, "I now take vitamin C."

The Finnish review of 21 vitamin C studies mentioned earlier showed that at doses of 1,000 milligrams a day, the vitamin consistently reduced the severity of cold symptoms. The average symptom-reduction score was 23 percent.

But what about all the vitamin C studies that have shown no benefit? They apparently gave too little vitamin C for too short a time. The studies that showed benefits involved at least 1,000

# Never Treat Children's Colds with Aspirin ━━━━━

In children under 18 who are experiencing significant discomfort from fever caused by colds, flu or chickenpox, do not give aspirin or its herbal equivalents, willow bark, meadowsweet or wintergreen. The combination of viral fevers and aspirin is associated with Reye's syndrome, a rare but potentially fatal illness that affects the brain and liver. Instead, place the child in a tepid bath. If you can't resist medication, give acetaminophen (Tylenol, Panadol, St. Joseph Aspirin-Free). When in doubt, call your child's physician.

milligrams a day from the first throat tickle until the cold had completely cleared up. Basically, there's a threshold below which vitamin C provides no benefit, but if you take more than a gram a day, it works.

Dr. Dick advocates taking 2,000 milligrams a day in four 500-milligram doses when you have a cold. A few other vitamin C advocates recommend 3,000 to 4,000 milligrams a day. But high doses of vitamin C can cause diarrhea; if diarrhea develops, reduce your dose.

**Try chicken soup.** Chicken soup apparently helps, but so do soups made without chicken. Eight hundred years ago, Egyptian rabbi/physician Moses Maimonides recommended chicken soup for the common cold. It's been a mainstay of folk medicine ever since. Florida researcher Marvin Sackner showed that chicken soup does indeed relieve nasal congestion better than plain hot water. His elderly mother, Goldie, though proud of her son, was reportedly miffed that he'd used chicken soup from a deli near his laboratory instead of her infinitely more therapeutic family recipe.

Stephen Rennard, M.D., chief of pulmonary and critical care medicine at the University of Nebraska in Omaha, did not make the same mistake. In a 1993 study, he confirmed chicken soup's benefits using a recipe handed down from his wife's grandmother. His test-tube experiment showed that chicken soup significantly reduced the inflammation-producing action of certain white blood cells. Surprisingly, the soup showed its beneficial effect even before the chicken was added, when it was simply vegetable soup containing onions, sweet potatoes, carrots, turnips and parsnips.

Many studies have shown that onions have anti-inflammatory effects, and Dr. Rennard found that when tested one at a time, all five vegetables had anti-inflammatory action. "I'm a mainstream physician," he says, "but plants were the original medicines. There's a lot of wisdom in traditional medical advice."

**Take herbs.** The immune-boosting herbs recommended for preventing colds, especially echinacea and goldenseal, also help treat them. Andrew Weil, M.D., professor of preventive medicine at the University of Arizona College of Medicine in Tucson and author of *Natural Health, Natural Healing,* suggests taking a dropperful of echinacea and/or goldenseal tincture in water four times a day whenever you have a cold. You might also add the tincture to chamomile or ginger tea, both which have mild immune-stimulating benefits.

**Look into Chinese medicine.** Chinese medicine considers the common cold to represent an invasion of the body by the elements wind and heat. An age-old formula known as Yin Chiao Chieh Tu Pien (*yin chow chee dew peein*) expels wind and heat from the respiratory tract. The formula works, according to Harriet Beinfield, a licensed acupuncturist who practices Chinese medicine in San Francisco and is co-author of *Between Heaven and Earth: A Guide to Chinese Medicine.* "It can really impress people who have not tried Chinese herbs," she says.

She says that at the first sign of a sore throat or runny nose, taking six tablets of Yin Chiao every three hours can keep symptoms from developing into a full-blown cold. Yin Chiao contains primarily honeysuckle and forsythia. It is available from many practitioners of Chinese medicine.

**Try a homeopathic remedy.** Homeopaths most frequently prescribe microdoses of *Allium cepa* (onion), *Euphrasia* (eyebright) and *Natrum mur* (salt) for the common cold. Other homeopathic medicines sometimes used include *Aconite* (monkshood), *Bryonia* (wild hops), *Belladonna* and *Phospho-*

# Colds: Civilization's Illness

What happens to cold viruses when no one has a cold? "Someone always has a cold," explains Elliot Dick, M.D., chief of the Respiratory Viruses Laboratory at the University of Wisconsin at Madison. "If not, the virus dies out."

Dr. Dick proved this with a series of studies at the McMurdo Sound U.S. Research Station in Antarctica. A small group of scientists stay there year-round and have no contact with the outside world for the entire (very long) Antarctic winter. In a typical year, when the summer people depart, one or two colds remain among the winter group and spread around the station. But after a while, everyone catches those colds and gains immunity to those viruses. With no susceptible people left to infect, those colds simply die out. No one at the station catches any more colds until the following spring, when outsiders return and bring new ones in. In other words, for colds to survive, cold viruses need a reasonably large number of people, some of whom are transients.

Cold viruses infect only humans and a few species of monkeys. When the viruses first appeared, they must have struggled for survival in monkey bands and early hunter-gatherer societies, which were small, fairly isolated and self-contained. Then cold viruses got lucky: Humans developed civilization. Large numbers of people settled down together and began traveling to neighboring settlements, producing the perfect environment to keep colds spreading from person to person. Colds have been humanity's leading illness ever since.

*rus.* To use these medicines, follow package directions. (For a more detailed description of these treatments and others, see Homeopathy on page 259.)

**Think zinc.** When three-year-old Karen Eby of Austin, Texas, was diagnosed with leukemia in 1978, her physician suggested zinc supplements to stimulate her immune system. Karen swallowed her zinc tablets whole, but one day she had a cold and sucked them instead. Soon after, her cold vanished. Karen's father, George, became intrigued, and he persuaded some researchers to test zinc as a cold remedy. Compared with a group of people with colds who took a placebo, those who sucked on one 23-milligram zinc gluconate lozenge every two hours experienced significantly briefer colds.

Several other studies have also shown that zinc relieves cold symptoms—but only if you start sucking on zinc gluconate at the first sign of a tickle in the throat. Unfortunately, zinc gluconate tastes terrible. Supplement makers now offer flavored zinc lozenges that mask some of its taste.

"I use a zinc/peppermint combination that I buy at my local health food store," says zinc researcher William Halcomb, D.O., of Mesa, Arizona. "Or just suck on a mint Lifesaver while you suck on the zinc." In addition, you should suck the lozenges after eating. "On an empty stomach, they can cause nausea," Dr. Halcomb says.

**Experiment with dairy foods.** A good deal of folklore suggests that milk and dairy products spur nasal mucus production and increase the severity of colds. Nutritionists have generally dismissed this notion as a myth, but some physicians insist that a dairy-free diet reduces the risk and severity of colds, flu and sinus and ear infections.

"Dairy is a tremendous mucus producer and a burden on the respiratory, digestive and immune systems," says Christiane Northrup, M.D., a gynecologist in Yarmouth, Maine, who specializes in natural medicine. "Eliminate dairy foods and you suffer less from colds."

One scientific study supports her view. It shows that a chemical in milk triggers the release of histamine, which triggers runny nose and nasal congestion. Next time you have a cold, cut down on dairy products and see if the change helps.

**Listen to your body.** "Feed a fever, starve a cold." Or is it "Starve a fever, stuff a cold"? You hear it both ways, but the fact is, you shouldn't starve or stuff either one. Colds often suppress appetite, and some people say that eating lightly or drinking only vegetable juices speeds their recovery. Eat well if you feel hungry. Refrain if you don't.

## CHAPTER 6

# COMPANIONSHIP

*One Plus One Equals Better Health*

In the early 1970s, Leonard Syme, Ph.D., found himself gazing in disbelief at raw data from a study he was co-ordinating on ethnic Japanese men's risk of heart attack.

"Japan has the lowest rate of heart disease in the industrialized world," says Dr. Syme, professor of epidemiology at the University of California at Berkeley School of Public Health. "Twenty years ago, most epidemiologists, myself included, were convinced that what protected them was their low-fat diet. We all believed that dietary fat explained why Japanese men who immigrated to the United States had a substantially higher rate of heart disease. When they moved, they began eating a more American, higher-fat diet, and fairly quickly, their rate of heart disease increased two- to fivefold."

Simple—or so Dr. Syme thought until he examined the data on heart disease in 17,000 ethnic Japanese men living in Japan and California. "We looked at men in both places who had the same cholesterol levels, a strong indicator of their dietary fat consumption, and the California Japanese had five times as much heart disease. Then we compared men with the same blood pressure, smoking habits and every other recognized risk factor. Compared with Japanese men in Japan, the California Japanese had two to five times as much heart disease. I had no idea why."

## Hearts Love Friendship

Across the country in Roseto, Pennsylvania, Stewart Wolf, M.D., and John Bruhn, M.D., stumbled on a similar heart disease surprise. The men of Roseto had a lifestyle that was indistinguishable from that of men in nearby East Stroudsburg. They smoked as much, were just as sedentary and ate a diet just as high in fat. But their death rate from heart disease was substantially lower—Roseto men in their fifties had 80 percent fewer heart attack deaths, and for men over 65, the figure was 60 percent lower.

Since none of the standard risk factors could explain this astonishing difference, what could? "Companionship," Dr. Syme says. "Close social ties."

Dr. Syme's quest for answers to his unexpected research finding took him to Japan, where he met with Japanese epidemiologists. "Japanese society," he explains, "is organized around social networks much tighter than what we have in the United States. Even with increasing Westernization, Japanese people still have very close ties to their families, neighborhoods and jobs. To Americans, that looks claustrophobic, like an invasion of privacy. But to the Japanese, our mobile, individualistic lifestyle looks terribly lonely, rootless and isolated."

Dr. Syme began to wonder if social isolation might explain his study's odd findings. In addition to eating more fat when they moved to the United States, Japanese immigrants also became more isolated from their traditional social support networks.

In 1974, Dr. Syme and Lisa Berkman, Ph.D., professor of epidemiology and public health at Yale University (who was then a graduate student) investigated the health impact of social support by unearthing a 1965 survey of 6,928 residents of Alameda County, California, that asked about their marital status, contacts with family and friends and membership in civic, social and religious organizations. Then they used the Alameda County death registry to see who in the sample had died during the intervening nine years. The results were striking. The more social connections the survey takers reported in 1965, the less likely they were to die—not just from heart disease but from all causes.

Compared with those reporting the most social ties, those claiming the fewest had twice the death rate.

## Isolation Harms Health

"Social isolation," Dr. Syme says, "must be considered a significant risk factor for serious illness. By the same token, close social ties must be considered protective." The Barbra Streisand song says, "people who need people are the luckiest people in the world." They're also the *healthiest*.

Close social ties also explain the remarkably low rate of heart disease in Roseto. The town was founded in 1882 by a close-knit group of immigrants from southern Italy. Over the decades, they retained their traditions of family closeness, devoted churchgoing, neighborliness, three-generation households, membership in particular social organizations and marriage to other Italian-Americans, often people from Roseto or towns nearby. The same could not be said for East Stroudsburg, which was a more fragmented "American" town.

Over time, of course, even close-knit Roseto became Americanized. Starting in the 1950s, young people began leaving, three-generation households gave way to more one-generation nuclear families, and suburbanization took more residents to new homes on the outskirts of town. This largely destroyed the culture around Roseto's main street, Garibaldi Avenue, where neighbors had traditionally kept their doors open and frequently dropped in on one another. As the community's tight social structure slowly unraveled, its death rate from heart disease rose, but Roseto's residual cohesion kept its death rate considerably below East Stroudsburg's.

A lack of social ties also helps explain why Type-A behavior—the high-stress lifestyle characterized by ambition, hostility and time pressure—puts people at increased risk for heart disease, says Dr. Syme. "What kind of people are socially isolated? One obvious group is the hard-driving type whose preoccupation with achievement leaves little if any time for family, friends and other social connections," he says. "Type-A individuals are isolated, and not surprisingly, they're at high risk for heart disease."

Companionship may also explain why women live, on average, about seven years longer than men. The conventional wisdom is that many male-dominated occupations put men in harm's way. True, but in addition, men tend to have fewer close social ties than women.

A fundamental social connection for both men and women is marriage, and having a reasonably happy one is a major boon to health. Studies dating back to the 1940s show that single, widowed or divorced men have a death rate twice that of married men. And single, widowed or divorced women have a death rate 50 percent higher than their married counterparts.

More recently, a ten-year study of more than 7,500 adults by epidemiologists at the University of California's San Francisco Medical Center showed that compared with married men, single men of the same age were more than twice as likely to have died from all causes. Even when single men live with a family member or a friend, their death rate is still substantially higher than married men's.

"The relationship between social isolation and early death," says David Spiegel, M.D., professor of psychiatry at Stanford University and director of the university's Psychosocial Treatment Laboratory, "is as strong statistically as the relationship between dying and smoking or having high cholesterol. Numerically at least, it may be as important for health to have a strong network of family and friends as it is to stop smoking or reduce your cholesterol level. But for a factor so strongly related to health and longevity, medical science has greatly underestimated the value of social support."

## How Companionship Keeps You Healthy

The value of social support has been hiding in plain sight for so long that it's amazing it took researchers so long to discover it. "From the day we are born," Dr. Spiegel says, "social support is essential to human survival. We have a more prolonged period of helplessness and dependency than any other mammal. For years, we must rely fully on our parents' physical and social skills."

Thousands of years ago, humans also discovered the survival advantage of organizing themselves into clans, tribes, villages, cities and nations. Many other animals are stronger, faster and endowed with more acute senses. But thanks to language and symbols, we humans have a unique ability to engage in complicated interactions, advance the common good and protect ourselves from predators—both animal and human. As a result, we have populated the entire habitable earth. Our clichés tell the tale: "There's strength in numbers." "Two heads are better than one." "One for all, and all for one."

But only since the advent of psychoneuroimmunology—the study of how emotions influence the central nervous system and the immune system—have scientists come to appreciate the fact that "all for one" means more than simply everyone working toward a common goal. It also means that the "all" has profound physiological impact on the "one."

In the 1940s, when researchers first documented the "marriage bonus" on health, they speculated how a stable home life might contribute to health and longevity.

*Nutrition.* Married people, especially those with children, are more likely than singles to eat healthfully.

*Bad habits.* The social support provided by marriage helps people avoid—and quit—bad habits, particularly smoking, excessive drinking and overeating.

*Risk-taking.* This one relates to men, who, in general, take more risks than women. Compared with single men, husbands and fathers are less likely to drive race cars, skydive and engage in violent crime and other reckless pursuits that might risk their lives.

*Medical care.* Finally, spouses often encourage each other to seek medical care. Loners may neglect to obtain care until diseases have progressed to the point where they are difficult to treat. Spouses also tend to have a family physician and get regular screening for things like heart disease and breast and colorectal cancer.

All these points have merit, but they represent only part of the story. Close social ties to spouses, friends, relatives and community organizations also enhance the immune system. Just as exercise conditions our muscles to handle heavier loads, social interactions condition the immune system so we experience less illness and recover more quickly from diseases we can't avoid.

## Your Immune System Needs Friends

In recent years, several studies have shown that social isolation releases a flood of stress hormones into the blood that triggers many psychological and physiological changes, including increased heart rate, impaired immune function, difficulty metabolizing sugar and feelings of depression and anxiety ranging from simple tension to panic.

"These hormones normally ebb and flow," Dr. Spiegel explains. "But when stress becomes chronic, they remain consistently high, potentially impairing the body's ability to heal." On the other hand, well-developed social networks dam the flood of stress hormones, minimizing their presence in the bloodstream and allowing the body to cope with stress more effectively and heal more efficiently.

At the Ohio State University College of Medicine in Columbus, virologist Ronald Glaser, Ph.D., and psychologist Janice Kiecolt-Glaser, Ph.D., compared the immune function of 38 married women with that of 38 women who had been separated from their husbands for up to six years. The married women had better immune function and reported better health—fewer and briefer illnesses. Among the separated women, those who felt "better off" divorced had better immune function than those who felt lonely and depressed.

In another study, Dr. Glaser and Dr. Kiecolt-Glaser surveyed a large group of medical students about their social connections and then took blood samples from them during exams, when they were all under considerable stress. The students who were relatively isolated showed high levels of stress hormones. But those who reported extensive social networks showed significantly lower levels.

## The Magic and Medicine of Support Groups

In 1981, at age 58, New York clinical psychologist Mark Flapan, Ph.D., developed strange symptoms. His hands and feet swelled up. Cool breezes turned his fingers blue. And his skin became darker in color and oddly tight. A rheumatologist finally diagnosed him as having a disease he and his wife, Helene, had never heard of—scleroderma, literally, hardening of the skin.

"We read some medical journals," Helene recalls, "and immediately felt devastated. They all said scleroderma was rapidly fatal. We thought Mark would die."

Desperate, Dr. Flapan consulted other rheumatologists and finally found one who said the journals were wrong, that the disease was not a death sentence and that many people with scleroderma had mild cases and lived full lives. Who were these people? The Flapans decided to find out.

They contacted a large number of New York–area scleroderma patients through their rheumatologists and invited them to a meeting at their apartment. At first only a few people showed up, but as word spread, the group grew. Today, the Flapans coordinate two organizations—the New York Scleroderma Society, whose nine meetings a year attract more than 100 people, and the Scleroderma Federation, a national organization with 20 chapters around the country and affiliates around the world.

"The support group meetings are a big help emotionally," Helene Flapan says. "Newly diagnosed scleroderma sufferers and their families always arrive very scared because they've usually heard only the worst, that this is a crippling, disfiguring, fatal disease. They see some people in a bad way. But others look fine, and they realize that things may not be so bad after all. It's very comforting."

It's also typical of support groups, which number "in the millions," according to Edward Madara, director of the American

(continued on page 108)

# The Healing Power of Pets

You've seen the bumper stickers: I ♥ my dog. Right there where you'd expect the word love, there's a goofy red heart. Well, it turns out it's not so goofy. There's scientific evidence that your pet really is good for your heart.

About 15 years ago, researchers at Brooklyn College in New York stumbled on an unexpected health bonus: Independent of all other medical and lifestyle factors, men who'd had heart attacks were more likely to survive if they had pets. Since then, many studies have shown that having a cat purr in your lap reduces blood pressure as effectively as many medications. Gazing at a fish tank is as relaxing as some pharmaceutical tranquilizers. And compared with those who have no pets, pet owners make fewer trips to the doctor.

Not too long ago researchers at Baker Medical Research Institute in Prahan, Australia, compared blood pressure and cholesterol levels in 784 pet owners and 4,957 people who had no pets. The pet owners' levels were significantly lower, suggesting that pet ownership may help prevent heart disease.

Dog owners must walk their dogs, which is an excellent way to get regular, moderate exercise. But owners of cats, birds, fish and iguanas show similar health benefits, so there has to be more to the pet advantage than just exercise. Increasingly, researchers believe that pet companionship provides many of the benefits of close human ties.

Federal law now says that elderly or handicapped residents of federally subsidized housing must be permitted to keep pets. In addition, pet-facilitated therapy (PFT) programs, in which pet owners volunteer to visit regularly with their pets, are fixtures in many of the nation's pediatric hospitals and nursing homes.

In one study, Patty Beyersdorfer, R.N., and Donna Birkenhauer,

R.N., took PFT one step further—into the Alzheimer's disease care unit of Maple Knoll Village, a nursing home in Cincinnati. Thirty minutes a week for five weeks, the two nurses took two adult golden retrievers to visit the 18 residents, who ranged in age from 65 to 95.

The dogs were an instant hit. Residents who were chronically agitated became noticeably calmer around the dogs. Those who were withdrawn came out of their shells and fed, brushed and petted the retrievers. Residents who'd become silent began talking either to the dogs or about them with staff and other patients. And two of the people with Alzheimer's delighted in walking the dogs up and down the hall. As an added bonus, the staff reported increased job satisfaction on days when the dogs visited.

Of course, some people dislike animals, and others are allergic or have medical reasons why they cannot care for pets. But if you enjoy having a pet, the relationship is as health-enhancing as other close social ties.

Dogs may even be able to do something human companions cannot—predict medical emergencies. In folklore, dogs are famous for running for help and barking when their owners are in danger. British veterinary researcher Andrew Edney, D.V.M., has discovered that they also have an uncanny ability do the same thing shortly before their owners experience medical emergencies.

Dr. Edney reviewed stories involving 121 dogs who exhibited unusual behaviors up to 45 minutes before their owners had seizures or diabetic crises. They barked, jumped up and down, physically pushed their owner to lie down and herded others in the household into the person's presence. Dr. Edney does not know how dogs sense impending emergencies, but his study certainly gives new meaning to the phrase "man's best friend."

Self-Help Clearinghouse (ASHC) in Denville, New Jersey. They encompass everything from tiny knots of people coping with problems you never heard of—5P syndrome, porphyria and phenylketonuria—to the tens of thousands of Alcoholics Anonymous fellowships that hold meetings in virtually every community around the country. "Support groups reduce isolation," Madara explains. "They're empowering and comforting. They teach practical coping skills. Sometimes they change laws and public perceptions. And usually, they're free."

Support groups turn life wonderfully upside-down. They take illnesses and other trying experiences that usually leave people feeling isolated and turn them into the sole criterion for membership. "Doctors and psychologists can't be all things to all people," Madara says. "When you sit down with those who have shared your experience—no matter whether it's multiple sclerosis, an unfaithful spouse or a recent cancer diagnosis—you feel a sense of comfort and closeness no professional relationship can match." Support groups also encourage participants to help each other, which helps them feel more competent and effective in the world.

What happens when someone in a support group for, say, cancer, goes downhill and dies? Do the other members get so demoralized that the group loses its value? Dr. Spiegel investigated this question in his group for women with advanced breast cancer.

"Members were, of course, saddened when someone passed away. But we found that they were not scared by each other's medical problems because dying was something each of them was worried about anyway." Support groups become even more valuable in the face of life-threatening illness because they provide a safe place for people to discuss their fears.

Several studies have documented support groups' effectiveness, but Madara says their continuing existence and steady growth is proof enough for him. "People vote with their feet," he says. "The groups continue only as long as the participants feel they help them."

Madara's organization, which began as the New Jersey Self-Help Clearinghouse in 1978 and went national in 1989, tries to keep tabs on the Garden State's approximately 4,000 support groups. Each year, Madara estimates, about 500 new groups form throughout New Jersey, and about 300 die. Madara says he believes the New Jersey figures reflect a national trend toward slow, steady growth in support groups. Many well-known national organizations began as support groups—Mothers Against Drunk Driving, the Multiple Sclerosis Society and the Association for Retarded Citizens, to name just a few.

Anyone in the United States can contact Madara's ASHC and get information about how to find groups near them by sending a self-addressed, stamped envelope to 25 Pocono Road, St. Clares–Riverside Medical Center, Denville, NJ 07834.

But what if no group exists? The ASHC can help you start one. "We help people launch groups all the time," Madara explains. "Not too long ago, a woman with serious postpartum depression called looking for a support group, but there weren't any. We helped her start one and get a little publicity in her local paper. Now Depression After Delivery has 70 chapters nationally."

## Rx: Reach Out and Touch Someone

For people facing serious challenges, emotional support from a spouse, friends, family members or a support group can feel like a real lifesaver. Dr. Syme's studies of ethnic Japanese men and the studies of Roseto, Pennsylvania, by Dr. Wolf and Dr. Bruhn show that social ties really do save lives. Those investigations represent only a small fraction of the research showing that in addition to bolstering the immune system, companionship has an enormous number of practical health benefits.

*Arthritis.* Nurse and health educator Kate Lorig, R.N., Dr.P.H., investigated the Arthritis Self-Management Program (ASMP) at Stanford University. The combination class and support group meets weekly for six weeks, though some participants continue to get together afterward. Dr. Lorig analyzed the medical records of 401 participants over a four-year period and then surveyed them about their health. Medically, the average participant was 9 percent more disabled after four years, yet compared to when they entered the program, they reported 20 percent less pain and 40 percent fewer physician visits.

*Asthma.* In 1993, physicians at Northern California medical facilities operated by Kaiser Permanente, a large health maintenance organization, recruited 323 adults with moderate to severe asthma and assigned them to one of four groups. One group got the usual care. The others received written information about asthma, one-on-one instruction about asthma or information in the context of a support group.

After two years, those who received the usual care or just written information showed a small reduction in asthma-related medical visits, but the people who received face-to-face instruction or participated in the support group registered a major reduction. The greatest decrease in medical visits was recorded by those in the support group. Support group participation cut their asthma-related doctor visits almost in half.

*Cancer.* Stanford University's Dr. Spiegel used to scoff at the notion that social support could extend life, but his own research changed his mind. In the late 1970s, he divided 86 women with advanced breast cancer into two groups. One group received standard medical care and the other got standard care plus participation in a weekly 90-minute support group that he led. Dr. Spiegel theorized that the support group would improve the participants' ability to cope with their illness, but he had no expectation that it would extend anyone's survival. Surprisingly, it did. After ten years, 83 of the 86 women had died, but those in the support group lived twice as long—an average of 37 months compared with just 19 months for those who received only standard care.

Dr. Spiegel's findings have been corroborated by Fawzy I. Fawzy, M.D., professor of psychiatry and biobehavioral sciences at the University of California at Los Angeles School of Medicine. Dr. Fawzy recruited 68 people with malignant melanoma (skin cancer) and invited half to participate in a 90-minute group once a week for six weeks. In the group, people received emotional support, information about melanoma, and nutrition and stress-management tips. Compared with melanoma patients who received just standard medical care, those in the support/education group showed less fatigue and depression and better coping abilities.

Six years after Dr. Fawzy completed this study, he learned of Dr. Spiegel's research and tracked down his participants to see if those in his group had survived any longer. Despite the brevity of his group (just six weeks), they had: Among the patients who received only standard care, ten had died, but among his group participants, there were only three deaths.

A support group is an integral part of both Dr. Michael Lerner's Commonweal Cancer Help Program and Dr. Harold Benjamin's Wellness Community. (For more details on these two cancer support groups, see Complementary Cancer Care on page 115.)

*Childbirth.* Pregnant women who have a husband, friend or relative in the delivery room with them have lower rates of cesarean section than women who give birth alone. They also require less pain medication and give birth to babies who require less medical assistance. These results come from the University of Leeds in England, where researchers analyzed the results of 20 studies that investigated factors affecting delivery complications and birth outcomes. In recent years, obstetricians have been trying to minimize cesarean sections because they are medically riskier than vaginal birth and cost a great deal more. Researchers found that while several medical interventions reduce the need for C-sections, the one with the greatest impact is companionship for the mother in the delivery room.

*Heart attack.* Yale researchers (including Dr. Berkman, coauthor of the influential Alameda County study that linked support to longevity) surveyed 2,500 elderly men and women, asking how many people they could count on to discuss their problems or help them make difficult decisions—zero, one, or two or more. Over time, nearly 200 of the people who took the survey were hospitalized with heart attacks.

In the six months following hospitalization, those with the fewest people they could count on had three times the death rate of those with the most support. Among those claiming no support, 38 percent died in the hospital. Those with one support person had a 23 percent death rate. And among those with two or more support people, only 12 percent died.

*Heart disease.* Dean Ornish, M.D., president of the Preventive Medicine Research Institute in Sausalito, California, has accomplished something cardiologists long thought was impossible—his nondrug, nonsurgical program based entirely on Nature's cures reverses heart disease, shrinking the plaques on his participants' coronary arteries and giving them a new lease on life. (For the full details, see Ornish Therapy on page 368.)

In addition to prescribing an ultra-low-fat diet, yoga, meditation and regular moderate exercise, Dr. Ornish has all the therapy participants take part in a support group that meets regularly.

"The support group meetings are powerful experiences," Dr. Ornish explains. "They help break down the barriers that keep people feeling isolated. Not that people tell all their secrets; no one is totally open. But people open up considerably about their hopes and fears. If you can never show who you really are, warts and all, it's isolating and very stressful."

*Longevity.* In a six-year study reported in 1994, George Kaplan, Ph.D., of the California Department of Health Services' Human Population Laboratory in Berkeley, tracked 2,503 Finnish men ages 42 to 60. Compared with married men who reported the most friends and memberships in social clubs and organizations, single, divorced or widowed men with the fewest such social ties were twice as likely to die from all causes. A separate analysis of relationship satisfaction showed that the men who rated their social connections least nurturing had almost twice the death rate of men who called their relationships fulfilling.

*Stroke.* In a 1993 study, Duke University researchers studied 46 people hospitalized in Durham, North Carolina, for strokes. They determined that 8 had little social support, 24 had a moderate amount and 14 had a great deal. Then they correlated the patients' social support with their recovery after six months. Those with the most support recovered significantly more quickly and fully—even those who had the most severe strokes.

The phone company ads urge us to "Reach out and touch someone." What they fail to mention is that by doing so, we also help ourselves. Have you called your mother lately? Do it now. She'll feel better, and your own immune system will benefit. Have you been meaning to track down that long-lost high school friend? Do it now. And what about that family reunion you'd like to attend but just can't find the time? Make the time. Go. Everyone there may look a little older—but their very presence helps them, and you, stay in the best of health.

## How to Be Supportive

If a friend or loved one becomes seriously ill or needs support for any reason, Dr. Spiegel offers these suggestions.

**Get real.** Support means genuine caring. Meaningful support involves more than superficial contact. Concrete actions speak much louder than good wishes.

**Banish secrets.** Families often want to protect each other from bad news, but hiding a person's illness is quite stressful for everyone who keeps the secret, and it cheats close friends and relatives of the opportunity to support the affected person.

**Include the children.** If they sense they're being excluded, they may feel disrespected or blame themselves for having caused the problem. Explain the situation in terms they can understand. For a young child, it's enough to say, "Grandpa is very sick, and we're afraid he might die." An older child may be interested in more details. Encourage them to be supportive by visiting, talking with the person and doing anything that helps them feel part of the group support effort.

**Be selective.** There's no need to tell everyone you know about the situation. It takes too much time and energy that's best spent supporting the sick person. On the other hand, word travels fast, and no one likes to feel shut out. Designate one or more people to dispense relevant information to well-wishers who are not in the person's inner circle.

**Be specific.** If you say, "Call me if there's anything I can do," chances are your phone won't ring, because few people like to ask for help. Instead, say, "I'd really like to help in some way. I could cook a meal for you over the weekend or take you to any doctor's appointment on my day off." Quite often it's the little things that help most, such walking the dog, taking the kids to school, doing laundry or shopping.

**Offer to help with research.** Many diseases, but particularly cancer, confront people with many choices they rarely feel competent to make without doing research. But sick people may not have the energy, and even if they do, it helps to discuss options with others who are also well-informed. Offer to gather information and help the person sort through it. For free cancer information, call your local office of the American Cancer Society. For heart disease, call the American Heart Association. For other conditions, ask your physician for a referral to a social worker or a self-help group.

**Listen.** Try to draw the person out. If you have a flair for entertainment, fine—tell jokes and try to cheer the person up. But don't overdo it. No amount of cheerfulness can take a person's mind off a serious illness or other life crisis. Acknowledge the gravity of the situation and invite the person to talk about it.

**Be firm.** When you get sick, make your own decisions. When a loved one gets sick, support that person's decisions. One of the most shocking things about illness is the feeling that you've lost control over your life. Making as many decisions as you can helps re-establish that precious sense of control. When loved ones are ill, assuming that they are mentally competent, help them weigh their options, but encourage them to make their own decisions and support them, even if you disagree with what they decide. Don't say, "You should . . . " No one likes to feel that they're being ordered around. Instead say, "Have you considered . . . ?" If you get cancer and immediately switch to an ultra-low-fat vegetarian diet, fine, that's your right. But if your mother develops cancer and wants to keep eating ice cream and cheesecake, that's her right.

**Feel your emotions.** There's no need to keep a stiff upper lip. A hug and a few tears often go a long way toward showing the person that you truly care.

## CHAPTER 7

# COMPLEMENTARY CANCER CARE

## Natural Therapies Gain New Respect

Rita Arditti, Ph.D., of Boston had no idea she would become a quiet pioneer in cancer care when she was diagnosed with breast cancer at age 39. The year was 1974, and lumpectomy, removal of only the tumor, was not yet offered in this country. So the molecular biologist had a modified radical mastectomy—removal of the breast and nearby lymph nodes, followed by radiation.

Five years later Dr. Arditti's cancer recurred in her lungs. Her doctors advised removal of her ovaries to suppress production of the tumor-stimulating hormone estrogen. (The estrogen-suppressing drug tamoxifen was not yet available.) Dr. Arditti had the surgery, and her lung tumors disappeared.

"I felt very thankful, of course," she explains, "but I did some research and decided there was more to treating cancer than what my oncologist prescribed. Some studies suggested that a diet high in animal fats increased risk of breast cancer. Red meats contain the most fat, so I stopped eating them."

It was a modest lifestyle change—and one that, at the time,

many oncologists would have dismissed as unnecessary or "quackery"—but it may well have contributed to Dr. Arditti's long-term survival. "I knew that vegetarianism and other unconventional approaches to cancer were controversial, but I felt they were often criticized unfairly," she recalls. "Medicine is very conservative. As a scientist myself, I know it's not always the best ideas that get the recognition, especially if they rock the boat."

## Questing for Healing

In 1983, Dr. Arditti had a second recurrence—in the lymph nodes around her neck. By then tamoxifen was available, and her oncologist recommended it to suppress the small amount of estrogen her adrenal glands and fat tissue produced. Again her cancer regressed, and again she was thankful for conventional treatment. But with two recurrences, Dr. Arditti knew her risk of another was quite high.

By this time more studies had linked dietary fat to cancer, and *Recalled to Life,* a first-person account by a noted physician, recounted how an ultra-low-fat macrobiotic diet appeared to have sent his "terminal" prostate cancer into remission. Dr. Arditti adopted macrobiotics, reducing her fat intake even more by adopting an all-plant diet of fruits, vegetables, beans and grains, with no meat, poultry, fish or dairy products. She also began looking for other unconventional cancer therapies.

A year later she found the Commonweal Cancer Help Program, a week-long retreat for cancer patients in Bolinas, California, north of San Francisco. Commonweal does not treat cancer. In fact, to attend, participants must be under the care of an oncologist. Instead, the pioneering program uses four of Nature's cures—vegetarian diet, psychological support, moderate exercise and personal growth through the arts—to boost the health and well-being of people with cancer so they can cope more effectively with the disease and quite possibly live longer.

"If you're eating well, getting emotional support and moderate exercise and growing as a person, you become a healthier

# How to Avoid Cancer Quackery ━━━━━

Right this way for your snake oil preparation . . . step right up.

In your rational mind, you'd never fall for it, but people's desperation levels tend to cloud their best judgment once they've been diagnosed with cancer. And there are always people to tell convincing tales about how some exotic, new and usually expensive remedy did the trick for them. Testimonials support many complementary therapies, but stories are not scientific studies. When you're investigating complementary therapies, how do you protect yourself from the snake oil salesmen? Here are a few tips.

**Beware of any practitioner who claims to "cure" cancer.** Some individuals may swear they've been cured, but no complementary therapy has been shown to be reliably curative.

**Beware of practitioners touting "secret formulas."** Secrecy increases risk of exploitation. Know what you're using before you try it.

**Do some research.** *Choices in Healing: Integrating the Best of the Conventional and Complementary Approaches to Cancer* by Michael Lerner, Ph.D., contains extensive analyses of several therapies, with clear descriptions of any scientific studies that have evaluated them.

**Evaluate the practitioner.** This is not easy, but before you consent to any complementary treatment, make sure you feel comfortable with its provider. Ask about credentials. Some practitioners are physicians; others are not. Ask about the practitioner's philosophy and request copies of any studies that have evaluated the therapy.

**Evaluate the staff.** Get a feel for their experience, compassion and professionalism.

**Ask for referrals to satisfied clients.** Ask practitioners to put you in touch with people who have benefited from their therapies. Call several and ask about their experiences.

**Ask about cost.** According to a 1990 report by the Congressional Office of Technology Assessment, complementary therapies cost from $3,600 to $52,000. (For comparison, in 1994 a week at the Commonweal Cancer Help Program cost $1,280, and The Wellness Community (TWC) programs are free.)

cancer patient," explains Michael Lerner, Ph.D., a former Yale psychology professor who founded Commonweal in 1976 with Rachel Remen, M.D., a Sausalito, California, physician/psychotherapist. "You're not healthy, of course, because you're dealing with cancer, but compared with cancer patients who don't improve these areas of their lives, you're healthier. Many studies show that healthier cancer patients often respond better to conventional care and have better treatment outcomes—enhanced quality of life and sometimes longer, healthier, disease-free survival."

## The Wave of the Future

Welcome to a major innovation in cancer care, a new, more comprehensive philosophy that combines the best of conventional oncology with the most effective "complementary" therapies. Until recently, the approaches used at Commonweal, as well as at an increasing number of the nation's leading cancer centers, were called alternative, unorthodox or unconventional—when they weren't dismissed as outright quackery, that is. The recent name change to "complementary" signals not only their increasing acceptance by mainstream oncologists but also the crucial idea that they do not replace standard medical care; rather, they add to it.

Dr. Lerner began investigating complementary cancer therapies more than ten years ago when his father was diagnosed with non-Hodgkins lymphoma. Dr. Lerner suggested combining mainstream treatments with some of the alternative healing arts he valued for his own well-being: vegetarianism, yoga and massage. But the elder Lerner declined, arguing that he knew of no persuasive evidence that they worked. Dr. Lerner had to agree, and he lamented the lack of scientific information about them.

Then as Fate would have it, Dr. Lerner was awarded a MacArthur Foundation "genius" grant ($50,000 a year, tax-free, for five years). He decided to use the money to conduct his own scientific investigation of complementary cancer care around the world.

In 1994, his decade-long inquiry culminated in the publication of *Choices in Healing: Integrating the Best of Conventional and Complementary Approaches to Cancer.* His conclusion: No single complementary therapy or combination of them reliably cures cancer. In fact, he says, "mainstream oncology clearly has the best track record of treatment success. But a growing body of scientific evidence suggests that several complementary approaches have real value for many cancer patients."

Dr. Lerner's view is controversial. Some oncologists still dismiss all complementary therapies as the work of medical charlatans, but a growing number now support people with cancer who explore the complementary therapies in addition to standard care.

"Despite our many successes with surgery, chemotherapy, radiation and other conventional cancer treatments, we doctors have still not conquered most cancers," explains oncologist Laurens P. White, M.D., clinical professor at the University of California's San Francisco Medical Center and past president of the California Medical Association. "It's a mistake for doctors to dismiss other approaches as nonsense. As long as unorthodox approaches are used in complementary fashion, most do no harm, and there's growing evidence to suggest that some have value."

"For the last five years or so, a new view of cancer care has been slowly emerging in mainstream oncology: the belief that it's time to combine the best of conventional medicine with the best of the complementary therapies," says Julia Rowland, Ph.D., assistant professor of psychiatry at Georgetown University Medical Center in Washington, D.C., and director of psycho-oncology at the Vincent T. Lombardi Cancer Center there. "Twenty years ago, this combination approach would have been attacked as 'radical,' but since then, a great deal of research has shown that things like emotional support, diet and exercise play important roles in maintaining health and recovering from many serious illnesses. Now this new understanding is being incorporated into oncology, and in my opinion, it's good news for cancer patients."

## Support Groups Save Lives

"Psychologists who specialize in cancer have known for years that emotional support reduces the tremendous stress of having cancer and helps people cope better with the illness," Dr. Lerner explains. "But most oncologists discounted the importance of social support. Now that's all changed. These days it's difficult to be diagnosed with cancer and not have your oncologist or some other health-care provider suggest that you enroll in a support group—thanks to the Spiegel study."

The Spiegel study was conducted by David Spiegel, M.D., professor of psychiatry at Stanford University and director of the university's Psychosocial Treatment Laboratory. In the late 1970s, he divided 86 women with advanced breast cancer into two groups. One received standard medical care; the other received standard care and participated in a weekly 90-minute support group led by Dr. Spiegel.

Dr. Spiegel theorized that the support group would improve the participants' ability to cope with their illness, but he firmly believed that it would not extend anyone's survival. Surprisingly, it did. After ten years, 83 of the 86 women had died, but those in the support group lived twice as long—an average of 37 months compared with just 19 months for those who received only standard care.

Dr. Spiegel's findings have been supported by Fawzy I. Fawzy, M.D., professor of psychiatry and biobehavioral sciences at the University of California at Los Angeles School of Medicine. Dr. Fawzy found 68 people with malignant melanoma (skin cancer) and invited half of them to take part in a 90-minute group once a week for six weeks. Members of this group received emotional support, information about melanoma and nutrition and stress-management tips. Those in the support/education group experienced less fatigue and depression and had better coping abilities, compared with those who received just standard medical care,

Six years after completing this study, Dr. Fawzy learned of Dr. Spiegel's research. He tracked down the participants in his study to see if those in his support group had survived any longer. Despite the fact that his group lasted just six weeks, he found that among his group participants, there were only three deaths, while among the people who received only standard care, ten had died.

Many studies have correlated divorce, bereavement, job loss and other isolating emotional stresses with depression of the immune system's ability to protect the body from disease. Other studies have shown that social connections—close ties to friends, family, organizations and support groups—bolster the immune system and help protect the body from stress and illness. (For more on the benefits of social ties, see Companionship on page 99.)

Even without formal support groups, the same appears to be true for cancer survival. A 1990 report by epidemiologists Peggy Reynolds, Ph.D., and George Kaplan, Ph.D., at the University of California at Berkeley, culminated 17 years of study that surveyed the lifestyles of a large group of people with cancer. The results showed that compared with those who had the most social support, those with the least were more than twice as likely to die.

"Support group participation doesn't guarantee survival. Nor does being a loner doom cancer patients to rapid demise," explains Dr. Lerner, whose Commonweal program includes a twice-daily support group for all participants. "But given the mounting evidence that support groups may extend survival, it would seem prudent to participate. If I had cancer, I'd join a support group. I would also spend more time with the people I cherish."

Memorial Sloan-Kettering Cancer Center in New York City is just one of many comprehensive cancer centers around the country that now sponsor support groups for people with cancer. "For breast cancer, we have groups for women with local and advanced disease, pre-and post-mastectomy groups, groups for those coping with chemotherapy—all sorts of options," says Mary Jane Massie, M.D., an attending psychiatrist at the cancer center and professor of clinical psychiatry at Cornell University Medical Center. "Despite the studies showing extended survival, support groups' contribution to longevity still remains unclear. But there's no question that they help people cope with the emotional distress of having cancer. Improved coping is good for the immune system, so it certainly can't hurt your survival."

"I've never been big on groups, but when you have cancer, things change," says Clyde Childress, 71, a retired San Rafael, California, photographer with prostate cancer who attended the Commonweal program in 1993. "I was amazed how everyone— myself included—came out of their shells in the support group. It was very moving."

In addition to Commonweal, many other organizations around the country sponsor support groups for cancer patients. One of the largest is The Wellness Community (TWC), a national network of 13 support centers for people with cancer and their families. Founded in 1982 by psychologist Harold Benjamin, Ph.D., of Santa Monica, TWC has provided free emotional support to more than 25,000 people with cancer and currently serves more than 1,700 each week.

Other support centers for people with cancer are local programs. One such center is the Cancer Support Community in San Francisco, which attracted Anne Simons, M.D., assistant clinical professor of family and community medicine at the University of California's San Francisco Medical Center and author of *Before You Call the Doctor*, shortly after she was diagnosed with breast cancer in 1991. "It's never easy to deal with cancer," the 41-year-old mother of two explains, "but being in a group makes it easier. And the studies showing survival benefits are pretty impressive."

## The Benefits of Vegetarianism

Support groups represent one of four complementary therapies that Dr. Lerner calls "the health-promoting quartet." The other three are vegetarian diet, moderate exercise and the opportunity for personal growth through artistic expression. "All four are inherently good for the body and soul," he explains.

"All four help cancer patients become healthier and cope more effectively with their disease."

After support groups, vegetarianism has been the most extensively researched. (For the full details on the healing powers of a meatless diet, see Vegetarianism on page 409.) Vegetarianism does not cure cancer, but many studies show that a diet high in red meat is associated with increased cancer risk, a diet high in fruits and vegetables reduces risk, and people with cancer who adopt a vegetarian diet survive longer than those who continue to eat meat.

Several studies add to the enormous medical literature showing that meat-eating increases cancer risk.

In a 1994 report, Paolo Toniolo, M.D., director of the epidemiology program at New York University Medical Center in New York City, examined the dietary histories of 14,000 New York City women from 1985 through 1991. Compared with the women who ate no red meat (including beef, veal, lamb, pork and lunch meats), those who reported eating red meat every day had nearly twice the risk of developing breast cancer.

There's also some evidence that meat contributes to lung cancer risk. Not just smoking—smoking plus a diet full of meat. A 1993 study by National Cancer Institute (NCI) researchers surveyed the diet histories of 1,450 women smokers from 1986 through 1991. During that period, 429 developed lung cancer. Compared with those who ate the least meat, the women who ate the most were more than six times more likely to develop lung cancer.

A 1994 study by James Mann, Ph.D., professor of nutrition at the University of Otago in Dunedin, New Zealand, compared the health of 5,000 meat-eating men with that of 6,100 vegetarians, whose average age was around 40. Cancer and heart disease tend to strike after age 50, but even in this younger population, the vegetarians enjoyed significant protection. They had 28 percent less heart disease and 39 percent less cancer than the meat-eaters.

Finally, for a 1993 study, Edward Giovanunucci, M.D., Sc.D., professor of medicine at Harvard Medical School, analyzed diet information from 51,529 male health professionals who had been followed for seven years. All dietary fats increased their risk of prostate cancer, but "red meat represented the food group with the strongest association."

Meanwhile, as consumption of fresh fruits and vegetables increases, risk of every major cancer decreases.

Gladys Block, Ph.D., formerly an epidemiologist at the National Cancer Institute and now professor of epidemiology and nutrition at the University of California at Berkeley School of Public Health, analyzed nearly 200 studies of diet and cancer risk. Every study showed that fruits and vegetables protect against all the major cancers—breast, ovarian, cervical, lung, colon, throat, oral, stomach, bladder, pancreatic and prostate. "Compared with those who consumed the fewest fruits and vegetables, those who consumed the most had only about half the cancer risk," Dr. Block explains.

## Reach for Those Veggies

The NCI does not publicly advocate vegetarianism, but it urges Americans to "strive for five"—five daily servings of fruits and vegetables. Scientists believe that fruits and vegetables help prevent cancer because they are high in antioxidant nutrients—particularly vitamins A, C and E and the mineral selenium. (Antioxidants are nutrients that protect the body against naturally occurring oxygen ions—highly unstable molecules that harm cells.)

Some scientists believe that taking antioxidant supplements can also help prevent cancer. Dr. Block says that it's okay to take a supplement. But an even better choice is to get your nutrients at the supermarket by stocking up on fruits and vegetables. "Supplements' value in preventing cancer is controversial," she says, "but the benefits of fruits and vegetables are very clear."

Does vegetarianism help those who are already diagnosed with cancer? The jury is still out, but intriguing research suggests that the answer is yes.

James Carter, Ph.D., chair of the Department of Nutrition at the Tulane University School of Public Health in New Orleans, investigated the effect of a strict vegetarian diet (no red meat, poultry, fish or dairy products) on survival times for people with pancreatic cancer, one of the least treatable and most rapidly fatal cancers. According to NCI statistics, the average person with pancreatic cancer survives about 6 months after diagnosis. But among those who followed the strict vegetarian diet, average survival time was 17 months—more than twice as long.

At the University of Hawaii's Cancer Research Center in Honolulu, researchers studied how diet affected the survival of 675 men and women with lung cancer. Compared with those who ate the fewest fruits and vegetables, those with lung cancer who ate the most of these foods survived almost twice as long.

The Wellness Community's national network of cancer support groups teaches nutrition seminars for people with cancer and encourages a low-fat diet with less meat and more fruits and vegetables. Dr. Arditti, now a 20-year breast cancer survivor, can't be certain that her adoption of vegetarianism after her first recurrence has contributed to her longevity, "but I believe it has," she says. "It certainly hasn't done me any harm."

## The Benefits of Exercise

Intriguing research also suggests that exercise decreases cancer risk. In 1987, Rose Frisch, Ph.D., associate professor emerita of population sciences at Harvard University, surveyed more than 5,398 women ages 21 to 82. In every age group, regular exercise was associated with less risk of cancers of the breast, uterus, cervix, ovaries and vagina. For breast cancer, regular exercise cut risk in half.

A 1994 study of California women showed that regular moderate exercise can reduce women's risk of premenopausal breast cancer by as much as 60 percent. Leslie Bernstein, Ph.D., professor of preventive medicine at the North Cancer Center at the University of Southern California in Los Angeles, surveyed the lifetime exercise habits of 545 California women with breast cancer that was diagnosed before they were 40 and those of a comparison group of similar women who did not have cancer. Exercising four hours a week—in such activities as jogging, swimming and tennis—produced the most striking reduction in breast cancer risk. But as few as two hours of exercise a week also proved significantly beneficial.

Moderate exercise stimulates the immune system, Dr. Lerner explains, and elevates mood, which also boosts immune function. "Unfortunately, to my knowledge, no studies have evaluated the effect of exercise on cancer survival," he says. "But if I had cancer, I would get regular exercise. I would do more yoga and take long walks."

Steena Eaton of New York City embraced exercise as a complementary cancer therapy after she was diagnosed with breast cancer at age 54. Never much of an athlete, the occupational therapist spent a week at Commonweal in 1988. During her free time she felt oddly drawn to the ocean about a 20-minute walk from the inn where participants stay. "I swam in the ocean at Commonweal and found it physically invigorating and emotionally comforting," she recalls. She's been ocean swimming ever since at New York area beaches.

After her week at Commonweal, Dr. Arditti began doing yoga regularly, and she continued it for many years. (She recently switched to more strenuous aerobics.) In addition, she takes long walks, especially when vacationing in New Hampshire or Newfoundland.

## Art for Healing's Sake

There aren't any studies showing that personal growth through artistic expression extends cancer survival, but Dr. Lerner believes that it's healing. To some people, "healing" and "curing" mean the same thing. In fact, they are quite distinct.

"Curing," Dr. Lerner explains, "is what physicians hope to do—eliminate the disease and allow recovery. Healing is what patients must do for themselves. Healing is a deeply personal inner process of becoming whole again." Commonweal leaves curative efforts to the oncologists. Unfortunately, oncology often gives short shrift to healing, leaving many people with cancer feeling emotionally shortchanged, even if they recover.

"In our program," Dr. Lerner says, "as soon as we start talking about the difference between curing and healing, people's eyes light up. Though we don't treat cancer, I believe that the work we do on healing optimizes people's potential for recovery. It minimizes stress, fosters social support and improves quality of life. Several studies have associated these changes with improved treatment outcomes, not only in cancer but in other serious illnesses, such as heart disease, as well. Many people with cancer have told me that drawing, painting, sculpture, writing and music have helped them cope. If I had cancer, I would get more involved in writing and music."

The nation's major cancer centers have not added acupuncture, exercise workouts, music lessons and classes in vegetarian cooking to the support groups they already sponsor—at least not yet. But they are less and less likely to discourage them. Olive Soriero, M.D., former assistant clinical professor of gynecological oncology at Stanford University Medical Center and now a staff member at St. Vincent's Hospital in Indianapolis, sums up the view of an increasing number of oncologists this way: "I'm all for my patients improving their diets, getting moderate exercise, trying unorthodox treatments and doing whatever they can to grow and find inner peace—as long as they don't abandon conventional medicine to pursue them."

## The Chinese Connection

There's also a dearth of Western scientific research on the effects of Chinese medicine on cancer. Chinese physicians claim considerable success in treating many cancers, but most American scientists look askance at their research methods and question their conclusions. Nonetheless, Dr. Lerner believes acupuncture and Chinese herbal medicine both have value for people with cancer. "I've heard from dozens of cancer patients that they help relieve the nausea of chemotherapy. If I had cancer, I would explore them," he says.

# Conventional Medicine Doesn't Have All the Answers

Critics of the complementary therapies often charge that their practitioners prey on the unsophisticated and trick them into abandoning conventional cancer care for snake oil. In some cases this is true, but the few studies of this question show that most people who opt for complementary therapies are people like Dr. Arditti.

They have above-average levels of education, and only a small proportion (about 15 percent) abandon mainstream oncology. The vast majority (85 percent) use complementary therapies in addition to conventional cancer care or after having exhausted what mainstream oncology has to offer or because they feel that complementary approaches include a sense of compassion that's missing from conventional care.

Those who question the compassion of conventional cancer care often accuse mainstream oncology of being too aggressive and too eager to use radical surgical procedures, radiation and chemotherapy drugs that sometimes cause severe side effects. The nation's leading physicians retort that Americans enjoy the best health care in the world. But the "best" oncology here may not be viewed the same way by oncologists in other countries.

"Oncologists in the United States and Europe all have access to exactly the same scientific information," Dr. Lerner explains. "Yet they treat cancer differently. Cancer care decisions are cultural as well as medical, and American oncology is the most aggressive in the world. American oncologists are comparatively quick to recommend extensive surgery and aggressive chemotherapy and radiation regimens."

Other equally technologically advanced cancer specialists treat the disease differently. German oncologists often combine Western medicine with herbal treatments. Japanese oncologists often combine Western cancer treatments with dietary approaches, acupuncture and other traditional Asian healing arts.

Sometimes, of course, aggressive treatment is life-saving. But other times it may be unnecessarily disfiguring. Consider breast cancer: The first treatment was radical mastectomy, introduced about 100 years ago by the American surgeon William Halstead.

It was a major improvement over no treatment, but it was also very aggressive. Radical mastectomy removes the entire breast, the surrounding lymph nodes and the underlying chest muscles, leaving survivors disfigured and with reduced arm strength. In the early 1980s, surgeons in England and Italy reported that breast-sparing surgery that removed just the tumor (lumpectomy) produced survival results as good as those of radical mastectomy—if the woman had radiation afterward.

For early-stage breast cancer, lumpectomy quickly became the standard of care in Europe. But radical mastectomy and modified radical mastectomy continued to be preferred by most American surgeons. The National Institutes of Health and the American Cancer Society have urged breast surgeons to treat early-stage breast cancer less aggressively using lumpectomy, but a study published in the *Journal of the American Medical Association* lamented that "breast-conserving surgery is not performed on the majority of women with early-stage cancer."

Meanwhile, European pioneers of less aggressive breast cancer treatment now suggest that for many women with early-stage disease, postlumpectomy radiation may not be necessary. Starting in 1981, Swedish researchers performed lumpectomies on women with early-stage breast cancer, then gave radiation to only half of them. The two groups' survival rates were so similar that the researchers called radiation "overtreatment in about 80 percent of patients." Yet American women who have lumpectomies are routinely told that radiation is a standard part of treatment.

When Shelley Sorenson, a 36-year-old San Francisco librarian, was diagnosed with early-stage breast cancer, she was treated with lumpectomy, radiation and chemotherapy. Her oncologist also urged her to take tamoxifen, a drug that reduces risk of recurrences. But tamoxifen also impairs fertility, and Sorenson, who had no children, wanted to keep that option open.

"I agonized over the decision and finally decided not to take the tamoxifen, but I kept worrying that I'd made a bad decision," she recalls. Then she went to Commonweal, and in a seminar on cancer care, learned that even without tamoxifen, by European standards, she'd already been treated fairly aggressively. "That eased my mind," she says.

"I can't say which is 'best'—the American or European approach to treating breast cancer," Dr. Lerner says. "But once people understand that conventional oncology is practiced differently in the advanced countries, they realize that medicine is not monolithic, that there may be different ways to go. When an oncologist says, 'You really ought to do X,' patients can appreciate that they're hearing that doctor's best assessment. But that opinion is not necessarily the only way to view their situation."

## A Truce in the Cancer War

Until recently, the debate between conventional oncology and the complementary therapies has been an angry shouting match. The cancer establishment called complementary practitioners "quacks," while alternative practitioners dismissed surgery, radiation and chemotherapy as overly aggressive "cutting, burning and poisoning."

Now, thanks to researchers like Dr. Lerner and to assertive cancer patients like Dr. Arditti, the warring parties are negotiating a truce. "We still don't know that much about the complementary therapies," Dr. Lerner says. "They definitely need to be more thoroughly researched. But I'm optimistic that these studies will be conducted and that in the not-too-distant future, we'll know if any complementary therapies really help. I try to keep an open mind, but I believe that some, particularly emotional support, vegetarianism, exercise, personal growth and Chinese medicine, have real value for many people with cancer."

Dr. Arditti certainly agrees. She's beaten the odds. Today, fewer than half of people with breast cancer survive 20 years after diagnosis, but she is among them, cancer-free and healthy. Did her vegetarian diet, yoga, hiking and participation in Commonweal's support group contribute to her survival? "There's no way to know for certain," she says, "but they've certainly enhanced the quality of my life, and personally, I believe they've extended it. When people I know get cancer, I encourage them to explore complementary therapies in addition to the treatments their oncologists recommend."

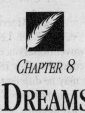

## CHAPTER 8

# DREAMS

## Therapeutic Theater in the Mind

**D**reams are magical, captivating, baffling and sometimes frightening. Throughout human history, they have helped people solve puzzling problems, gain profound insights, create great art and prevent and deal with serious illness.

Scientists still do not understand why we dream or what dreams mean. But since ancient times, virtually every culture on earth has believed that dreams carry important, though often obscure, messages for the waking world. Their meanings may never be crystal clear, but if you believe, as pioneering psychoanalyst Sigmund Freud did, that dreams are "the royal road to the unconscious mind," they are certainly worth contemplating. With a little preparation, you can remember your dreams, and with practice, you can use them to gain insight into your deeper self—and quite possibly feel healthier as a result.

## A Riddle Wrapped in an Enigma

Dreams have fascinated and troubled humanity since before the dawn of history. More than 3,000 years ago, as recorded in the Book of Genesis, Joseph won release from an Egyptian prison by successfully interpreting one of Pharaoh's dreams. The ancient Greeks believed that dreams were great healers. The sick slept in special healing temples in hopes of receiving therapeutic dreams from the gods. Inspired by an angel who visited him in a dream, the Muslim prophet Mohammed began writing the Koran. Native Americans and Australian Aborigines share a belief that dreams allow us to communicate with the spirit world of our ancestors. And Tibetan Buddhists draw no distinction between dreaming and waking. They consider all of life a dream.

Many of the world's greatest thinkers have pondered dreams. Taken collectively, their musings touch on just about every possibility for all those mental movies—rather like the contradictory images in many dreams. William Shakespeare considered dreams humanity's very essence: "We are such stuff as dreams are made on."

But the Greek philosopher Plato saw them as evil: "Our beastly and savage part, a terrible, fierce, lawless brood of desires." Another Greek philosopher, Herodotus, viewed dreams matter-of-factly as "comprised of matters in our thoughts during the day." Eighteenth-century British writer Charles Churchill dismissed them as meaningless "children of the night, bred of indigestion."

To Freud dreams represented "the imaginary gratification of unconscious wishes." And American writer-philosopher Henry David Thoreau considered dreams much more than that: "the very touchstones of our character."

Do dreams have meaning? Jonathan Swift, author of *Gulliver's Travels,* didn't think so: "Fools consult dream interpreters in vain." But a Jewish proverb says, "A dream left uninterpreted is like a letter left unread."

## Weird Science Close to Home

Despite all the energy great thinkers have invested in pondering dreams, scientists knew virtually nothing about the process of dreaming until 1952, when the world's first sleep scientist, Nathaniel Kleitman, Ph.D., professor of physiology at the

University of Chicago, assigned graduate student Eugene Aserinsky to monitor the eye movements of a group of sleepers. Years earlier, Dr. Kleitman had documented slow, rolling eye movements as people fell asleep. He theorized that eye movements throughout the night might provide a clue to the depth of sleep. Using sensors taped around subjects' eyes, Aserinsky and Dr. Kleitman recorded sleepers' eye movements and were astonished to discover that several times each night, the eyes ceased their slow rolling and darted back and forth wildly under the closed lids. Dr. Kleitman described the phenomenon as rapid eye movement (REM) sleep.

A few months later, Dr. Kleitman's lab assistant, William Dement, M.D., Ph.D., then a young medical student and now professor of psychiatry and behavioral science at Stanford University, director of the university's Sleep Disorders Center and chair of the National Commission on Sleep Disorders Research, discovered that sleepers who were awakened during REM sleep recalled dreams in vivid detail, but those awakened during non-REM sleep rarely recalled dreams. He concluded that REM sleep was dream sleep.

This discovery "jolted people," Dr. Dement recalls, "because the prevailing physiological view at the time was that the brain was more or less turned off during sleep." In subsequent studies, Dr. Dement showed that far from being quiet, the sleeping brain was quite active, and during REM sleep, it cranked up to levels of activity far more intense than those experienced during wakefulness.

Dr. Dement also discovered that people have four or five 90-minute sleep cycles each night—moving from light to progressively deeper sleep and finally into REM sleep before returning to light sleep again at the start of a new sleep cycle.

Periods of REM sleep grow progressively longer as the morning approaches. The dreams most people recall are the ones that occur during the final and longest REM period shortly before waking. The typical adult spends about two hours a night in REM sleep. Over an average life span, that works out to the equivalent of six years of dreaming and more than 100,000 dreams. For sighted people, these dreams are overwhelmingly visual, but those who are blind dream just as much, with auditory dreams predominating.

In addition to stimulating rapid eye movements, dreaming causes several other physiological changes. Heart rate and respiration increase. The sex organs become stimulated. Men develop erections, and women experience the vaginal changes of sexual arousal. The toes and fingertips move, but the major muscle groups become temporarily paralyzed (presumably to keep us from acting out our dreams). Dream paralysis does not always disappear upon waking. If you wake up in the middle of a dream, you may not be able to move for a few seconds.

## Whispers from the Subconscious

Why do we dream? No one really knows. For much of this century, the leading theory was the Freudian view that dreams preserved sleep. Freud theorized that the repressed urges that flood the mind in sleep would awaken us if not discharged as dreams. The question remains unanswered, but in 1994 Avi Karni, M.D., Ph.D., a researcher at the National Institute of Mental Health's Laboratory of Neuropsychology, demonstrated that dreams help consolidate memory. Dr. Karni trained subjects in a fairly challenging mental task—recognizing an object using only their peripheral vision. As their training progressed, participants' recognition ability improved markedly. Their recognition ability also improved after a good night's sleep. Dr. Karni wondered if dreaming might have something to do with it.

He divided newly recruited subjects into two groups and began to teach them the visual recognition task. During the process, one group was not allowed to dream. They were awakened as soon as they entered REM sleep. The other group was awakened during an equal number of non-REM periods. Those who did not dream showed no overnight improvement in recognition ability, but those who dreamed showed significant overnight improvement.

Dreams also appear to play some role in the brain's development. Newborns spend 50 percent of sleep time in REM sleep. For adolescents and most adults, REM sleep occupies 20 to 25 percent of the night. Among the elderly, REM periods drop to about 18 percent of sleep. Compared with those of normal intelligence, people who are severely retarded spend less time in REM sleep. REM sleep may also be disrupted by some mental illnesses and certain drugs, such as the antidepressant phenelzine (Nardil).

Those deprived of dreaming for a few nights by being awakened as they enter REM sleep tend to make up lost dream time as soon as they can have REM sleep again. But up to several months of REM deprivation does not appear to cause major mental health problems. In fact, some people notice relief from depression when deprived of REM sleep. Clearly, scientists still have a great deal to learn about why we dream.

But researchers have discovered where dreams come from. In 1977, sleep researchers J. Allan Hobson, M.D., and Robert McCarley, M.D., both professors of psychiatry at Harvard University, suggested that dreams come from a primitive part of the brain stem called the pons, which sits atop the spinal cord.

The cells of the pons fire steadily throughout the day, but during dreaming, their activity intensifies, becoming wild and erratic. Sudden, lightning-like nerve impulses travel up into the cerebral cortex, the part of the brain that reasons and generates emotions.

Scientists theorize that these bursts of neuroelectrical energy might be viewed as random dots appearing on a blank page. The cerebral cortex plays connect-the-dots and draws a picture that we experience as a dream. "The brain always tries to impose meaning on any signals it receives," Dr. Hobson says. "Dreams are the stories the cortex develops to impose structure on the nerve impulses that flood it during the night."

Dr. Hobson doubts that dreams mean anything. He considers them nothing more than cerebral dust clouds raised by random nerve firings in the pons and dismisses interpretation attempts as "a fool's errand." He asks, "If dreams are so all-fired important, why do we forget them so easily?"

His views are echoed by Francis Crick, Ph.D., the British scientist who shared a Nobel Prize for discovering the structure of DNA, the molecule that contains the genetic code. In 1983, Dr. Crick proposed dreams as "the wastebasket of the brain," the final resting place for discarded ideas and fantasies. He warned against focusing too intently on dreams, saying that people might be better off forgetting them.

## The Creative Power of Dreams

Distinguished as these scientists are, their view doesn't square at all with the dozens of cultural traditions worldwide that revere dreams as divine or personal messages, nor with the views of most psychologists (both Freudians and non-Freudians), nor with the findings of most sleep/dream scientists: "I disagree with the random-firing theory," says Stanford's Dr. Dement. "I cannot accept that dreams are merely a product of neurological chance."

The fact is, dreams have inspired great art, solved major problems, warned of illness and misdiagnosis and helped people cope with major life stresses.

Two of the most important discoveries in nineteenth-century chemistry were inspired by dreams. During the 1860s, Russian chemist Dimitri Mendeleev spent years trying to classify all the elements according to their atomic weights and reactivity patterns, but to no avail. Then one night in 1869, he "saw in a dream a table where all the elements fell into place." Upon waking the next morning, he drafted the Periodic Table of Elements. Around the same time, German chemist Freidrich August Kekulé von Stradonitz was equally frustrated by his inability to figure out the molecular structure of benzene. While dozing by his fireplace, he dreamed he saw a snake grab its own tail. Upon waking, he realized that benzene must be a ring, a discovery that was a major breakthrough in organic chemistry.

The story for *The Strange Case of Dr. Jekyll and Mr. Hyde* came to Robert Louis Stevenson in a dream. He woke up and jumped to his desk; he drafted the whole novel in less than a week.

Noted psychologist Carl Jung owes his idea of a "collective unconscious" to a dream in which he wandered around a strange yet oddly familiar mansion discovering art and artifacts from every age of human existence.

Elias Howe invented the sewing machine thanks to a dream. After failing to develop a working model in which the eye of the needle was in the middle of the shank, he had a dream that he was captured by a tribe of spear-wielding Africans whose king sentenced him to death for failing to perfect his machine. As he was led to his execution, Howe noticed that his captors' spears had eye-holes near their points. He redesigned his needle with an eye near the point and soon had a working sewing machine.

Golfer Jack Nicklaus claims that a dream insight led him to change his grip and swing, improving his game by several strokes overnight.

Mozart and Beethoven are only two of several great composers who found musical inspiration in their dreams. This tradition continues today. Singer-songwriter Billy Joel says, "All the music I've ever written comes from my dreams." He pays homage to his nighttime Muse in his album *The River of Dreams*.

Dr. Dement quit smoking because of a dream. "I used to be a heavy smoker," he explains. "One night I dreamed that I coughed up blood into a handkerchief. A radiologist friend showed me my chest x-rays. I could see a large tumor. All of a sudden a wave of incredible sadness washed over me. I realized I had only a little while to live and would not survive to see my children grow to adulthood. Then I woke up and realized that I didn't have lung cancer, that I'd only been dreaming. I felt incredible relief, as though I'd been reborn. I never smoked another cigarette. That dream saved my life."

Author William Styron owes one of his novels to a dream: He wanted to write about the Holocaust but could not settle on an approach. "Then one night, I dreamed that a young woman I used to know was at my door," he recalls. "She opened it and I saw concentration camp numbers tattooed on her arm. Suddenly the story came to me. When I woke up, I wrote the first page of *Sophie's Choice*."

## The Healing Power of Dreams

California psychologist Patricia Garfield, Ph.D., author of *Creative Dreaming*, discovered the diagnostic power of dreams when she fell on her left arm in 1988. Her doctor assured her that her arm was sprained, not broken. Ten days later, Dr. Garfield dreamed that her arm was broken. She demanded x-rays, which revealed a fracture. This experience led her to write *The Healing Power of Dreams*.

Dr. Garfield says that some dreams may provide an early warning of illness, and she advises consulting a physician if you dream that you're in pain or freezing or burning, or if you dream of animals becoming injured or dying or of buildings getting damaged or destroyed.

Dr. Garfield's experience dovetails with a study of dreams among those with suspected heart disease. Robert C. Smith, M.D., professor of psychiatry at Michigan State University in East Lansing, asked patients with suspected heart disease to record their dreams for a year. Then Dr. Smith evaluated their hearts, using sophisticated tests. Those with the most damaged hearts reported the most nightmares and other bad dreams.

## Quest for Meaning

Some dreams certainly communicate clear messages, but most, if we recall them at all, are collections of fleeting, surreal images that might mean almost anything—or nothing. Some dream interpreters have constructed elaborate lists of dream symbols and what they supposedly mean, but Alex Lukeman, author of *What Your Dreams Can Teach You*, argues that dream symbols are best understood in personal terms.

A dream of an airplane trip might suggest work anxieties to a flight attendant, exciting new possibilities to someone leaving an unsatisfying relationship, death to a person with a serious illness or a desire to visit family to someone who feels lonely—or it could be a nightmare to someone who fears flying.

Noted dream interpreter (and cigar lover) Sigmund Freud

once dismissed the notion that every dream image of a tubular object symbolized a penis by saying, "Sometimes a cigar is just a cigar."

Lukeman agrees, and he urges people who are interested in using dreams to commune with their unconscious minds to steer clear of pat symbol interpretations. "Only you can ultimately interpret the meaning any dream has for you," he says. To do that, the first step is to recall your dreams.

## How to Recall Your Dreams

Everyone dreams. The issue is not, as Shakespeare put it in Hamlet, "to sleep, perchance to dream," but rather "to dream, perchance to remember." Some people recall their dreams vividly without any special effort. Others retain a few fleeting images or nothing at all. But no matter how well—or poorly— you have recalled your dreams in the past, if you'd like to remember them, you can. It's a simple matter of self-training. Dream recall is surprisingly easy. Here's how Lukeman and Stanford University dream researcher Stephen LaBerge, Ph.D., director of The Lucidity Institute in Portola Valley, California, suggest doing it.

**Get plenty of sleep.** Adequate rest is essential to good dream recall. In addition, those who feel well-rested cope better with brief wake-ups in the wee hours to record their dreams.

**Talk to yourself.** When you go to sleep, as you get comfortable in bed, declare aloud your intentions: "Tonight I'm going to remember my dreams."

**Capture memories quickly.** Place a pad and pen by your bed before you retire. Whenever you wake up, jot down as much as you can remember of your dreams. The next morning, write up your notes in story form, filling in any details you did not previously jot down. Some people find that using a flashlight rather than turning on a lamp helps them hold onto those fleeting dream memories. Or use a small hand-held tape recorder, the kind that records on microcassettes. Dictate what you recall and then write it up the next morning.

**Be still.** When you awaken to record your dreams, move as little as possible. Motion tends to dissipate dream memories.

**Don't hold out for the full picture.** Cling to any dream fragments you recall and jot them down, even if they do not make a coherent story. Over time, memories of disjointed images or scenes expand into memories of entire dreams.

**Keep a record.** Place your dream write-ups in a journal, with each dream dated and titled. Titles need not be elaborate; all they need to do is reflect the major event or prevailing mood of the dream. After the dream record, include a brief statement summarizing how you're feeling about your life—any significant preoccupations, accomplishments or stressors—and your first impression of what the dream might mean. Reread your dream journal periodically. Over time, you may see patterns emerge and gain new insights into the meaning of your dreams.

Because REM periods lengthen during successive sleep cycles, dreams occupy more of sleep as the night progresses and typically become more elaborate. Expect to experience longer dreams toward morning.

The easiest dreams to capture are the final ones of each night, the ones that occur shortly before you wake up. If you'd like to recall your dreams throughout the night, remember that REM periods occur approximately every 90 minutes. Try setting an alarm to wake you one or more times at multiples of 90 minutes from the time you retire.

If you've remembered your dreams only rarely, it may take a few months to develop consistent dream recall. Don't get frustrated. There's always another night.

## In Search of Healing Lucidity

Among the most profound, exhilarating—and healing—dreams are "lucid" dreams, during which dreamers realize they are dreaming and in some cases take control of their dreams to solve problems, overcome nightmares, gain personal confidence and heal emotional wounds and physical ailments.

Dr. LaBerge, the nation's leading authority on lucid dreaming, says that anyone who remembers dreams can learn to dream lucidly and reap profound personal rewards in the process.

Veiled references to lucid dreaming run through history like ghostly images in a recurring dream. During the fourth century, Aristotle wrote that while asleep, there is often "something in consciousness which declares that what presents itself is a dream." Eight hundred years later, St. Augustine recounted the tale of a Carthaginian physician who had a lucid dream that cemented his religious faith. The twelfth-century Spanish Muslim philosopher Ibn El-Arabi was the first to promote lucid dreaming: "A person must control his thoughts in a dream. The training of this alertness . . . produces great benefits."

But no one paid much attention to lucid dreaming until the mid-nineteenth century, when the Marquis d'Hervey de Saint-Denys, a French professor of Chinese, published his 1867 book, *Dreams and How to Guide Them,* an account of his lifelong hobby of dream recording that touted lucidity as the most exhilarating form of dreaming. Saint-Denys' book helped inspire Freud's seminal 1900 work, *The Interpretation of Dreams.* "There are some people who are quite clearly aware that they are asleep and dreaming, and who thus seem to possess the faculty of consciously directing their dreams," Freud noted. The term "lucid dreaming" was coined in 1913 by Dutch psychiatrist Frederik Willems van Eeden, who published an account of 352 of his own dreams.

Still, most scientists remained skeptical of lucid dreaming because, for much of this century, the Freudian view dominated the discussion. Freud viewed dreams as seething cauldrons of irrationality, sexual urges and primitive impulses. If dreams were careening emotional roller coasters, how could any passenger control the ride?

Then in 1985, Dr. LaBerge published *Lucid Dreaming,* an account of his experiments proving that it's possible to be "wide awake while dreaming." His views remain controversial, but Dr. Dement, whose sleep laboratory hosted Dr. LaBerge's research, insists, "lucid dreaming is real."

In 1977, Dr. LaBerge was a Stanford graduate student in psychophysiology and an amateur "oneironaut" (*oh-NYE-roe-nawt*), from the Greek for "an explorer of dreaming."

Fascinated by his own dreams, he read some of the early works on lucid dreaming and experienced quite a few himself. But he knew that lucid dreaming would remain forever on the fringes of science until someone proved that dreamers could remain conscious while dreaming.

Dr. LaBerge came up with a way to do it. "Several dream studies had shown a precise correspondence between the direction of dreamers' observable eye movements and the direction they report 'looking' in their dreams. In one study, a dreamer was awakened during REM sleep after about two dozen back-and-forth eye movements. He reported that in his dream, he'd been watching a Ping-Pong game. It occurred to me that by moving my own eyes in a recognizable pattern, I might be able to send a signal to the outside world that I was having a lucid dream."

In early 1978, Dr. LaBerge went to sleep in the Stanford Sleep Laboratory with sensors taped around his eyes and a signal arranged with a research colleague—up-and-down eye movements. Toward morning, in the middle of a dream involving a vacuum cleaner, he realized he was dreaming because the instruction manual floated by him as if weightless. This was his chance. He imagined his hand moving up and down in front of his face and followed it with his eyes. In the morning, on the sensor trace, there were his up-and-down eye movements, marking the first time in history that a dreamer had consciously sent a message to the waking world.

Since that remarkable night, Dr. LaBerge has continued his lucid dream research as director of the Lucidity Institute in Portola Valley, California. With the help of a small group of oneironauts who have frequent lucid dreams, he's made a number of discoveries.

For one thing, dream time is remarkably similar to waking time. For more than 100 years, students of dreaming have believed that dreams happen in a flash, thanks to nineteenth-century dream researcher Alfred Maury, who had an elaborate novel-like dream of involvement in the French Revolution, culminating in his own beheading for treason. The guillotine blade fell—and Maury woke up to the discovery that his headboard had fallen on his neck. He deduced that his epic dream had taken only a second or two. Some dreams may occur in a moment, but when Dr. LaBerge asked lucid dreamers to count off 10 seconds while dreaming, their average estimate of 10 seconds was actually 13 seconds.

When dreamers dream of holding their breath, they actually hold their breath. Dr. LaBerge and other lucid dreamers used eye movements to signal that they'd begun a lucid dream and then held their breath in their dreams while hooked up to sensitive equipment that recorded their breathing. In each of 12 breath-holding dreams, the lucid dreamers actually held their breath.

During lucid dreaming, women frequently have sexual dreams and experience dream orgasms that produce physiological changes similar to waking orgasms. Men seem to experience sexual lucid dreams less frequently. When they do, their orgasms feel real, but unlike teenagers having "wet dreams," they do not ejaculate.

In dreaming as in waking, the brain's left hemisphere is more active during analytical thinking, while the right hemisphere is more active during artistic thinking. Dr. LaBerge and other lucid dreamers signaled that they were dreaming lucidly and then sang a song and counted to ten. Brain wave recordings showed that after the signal, their right brains were more active (during the dream song), followed by a shift to left-brain activity (during the dream counting).

Compared with waking daydreams, lucid dreaming is more like actually doing what you dream about. "When we had subjects imagine singing and counting," Dr. LaBerge explains, "neither task produced any consistent shifts in brain activity. But singing and counting during lucid dreams produced brain activity equivalent to that which occurs during actual performance of those tasks."

"Our studies," Dr. LaBerge says, "have amassed strong laboratory evidence that what happens in the inner world of dreams—especially during lucid dreams—can produce physical effects on the dreamer's brain as real as those produced by corresponding events in the external world. Far from the view that dreams are 'airy nothings' devoid of reality and meaning, what we do—or leave undone—in dreams can affect us as profoundly as what we do—or don't do—in our waking lives."

## How to Dream Lucidly

There is no method guaranteed to produce lucid dreams, but here are several ways to increase the possibility.

**Set your alarm.** Lucid dreams seem to be most likely to occur during the longer REM periods of early morning, within two to three hours of waking. Set your alarm two to three hours earlier than usual, and you'll boost your chances of waking up in a lucid dream.

**Practice MILD.** MILD is Dr. LaBerge's acronym for "mnemonic induction of lucid dreaming." It's a simply memory aid that links one action to another, such as thinking "When I pass the supermarket, I'll remember to buy bread." "Before I developed MILD," Dr. LaBerge recalls, "I recalled less than one lucid dream per month. But using the MILD technique, I recalled an average of five." Here's how to practice MILD.

Several times each day, and anytime you wake up from sleeping, focus on your intent to dream lucidly. Say out loud, "The next time I'm dreaming, I want to recognize that I'm dreaming." "You must really intend to have a lucid dream," Dr. LaBerge says.

Practice memory induction while awake. Repeat to yourself: The next time I see X, I'll ask myself if I'm dreaming. Your Xs are your "mnemonic targets." Jot down four different targets per day, such as a dog, a bus, a piece of mail with a colored envelope and a woman pushing a baby carriage. Each morning commit them to memory. When you see one during the day, ask yourself: Am I dreaming? Of course, you're not, but this exercise prepares your sleeping mind to recognize lucidity cues.

Lucidity cues are experiences that would be odd or impossible in the external world: appearing in public naked, defying gravity, being underwater, meeting a dead relative or being suddenly transported back to first grade. As you dream, try to pay attention to things that appear unusual. When you notice one, think "I must be dreaming."

During the early morning, when you wake up from a dream, go over it in your mind several times until you have memorized it.

Then repeat your intention statement: "The next time I'm dreaming, I want to recognize that I'm dreaming."

Next visualize yourself back in the dream that you just had (and memorized), only this time see yourself realizing that you are dreaming.

Repeat the previous two steps several times.

**Invest in a lucid dream induction device.** Dr. LaBerge has developed three devices to promote lucid dreaming. The least expensive is the DreamLink. It looks like a large pair of thick sunglasses or an oversize sleep mask and has two tiny built-in lights and an alarm clock. Because dreams generally occur about every 90 minutes, you set the alarm for that interval, and every hour and a half the DreamLink's tiny lights flash over your closed eyelids. Sleepers can "see" these lights and use them as lucidity cues.

The NovaDreamer is more sophisticated. It looks like the DreamLink but contains photoelectric sensors that accurately detect the rapid eye movements of REM sleep. Whenever you enter a REM period, the NovaDreamer's lights flash.

The DreamLight is Dr. LaBerge's top-of-the-line lucid-dreaming inducer. In addition to detecting REM sleep, it contains a microcomputer that can produce many different lucidity cues, including flashing lights and tones. It also records the times of your REM periods and includes an alarm so you can wake up during them.

For a free catalog about any of Dr. LaBerge's lucid dream induction devices, contact The Lucidity Institute, 2555 Park Boulevard, Suite 2, Palo Alto, CA 94306.

## Lucid Dreaming with a Mission

People who have lucid dreams almost always enjoy and value them. "The times I've been dreaming and realized I was dreaming," says San Francisco illustrator Dan Hubig, "have been memorable, refreshing and exhilarating—among my best dreams."

Refreshment is reason enough to cultivate lucid dreaming. But lucid dreamers say they derive more profound benefits: preparation for challenges, problem-solving, overcoming nightmares, physical and emotional healing and even coming to terms with mortality. Here are some dream reports Dr. LaBerge has received from lucid dreamers around the country.

*Coming to terms with mortality.* A dreamer in Lauderhill, Florida, used a lucid dream to accomplish what many people consider impossible—overcoming the fear of death. "I found myself walking through a hell-like place. Since I was asleep in my bed, I realized that this could not be, that I must be dreaming. At that instant, I was stabbed in the back. Feeling the pain in my dream, I decided to see what dying would be like. I entered a catatonic state. I willed my dream soul to depart from my dream body. With my dream soul, I floated upward. It was a strange feeling to see my dream body beneath me. I felt an all-pervading peace and calm. I said to myself: 'If this is what dying is like, it isn't so bad.' From that day forward, I have had no fear of dying. I have even remained calm in life-threatening situations."

*Emotional healing.* Johann von Goethe, the eighteenth-century German poet, dramatist, novelist and statesman, once said, "There have been times I have fallen asleep in tears, but in my dreams, the most charming forms have come to cheer me, and I have risen fresh and joyful."

Perhaps he had healing dreams similar to this one, recorded by a woman in Portola Valley, California. "When my grandmother died, I was terribly unhappy. I decided to use her as a lucidity cue to ask how she was and tell her how much I loved and missed her. The next time she appeared in a dream, I felt so sad that I did not become lucid. For several days, I repeated: 'If I dream of Grams, I will remember that I'm dreaming.' The next time I saw her, she looked so vivid and real, it was hard to believe I was dreaming. But I realized that I was, and asked her how she was. She answered with some despair, 'Oh, darling, I don't know. I don't know where I am.'

"I felt elated that I'd made contact with her but also distraught that she felt disturbed. Two weeks later, I dreamed of her again and immediately realized I was dreaming. This time she said, 'I am not feeling so unsettled anymore.' She also said something I could not understand about existing fairly happily 'somewhere.' I hugged her a long time and told her I would always love her. Perhaps I truly contacted her spirit. Perhaps I simply spoke with my inner self. I don't know. But after those two dreams, something settled inside me. My deep sadness over her death began slipping away."

*Overcoming nightmares.* An estimated one-third to one-half of adults experience occasional nightmares. Factors that contribute to bad dreams include illness (especially fever), traumatic events (assault or earthquake), family and relationship problems and general emotional anxieties.

Psychotherapy while waking can help, but so can self-therapy during lucid dreaming. A woman in Fresno, California, was plagued by recurring nightmares of being chased by monsters. "Finally I decided I could not live fully while my fears had such power over me. I began dreaming, determined not to yield. I'd read somewhere that a fear could only be dissipated by friendliness and trust. So I made up my mind to be friendly. Suddenly I was faced with a large, nebulous monster. I was really scared. I almost turned and ran. But by sheer will, I stood my ground and let it approach. I said to myself, 'This is a dream, and if I forget it, I'll have to go through all of this again in another nightmare.'

"I smiled as sincerely as I could and spoke as calmly as I could, which was a big step for me—waking or sleeping fears usually leave me speechless. I said something like, 'I'm not afraid. I want to be friends. You are welcome in my dream.' As soon as I'd spoken, the monster became friendly. I was ecstatic. I woke up saying, 'I did it!' "

*Physical healing.* A lucid dreamer in Mount Prospect, Illinois, credits a healing dream with a remarkable recovery from a sprained ankle. Perhaps he would have gotten back on his feet just as quickly without the following dream, but he doesn't think so. "My sprained ankle was very swollen. It was difficult to walk. Then I had a dream that I was running. I realized that this couldn't be, so I must be dreaming.

"At this point, I began waking up and became conscious of the pain in my ankle. But I stayed in the dream by reaching for my dream ankle with dream hands. As I held my ankle in the dream, I felt a vibration that made me think of electricity. Amazed, I decided to throw lightning bolts all around my ankle. That's all I remember. But I woke up with no pain in my ankle, and I could walk on it with considerable ease."

*Preparation for challenges.* Another lucid dreamer in Mount Prospect, Illinois, was studying to become a professional French horn player but was bothered by performance anxiety. "Before going to bed I focused on my desire to dream of performing solo before a large audience without any nervousness or anxiety. On the third night, I had this lucid dream: I was performing a solo recital without accompaniment at Orchestra Hall in Chicago (a place I'd performed in an orchestra). I felt no anxiety, and I gained confidence with every note I played. I played perfectly a piece I'd heard only once before (and had never attempted to play in my waking life). I received an ovation, which added to my confidence.

"When I woke up, I made a quick note of the dream and the piece I'd played in it. While practicing the next day, I sight-read the piece, and remarkably, played it almost perfectly. Two weeks—and a few lucid dreams—later, I performed with the orchestra. For the first time in my life, nerves did not hamper my playing, and the performance went extremely well."

*Problem-solving.* Many lucid dreamers find that they can count on their dreams to help them solve problems. A woman in Hays, Kansas, reported this experience: "After I got pregnant, my husband and I began considering baby names. During one lucid dream, I had a baby in my arms and tried out various names by presenting the child to my parents: 'Mom, Dad, this is Chris.' 'Mom, Dad, this is Justin.' I tried many names and watched their reactions to them. Finally, I settled on a boy's and a girl's name. Unfortunately, I had other dreams that night, and when I woke up, I couldn't remember the two names.

"The next night, I entered a lucid dream and recalled that during my earlier 'name dream,' I'd mentioned the two names to a friend. I stopped the lucid dream I was having, and while still dreaming, called that friend and asked her the names. She told me. I immediately woke myself up and repeated the names several times aloud so that I would remember them in the morning."

A man in West Chazy, New York, owes his success as a computer programmer to lucid dreaming. "Whenever I have a new program to design, I dream I'm sitting in the kind of old-fashioned parlor that Sherlock Holmes had. I'm there with Albert Einstein—white bushy hair and everything. He and I are good friends. We talk about the program and do some flow charts on a blackboard. Once we think we've come up with a good one, we laugh. Einstein says, 'The rest is history,' and excuses himself to go to bed.

"I sit in his recliner and make some notes on a pad. I look at the notes and say to myself, 'I want to remember this when I wake up.' I concentrate very hard on the notepad and blackboard. Then I wake myself up. It's usually around 3:30 A.M. I grab the flashlight, pen and pad that I keep near my bed and start writing as fast as I can. I take these notes to work, and about 99 percent of the time, I design the program successfully from them."

Whether or not you experience lucid dreaming, the rewards of recalling and exploring your dreams can be profound. Even the researchers who doubt that dreams have meaning agree that dreams are among the mind's most amazing creations. Whether they are ultimately real or illusory is beside the point. They feel real while they last, and they often have great personal significance. Why waste two hours a night when the world of your dreams beckons with magic, mystery and healing potential beyond, well, your wildest dreams?

CHAPTER 9

# ELIMINATION DIETS

## When What You Eat Is Why You Hurt

After spending his teens with a chronically stuffed nose, Timothy Yaeger, of Newark, Delaware, was tested for allergies in 1976. "The allergist/immunologist told me I was allergic to ragweed, cat hair, dust and wheat. He urged me to have allergy shots and to stop eating all bread products." Yaeger was stunned: No bread? No pizza? No hamburger buns? No spaghetti? "That's right," the doctor replied, "if you want your symptoms to clear up."

"That's ridiculous," countered Tim's uncle, an internist who did not believe in food allergies. "Get the shots, but forget the nonsense about wheat." Yaeger followed his uncle's advice. The allergy shots helped his breathing, and he quickly forgot the recommendation to avoid wheat.

But Yaeger never felt quite right. During college, he had mood and energy swings, from depressed and lethargic to manic and hyperactive. Tests at the college health service turned up nothing. Yaeger began to doubt his sanity.

Then one day in 1983, Yaeger stumbled on a magazine article about food allergies. The list of possible symptoms included his. And a prime offender, the article said, was gluten, the protein in wheat and other grains that gives elasticity to dough made from them. Suddenly Yaeger recalled the allergist/immunologist's recommendation to avoid wheat. Maybe his uncle had been wrong.

Yaeger began shunning wheat. He ate oatmeal for breakfast, baked his own barley bread and avoided pastas. He felt a little better. Then he tried wheat again and immediately experienced a return of his symptoms. Maybe he was allergic to wheat. Or perhaps he was simply suggestible.

Yaeger consulted another allergist/immunologist, who asked him to fast for a few days, with water as his only sustenance. Then the doctor gave him capsules containing various foods and asked him to record his reactions. The capsules were unmarked, and Yaeger had no idea what they contained. Most caused him no problems, but a few triggered his symptoms. The offending capsules contained wheat, oats, barley and rye. The doctor diagnosed gluten intolerance and advised him to stop eating all four grains and anything made from them.

Yaeger vowed to do just that. "Of course, it was easier said than done," he recalls. "There's wheat in cereals, breads, pastas, baked goods—even most prepared sauces and soups. And just try telling your wife, mother, aunt or mother-in-law that you can no longer eat many of the dishes they enjoy serving. No one was obnoxious about it, but there was subtle pressure to eat what I shouldn't. Whenever I did, my symptoms came roaring back. After a while, I stopped fooling around. As long as I stick to my diet, I feel fine."

Yaeger's adjustment was not easy, but it was less difficult than you might think. "Instead of bread, I eat rice cakes. I still enjoy pasta, but I eat rice noodles. At restaurants, when friends order pizza, I have roast chicken. When they order sandwiches, I have a salad. And these days, there are plenty of books filled with substitutions for people who are gluten-sensitive."

## Asian Mystery Solved

Kelly Baron's strange illness began one morning when she woke with stomach cramps and diarrhea. The 45-year-old

Bridgeport, Connecticut, office manager dismissed her symptoms as just one of those things. But as the months passed, her symptoms occurred more frequently. She wrote them off to stress. She was unhappy at her job, and her favorite aunt had just died.

But Baron's symptoms persisted, and eventually she consulted her doctor. He could find nothing wrong and referred her to a gastroenterologist, who asked her if she'd traveled abroad recently. In fact, she'd spent a few weeks in Brazil shortly before her symptoms appeared.

The gastroenterologist diagnosed a parasitic infection, which is common in travelers, and prescribed metronidazole (Flagyl), a standard pharmaceutical. But the drug only made her feel worse. "In addition to diarrhea, I began having heart palpitations and shortness of breath. I felt exhausted and weepy. I lost my appetite and ten pounds. Before my illness, I was running six miles a day. But at that point, I could hardly take a walk around my neighborhood."

Next Baron consulted a holistic doctor, who told her that in addition to curing her parasitic infection, the medication also killed the beneficial bacteria in her intestines. He prescribed acidophilus capsules and large doses of vitamin C, along with other supplements. But this treatment provided scant relief.

At her wits' end, Baron took a vacation. While she was away, she felt much better, but upon her return, she got sick again. Convinced that her illness was a stress reaction to her job problems, she made a concerted effort to find a new job. She succeeded, but despite a major reduction in stress, her symptoms continued unabated.

Back she went to the gastroenterologist, who tested her for all sorts of parasites but found nothing. Another doctor suggested she might have a food allergy and advised her to eliminate common food triggers: wheat, yeast, dairy products and alcohol. But the elimination diet didn't help, so Baron's physician told her to cut out citrus, tomatoes and eggs. Her symptoms continued.

Fed up, Baron and her husband took a trip to Italy. While away, she decided to take a break from all food restrictions.

Miraculously, she felt fine, except for one day of symptoms. But when she returned home, her illness reappeared with a vengeance. "Am I crazy?" Baron wondered. "What was so different in Italy?"

Then she realized that to celebrate their return home, she and her husband had eaten at their favorite Japanese restaurant. She loved Asian food and ate it often, but in Italy, they'd had it only once—at a Chinese restaurant the day before her brief bout of symptoms. A light switched on. "It had to be soy," Baron realized. "Not only is it in soy sauce and tofu, but when I eliminated dairy, I substituted soy milk."

Baron eliminated all soy products from her diet and has felt fine ever since—except for one day when her old symptoms flared up again. She reflected on what she'd eaten the previous day and could come up with nothing containing soy. Then she recalled that she'd eaten tuna salad with mayonnaise. "Wouldn't you know, the tuna contained hydrolized soy protein and good old Hellman's had soy oil."

The problems Timothy Yaeger and Kelly Baron had with food are by no means rare. Millions of Americans are sensitive to wheat, milk and other foods, and food sensitivities may even play a role in two common, mysterious and disabling conditions—rheumatoid arthritis and multiple sclerosis. Yet this entire field is controversial. Like Yaeger's uncle, many physicians continue to insist that reports of food allergies are enormously exaggerated. They're right, but so are those who use diet modifications to recover from baffling illnesses.

## Food Allergy versus Food Intolerance

Much of the controversy surrounding food allergies stems from use of the word *allergy*. Most of the problems people call food allergies are not allergies. They're real. They're chronic. They may cause severe illness. And they involve reactions to specific foods. But they're not allergies. Rather, they are sensitivities or intolerances.

The distinction between an allergy and a sensitivity may seem trivial, but it's as real to allergist/immunologists as the distinction between the colors lime and teal is to a fashion designer.

In classic allergic reactions, such as hay fever, the offending substance (allergen) triggers a quick, predictable response based on specific actions of the immune system. For example, when microscopic grains of pollen enter the nostrils, some settle on a specific type of protein—immunoglobulin E (IgE)—that covers the outer membranes of special cells (mast cells) in the upper respiratory tract. In people who don't have hay fever, nothing happens. But in those who do, the IgE tells the mast cells to react to the pollen. The mast cells release histamine, which triggers allergy symptoms: nasal congestion, runny nose and itchy, watery eyes.

According to the American Academy of Allergy and Immunology, an estimated 5 percent of children and 2 percent of adults have similar reactions to foods. They usually come from families with allergies and asthma. In a true food allergy, eating even a tiny amount of the offending food, such as peanuts, quickly causes a severe reaction: hay fever symptoms plus possibly tongue swelling, abdominal distress and, in some cases, the most severe allergic reaction, anaphylaxis, which can be rapidly fatal unless treated on an emergency basis. Immediate-reaction food allergies were first documented more than 2,000 years ago by Hippocrates, the father of Western medicine, and became incorporated into immunology in the 1920s.

But the vast majority of those who have problems with one or more foods do not have true food allergies. Their reactions often develop gradually. They are not predictable, may not involve IgE and don't trigger release of histamine from the mast cells. Many people still use the term *food allergy* to describe them, but increasingly, these problems are called food intolerances or sensitivities.

## Why Foods Can Hurt

What we eat can certainly cause harm. The chapter on low-fat eating (page 291) demonstrates that fat is the chief villain in the American diet. Dietary fat contributes to risk of heart disease, stroke, many cancers, diabetes, obesity and chronic high blood pressure. The chapter on vegetarianism (page 409) shows how certain high-fat foods, particularly meats and dairy products, can contribute to all of the above, plus calcium loss and osteoporosis. And the discussion of Ornish therapy (page 368) explains how an ultra-low-fat vegetarian diet has achieved a feat that even the latest surgical techniques and pharmaceuticals cannot match—reversal of heart disease, the nation's leading killer.

Nevertheless, until about 20 years ago, most doctors and nutrition experts believed that, except for true food allergies that provoked immediate reactions, as long as food items were part of a balanced diet, they couldn't be harmful. And critics of the notion of food intolerances said, "We've been eating these plants for thousands of years. If they really caused harm, it would have been noticed long ago."

Don't look now, but food intolerances *were* noticed. The problem was that no one paid much attention. Gluten sensitivity, the first documented food intolerance, came to light 110 years ago. In 1888, the British physician S. J. Gee published a report describing several cases of what he called celiac disease—a chronic gastrointestinal condition that cleared up if those who had it stopped eating wheat, rye, barley and oats.

Dr. Gee's report had little impact for almost 50 years, until the late 1940s, when a food shortage at the end of World War II eliminated wheat from the Dutch diet for several months. Observant doctors noticed that many people with chronic upset stomach, bloating, diarrhea, abdominal pain and irritable bowel symptoms miraculously recovered and then relapsed when they returned to eating wheat.

An estimated 1 in 2,500 people has celiac disease, now usually called gluten intolerance. It often (but not always) runs in families, suggesting a genetic defect in the ability to metabolize this protein.

"We must remember that no one designed foods for human consumption," notes Jonathan Brostoff, M.D., director of the Allergy Clinic at Middlesex Hospital in London and co-author (with Linda Gamlin) of *The Complete Guide to Food Allergy and Intolerance*. "Our foods come from a pool of wild plants and animals that were domesticated by early farmers only 5,000 to 10,000 years ago, a blink of the eye in evolutionary terms. Unlike animals, plants can't run away from predators. But they have their own defenses: thorns, bitter taste and an array of chemical weapons against diseases, insects—and us. Plant breeding has removed some of these weapons, but by no means all."

No one knows how many people have food intolerances, but Dr. Brostoff estimates about 10 percent.

In general, common foods—wheat, milk, corn and eggs—are the most problematic. In recent years, as Asian foods and vegetarianism have become more popular, an increasing number of people, like Kelly Baron, are turning up with intolerance to soy. Initially, symptoms tend to be minor, but they grow more severe as time passes and may be provoked by an increasing number of foods. Often people don't even notice their symptoms for several years. Over time, they simply experience a slow decline in health and vitality and report vague, nonspecific symptoms that some mainstream physicians dismiss as "neurotic." Possible symptoms of food intolerance include indigestion, mouth sores, diarrhea, constipation, irritable bowel syndrome, bloating, flatulence, muscle and/or joint pain, headaches, mental fogginess and fatigue.

## Elimination Diets for Food Intolerance

"If you think you might have a classic food allergy or a food intolerance, start with a visit to your primary-care physician to rule out other possibilities, such as an ulcer or colitis," advises Anne Simons, M.D., assistant clinical professor of family and community medicine at the University of California's San Francisco Medical Center and author of *Before You Call the Doctor*. "Then consult an allergist/immunologist for skin tests and RAST—radioallergosorbent testing. Skin tests involve scratching the skin and introducing minute amounts of possible allergy triggers, such as pollen or peanuts. If a red welt develops, you're allergic to the substance. RAST uses blood samples to test for IgE reactions. Skin tests and RAST can diagnose classic allergies, but they are not all that useful for pinpointing food intolerances. To do that, you need an elimination diet."

Elimination diets limit food choices until you feel better. Once you do, you know you're intolerant to one or more of the foods you've eliminated. By reintroducing the foods you've eliminated one at a time over a period of weeks, you can often pinpoint your individual sensitivities and then avoid those foods or have them only once in a while. (Some food intolerances appear only with regular consumption.)

While you're observing an elimination diet, keep a diary of your feelings and reactions. Be as specific as possible. Stress, according to Dr. Brostoff, can make you more or less susceptible to foods you might be sensitive to, so it's helpful to have a record of your feelings as well.

The most rigorous elimination diet begins with a total fast—no food at all, just water for several days. Then you reintroduce foods one at a time, one a week until you begin to react. When you do, you eliminate that food and continue phased reintroductions. This rigorous elimination diet is efficient but hard to live with. That's why Dr. Brostoff developed a three-stage elimination diet, with common sensitivity triggers eliminated in Stages I and II and less likely triggers eliminated in Stage III.

*Stage I Elimination Diet.* The Stage I Elimination Diet is a no-junk-food diet. The following foods are allowed: vegetables, beans, whole-grain breads, potatoes, rice, milk, most cheeses, butter, noncaffeinated teas, most fresh fruits (the exceptions are listed below), fresh, unprocessed meats and fish, unsweetened juices and cereals without sugar or artificial coloring.

The following foods are not allowed: alcoholic beverages, foods prepared with alcohol, coffee, caffeinated teas, cola drinks, chocolate, sugar and artificial sweeteners and foods that contain them, vinegar, pickles, margarine, foods that contain additives, smoked meats such as bacon, ham and sausage, smoked fish, aged cheeses such as Cheddar and Brie, take-out food, restaurant food, bran, very salty foods, curries, pineapple and papaya.

# Fasting: Helpful or Hazardous?

Fasting might be called the ultimate elimination diet. *The University of California, Berkeley, Wellness Letter* sums up the conventional medical position on going without food and drink: "There's no danger in a 24-hour fast. Some religions call for occasional fasts, and some people derive satisfaction from fasting. But [longer fasts are] ineffective and risky. Fasting for more than two or three days becomes starvation."

The riskiness of fasting depends on how you define it. Complete abstinence from food and drink does indeed become hazardous to health after a few days. A healthy person can survive as long as a few weeks without food but only about three days without water.

Fasting for health and spiritual growth does not involve starvation but rather a major change in normal eating patterns. This type of fasting, sometimes called "modified fasting," typically involves eliminating solid foods and taking all nourishment in liquid form—water, broth or juices. It may also involve abstaining from all food by day and eating only at night, a practice followed annually by millions of Muslims around the world during the four-week fast of Ramadan.

Using this definition—diet modification, not abstinence—even extended fasts pose little threat of starvation. They are simply a different way to ingest nutrients. Many of the world's greatest thinkers reportedly fasted regularly for as long as 40 days: Moses, Jesus, Plato, Aristotle, Confucius, Hippocrates, Leonardo da Vinci and Gandhi, who has been quoted as saying, "Fasting brings spiritual rebirth."

Fasting's spiritual revelations are a matter of opinion, but on the physical side, a few studies have suggested intriguing health bene-

What do you look for while you're on this diet? It's possible that you'll feel worse for the first few days, because it's emotionally trying to stop eating familiar foods. In addition, if you regularly eat chocolate or drink coffee, caffeinated teas or colas, you may experience caffeine withdrawal effects during the first week. Symptoms include headache, sluggishness and constipa-

fits. Many fasters report increased energy and mental clarity. There appear to be two reasons for this. Digestion requires a good deal of energy, particularly the digestion of fatty meats and dairy products. That's why people often feel lethargic after a big meat meal. Water, broth and juices are low in fat and easy to digest, which frees up energy for other purposes.

A 1993 study showed that fasting also boosts levels of high-density lipoprotein (HDL), the "good" cholesterol that protects against heart attack. Researchers at Ben-Gurion University in Israel studied a group of Muslims during and after the fast of Ramadan. During their four-week fast, they ate and drank nothing by day, then had a large meal at night and sometimes a light snack before dawn. Much to the researchers' surprise, the Muslims' HDL levels were 30 percent higher during Ramadan than afterward, when they returned to eating normally.

Advocates also contend that fasting rids the body of toxins that accumulate in the digestive tract. Mainstream nutritionists scoff at this notion, but research suggests that a low-fat, liquid diet of fruit and vegetable juices eliminates common triggers of food intolerance and might relieve some people's sensitivity symptoms.

Some people should not fast: children, the frail elderly, pregnant and nursing women and people who are seriously underweight. In addition, those with chronic medical conditions should consult a clinical nutritionist before embarking on extended fasts. But if you're healthy and would like to try fasting for health and/or spiritual uplift, there's no medical reason why you shouldn't give a limited fast a try.

tion. You might also feel worse or experience cravings for forbidden foods because of your body's adjustment to not eating the foods you can't tolerate.

If you feel better, congratulations—one or more of the Stage I forbidden foods is probably causing your problem. To find out which one(s), begin by maintaining this diet for a month before you reintroduce anything, to give your system a rest from food reactions. Then reintroduce one forbidden food per week, and in your diary, record how it makes you feel. If any food triggers your symptoms, eliminate it, then reintroduce it some weeks later. If you become convinced that you're intolerant to a specific food, eliminate it for several months and then try it from time to time to see if you're still sensitive to it.

If you feel no better, proceed to Stage II. Maintain the Stage I diet right up to the time you begin Stage II.

**Stage II Elimination Diet.** During Stage II you must continue restricting all the foods that are forbidden in Stage I. Only the following foods are allowed: fresh vegetables, potatoes, beans, most fresh fruits (the exceptions are listed below), nuts you usually eat only occasionally, rice (unless you eat it often), vegetable oil, noncaffeinated teas, lamb, turkey, pork, duck and rabbit. All the meats you eat must be fresh and unprocessed.

You must also add the following to the list of forbidden foods: breads and grains, including wheat and bulgur, oats, rye, barley, rice (if you eat it often) and corn; corn products, including corn syrup, grits and polenta; beef; chicken; cheese; any kind of milk, including soy milk; butter; yogurt; oranges; margarine; eggs; all processed meats; lemons; limes; grapefruit; bouillon; yeast; peanuts; anything you normally eat every day or crave; mushrooms and aspirin.

Follow this diet for three weeks before you reintroduce anything. Continue to keep your diary. During the first few days of Stage II, adjustment to the diet may make you may feel worse.

If you feel better after three weeks, reintroduce one food per week to pinpoint your sensitivity(ies). If you feel no better, proceed to Stage III.

**Stage III Elimination Diet.** Most people discover their food intolerances during Stage I or II, but some need to try the rigorous Stage III regimen.

Stage III excludes everything except the following foods: celery, fennel, avocado, lettuce, rutabaga, watercress, spinach, alfalfa sprouts, okra, asparagus, rice, millet, buckwheat, turnips, parsnips, yams, sweet potatoes, plantains, wild rice, tapioca, chestnuts, chick-peas, pumpkin, bananas, pears, kiwifruit, mangoes, pomegranates, guavas, black currants, pumpkin seeds, macadamia nuts, pistachio nuts, cashew nuts, brazil nuts, pine nuts, olive oil, sunflower oil, safflower oil, turkey, duck, lamb, rabbit, goose and fish (except smoked fish or shellfish). In addition, if you typically eat any of the allowed foods more than once a week, exclude them.

Again, after following this rigorous diet for three weeks, begin introducing foods one at a time until you find your culprits.

Some people with food sensitivities find they must eliminate the offending items completely to remain symptom-free. Others find that after six months or so, they can eat foods to which they are sensitive occasionally without ill effects or with minor effects.

People with many food sensitivities sometimes find that they can keep their symptoms under control by using a "rotation diet," eating any given food item only once every four or five days.

Experiment and see what works best for you. If you still don't feel right after the three-stage elimination diet, consult a specialist in food sensitivities (see the organizations listed in Resources).

## Elimination Diet for Lactose Intolerance

Lactose is the milk sugar found in all dairy products. People with lactose intolerance have difficulty digesting it and experience stomach upset, diarrhea, gas and abdominal cramps.

Nursing mammals produce an enzyme—lactase—that allows them to digest their mothers' milk. After weaning, most mammals never drink milk again, and they lose the ability to produce lactase. Many humans also stop making lactase but continue to drink milk and consume dairy products throughout life. The result is lactose intolerance.

"Lactose intolerance," the University of California's Dr. Simons explains, "is most common among African Americans and

Asians, but many adolescents and adults of all races experience some degree of this problem, which usually remains unsuspected, undiagnosed and untreated. Anyone with chronic stomach upset and gas should suspect it."

To test yourself for lactose intolerance, eliminate all dairy foods from your diet for a few days and see how you feel. In addition to milk, yogurt, cheeses and ice cream, avoid milk solids and whey. (You'll have to read food labels carefully.) If you feel noticeably better, chances are you're lactose intolerant. Doctors can also test for lactose intolerance.

If you're sensitive to lactose, you have several choices.

*Go cold turkey.* You can refrain completely from eating dairy foods.

*Get a little culture.* You can try to eat yogurt, buttermilk and hard cheeses. Many people with lactose intolerance can consume these cultured-milk products without triggering symptoms.

*Call in the reinforcements.* You can buy milk and dairy products with added lactase. These products have become more widely available as lactose intolerance has been publicized. You can add your own lactase to milk using the over-the-counter lactase supplement Lactaid, which is available at pharmacies.

*Rely on substitutes.* You can use soy milk instead of cow's milk. Just don't try to use goat's milk; it also contains lactose, so it won't help the problem.

If you eliminate dairy products, be sure to get enough calcium by eating lots of low-fat cultured-milk dairy products and other foods rich in calcium: canned salmon, green leafy vegetables and tofu. You might also take a calcium supplement.

## Elimination Diet for MSG Intolerance

In 1968, a letter to the prestigious *New England Journal of Medicine* reported the occurrence of "two hours of numbness, weakness and heart palpitations" after eating at a Chinese restaurant. The doctor-correspondent speculated that the cause was the food additive used in many Asian cuisines, monosodium glutamate (MSG).

The wire services picked up the story, and newspapers from coast to coast warned of "Chinese restaurant syndrome." As medical reports of MSG reactions multiplied, new symptoms joined the list: headache, dizziness, nausea, diarrhea, depression, insomnia, rashes, rapid heartbeat, irregular heartbeat, mood swings, tremors and shortness of breath. Some people react immediately, while others develop symptoms up to 48 hours after consuming MSG.

Today many Chinese restaurants advertise "No MSG." "But Chinese restaurants are just the tip of the MSG iceberg," says George R. Schwartz, M.D., a Santa Fe, New Mexico, specialist in emergency medicine and toxicology and author of *In Bad Taste: The MSG Syndrome.* "More than 250 supermarket items contain MSG: Ac'cent, Lawry's Seasoned Salt, many condiments and most soup mixes, TV dinners and prepared dishes. And you'd be hard-pressed to find an airplane or fast food meal without it."

As reports of MSG syndrome piled up, the Glutamate Association, the trade group representing MSG manufacturers and users, protested that the additive was the innocent victim of overblown publicity. But over the last 25 years, MSG reactions have been implicated in many ailments: migraine headaches, depression, premenstrual syndrome and asthma attacks. One medical journal even advised doctors to rule out an MSG reaction before diagnosing heart attack.

MSG was first isolated from seaweed in Japan in 1908, and it enhanced the taste of food so noticeably that the Japanese called it aji-no-moto, "the origin of flavor." The use of MSG quickly spread throughout Asia, and after World War II it came to the United States, where studies showed that it stimulates the taste buds. It's now added to most processed foods. Most poultry stuffing mixes, for example, contain enough MSG to cause problems for the estimated 25 percent of Americans who are sensitive to the food additive, contends Dr. Schwartz.

To avoid MSG reactions, eliminate it from your diet. "Unfortunately, that's easier said than done," Dr. Schwartz explains. "Food labels do not necessarily list it. Instead, they might list 'textured protein,' 'hydrolyzed protein,' 'hydrolyzed vegetable protein,' 'yeast food,' 'sodium or calcium caseinate' or 'natural flavors,' all of which contain significant amounts of MSG. And watch out for any foods that come with 'flavor packets.' They usually contain MSG."

The Food and Drug Administration includes MSG on its list of additives "generally regarded as safe," but a study by Harvard researchers suggested that about 30 percent of Americans develop reactions to 5 grams of MSG, while 90 percent react to 10 grams. (One teaspoon of Ac'cent contains about 6 grams.) If you're MSG-sensitive, you can avoid it by eating a diet based on whole grains and fresh fruits and vegetables. Read labels carefully and avoid processed foods and fast foods. When planning to dine at Asian restaurants, call first and ask if they use MSG.

Many people who react to MSG are also sensitive to aspartic acid, an ingredient in the artificial sweetener NutraSweet and in Equal, the sugar substitute that contains NutraSweet. Try eliminating NutraSweet and see how you feel.

## Elimination Diet for Rheumatoid Arthritis

Until the mid-1980s, conventional medical wisdom held that diet had nothing to do with rheumatoid arthritis (RA), the most crippling form of joint inflammation, which affects more than two million Americans. Then reports began appearing that dietary changes relieved some pain and swelling in some people with RA.

A turning point came in 1991, when researchers at the University of Oslo, Norway, placed 53 people with RA on a ten-day fast, during which they consumed only noncaffeinated teas, vegetable juices and garlic-vegetable broth. Then study participants began to eat solid foods, but they abstained from meats, fish, eggs, dairy products, citrus fruits, salt, strong spices, preservatives, alcohol, caffeinated beverages and all foods containing gluten (wheat, barley, oats, rye).

Other foods were introduced one at a time every other day. If any participant reported joint pain, stiffness or inflammation, the food that was just introduced was eliminated for a week and then reintroduced. If symptoms recurred, it was eliminated entirely. After several months, participants' symptom scores were compared with those of people with RA who made no diet modifications. The elimination-diet group reported significantly less pain, fewer swollen joints, less morning stiffness and greater grip strength. Other studies have produced similar results.

Researchers are not sure why dietary changes relieve the symptoms of RA—and the more common osteoarthritis, which affects more than 16 million Americans. Some say that a high-fat diet increases levels of stimulatory prostaglandins, chemicals in the body that trigger inflammation. Others contend that people with arthritis are sensitive to certain foods, specifically plants of the nightshade family: tomatoes, eggplant, white potatoes and peppers (except the spices black and white pepper). And some assert that cooking robs foods of as-yet-undetermined constituents that protect the joints of sensitive individuals.

The debate over why dietary changes relieve arthritis symptoms will no doubt rage for years. But if you have arthritis, try reducing your fat intake. (For details on how to do this, see Low-Fat Eating on page 291.) It might also help to cut out nightshade foods and eat more fresh, raw fruits and vegetables.If these changes do not provide sufficient relief, try the three-stage elimination diet described earlier to help you pinpoint the particular foods to which you're sensitive.

Other studies suggest that taking about a tablespoon a day of olive oil, fish oil (which contains omega-3 fatty acids) or evening primrose oil (gamma-linoleic acid) also helps relieve arthritis symptoms after a period of about six months.

## Elimination Diet for Multiple Sclerosis

Multiple sclerosis (MS) is a baffling, heartbreaking, chronic illness of the nervous system that affects an estimated 350,000 Americans, about 60 percent of them women. Two-thirds of people diagnosed with MS are between the ages of 20 and 40.

In MS, the protective myelin sheath that covers the major nerves breaks down, causing neuroelectrical malfunctions and an enormous array of possible symptoms, from minor weakness to paralysis. In most people with MS, the symptoms come and go. After each attack, or exacerbation, some people return to normal, while others experience residual disability.

Scientists are not sure what causes MS, but there are two major theories: MS often appears in clusters, leading some experts to theorize that a virus or viruslike microorganism is the culprit. Others believe that MS is an autoimmune disease. In this view, the immune system mistakes the myelin sheath for a threatening invader and attacks it.

A third theory has also been proposed, but it has received scant attention from conventional medicine. It links MS to a high-fat diet. Its originator, Roy L. Swank, M.D., Ph.D., professor emeritus of neurology at Oregon Health Sciences University in Portland and author of *The Multiple Sclerosis Diet Book*, claims impressive results in treating MS with a low-fat elimination diet.

In the late 1940s, when Dr. Swank, now in his eighties, first became interested in MS, scientists were puzzled by the observation that the disease was more prevalent in countries farther from the equator. Rates in the United States, Canada, England, Scandinavia, Germany and Switzerland were higher than rates in Mexico and southern Europe. But a half-century ago, MS statistics were sketchy in most countries—except Norway, which had instituted one of the first comprehensive disease-reporting systems.

Dr. Swank looked at MS there, expecting to find more cases in northern Norway than in the southern part of the country. Instead he found a completely different pattern. The MS rate was low along the entire north-south Norwegian coast but considerably higher inland. What could account for this difference?

Using Norwegian diet surveys, Dr. Swank determined that the farm-based inland population ate a diet considerably higher in saturated fat (meats and dairy products) than the fishing-based coastal population. Intrigued, he reinterpreted the strange geographic distribution. All the northern countries with high MS rates also consumed more saturated fats than the southern countries with low MS rates.

How could dietary fat trigger MS? The answer is not entirely clear, and mainstream medicine remains unconvinced, but studies by Dr. Swank and others suggest that the blood of people with MS lacks a specific—and as yet undiscovered—component. The combination of this deficiency and a high-fat diet causes myelin damage and changes in blood flow through the brain.

To test his theory, beginning in 1950 (decades before dietary fat was linked to cancer, heart disease and other ills), Dr. Swank recruited 150 people with MS, placed them on a diet low in saturated fats and compared the course of their disease to that of a control group of people with MS who ate an unrestricted diet. After 20 years, those on the Swank diet experienced substantially fewer exacerbations, with fewer deaths and less disability. Their blood cholesterol levels also fell to an average of less than 150, substantially reducing their risk of heart disease.

Dr. Swank's book discusses his diet in detail, but briefly, here's what it involves.

For the first year, absolutely no red meat and no dark meat of chicken and turkey is permitted. After that, red meat must be lean and kept to a minimum, never exceeding one three-ounce serving a week. The following high-fat meats are forbidden: bacon, lunch meats, salami, frankfurters (including chicken and turkey franks), sausages, duck, goose and spareribs.

Saturated fat consumption must never exceed 15 grams (three teaspoons) a day. All processed foods containing saturated fat must be eliminated.

Nonfat dairy products are permitted. Other dairy products are largely forbidden.

Up to ten teaspoons a day of the following oils are permitted: safflower oil, sunflower oil, corn oil, cottonseed oil, soybean oil, sesame oil, wheat germ oil, linseed oil, peanut oil and olive oil. Margarine, butter, shortening, lard, coconut oil, palm oil and all hydrogenated or partially hydrogenated oils are forbidden, as well as all commercial products containing hydrogenated or partially hydrogenated oils.

Canned foods are permitted as long as they contain no forbidden fats.

Breads are permitted, but chips, cookies, cakes, muffins, biscuits and other baked goods prepared with forbidden fats are not.

All fruits and vegetables are permitted, but olives and avocados must be limited because of their relatively high fat content. Fruit and vegetable juices are permitted. Canned and frozen fruits and vegetables are permitted unless they are prepared with forbidden fats.

Egg whites are permitted. Three whole eggs are permitted each week, but no more than one egg a day.

Sugar should be limited. Chocolate and coconut products are forbidden.

Beverages containing caffeine must be limited to a combined total of no more than three a day—one cup of coffee, one cup of tea and one glass of cola.

Despite Dr. Swank's claims of significant benefit, his diet remains on the fringes of MS medicine. According to a 1992 report by the Therapeutic Claims Committee of the International Federation of Multiple Sclerosis Societies, it causes no harm, but "there appears to be no generally accepted scientific basis for use of this therapy. It has never been tested in a properly controlled clinical trial." Nonetheless, if you have MS, it can't hurt to try the Swank diet. Even if you notice no change in your MS symptoms, the low-fat diet can reduce your risk of cancer and heart disease.

## CHAPTER 10

# EXERCISE

### Even a Little Is Terrific for Your Health

You're always busy. You don't have time to exercise. Your life is a hectic whirl. By the end of the day, you don't have the energy to exercise. Of course, you've tried to exercise, but you've never been able to stick with it. You don't like to perspire. The local health club is expensive and snobby. And with your less-than-perfect body, you'd feel embarrassed to be seen there. Your home is too small for fancy equipment. You already have a cross-country ski machine gathering dust in your basement. Whenever you look at it, you don't feel motivated, you feel guilty. Instead of working out, you'd rather just curl up with a good book and not even *think* about exercise.

Fine. Curl up with this chapter—and free yourself from all the myths and emotional obstacles that have kept you from getting in better shape. The fact is, you don't have to spend half your life sweating buckets at fancy health clubs to reap major physical and emotional benefits from exercise. All it takes to improve health and fitness—and look and feel a whole lot better—is to incorporate just a little more physical activity into your daily life. You hardly have to break into a sweat.

169

## No Pain, Everything to Gain

Ridiculous, you say? Not at all. Just the latest findings from the nation's leading exercise researchers. "The fitness gurus used to insist that we had to punish ourselves with strenuous aerobic exercise for at least 30 minutes three times a week to become fit and healthy," says Bryant Stamford, Ph.D., director of the Health Promotion Center at the University of Louisville School of Medicine in Kentucky and author of *Fitness without Exercise*. "But the latest studies show major health benefits from exercise so modest that it doesn't even feel like a 'workout.' "

Impossible, you say? Consider the research.

Strolling a 20-minute mile—that's a leisurely lap or two around the typical mall—significantly decreases blood pressure and cholesterol, lowering risk of heart attack, stroke and high blood pressure. That's what John Duncan, Ph.D., associate director of the Cooper Institute for Aerobics Research in Dallas, discovered in a study of 102 women ages 20 to 40. "For exercise to improve your health, you don't have to wind up panting," Dr. Duncan says. "To reduce cholesterol and blood pressure, low-intensity exercise works quite well. The more out of shape you are, the more you benefit."

A study at the Mary Imogene Bassett Hospital of Columbia University in Cooperstown, New York, showed the same results. Ann Nafziger, M.D., co-director of the Clinical Pharmacology Research Center there, placed 344 women ages 20 to 69 on a program of low-intensity exercise just twice a week. It reduced their blood levels of total cholesterol and raised levels of HDL, the "good cholesterol," thus reducing their risk of heart disease.

In yet another study, Barry Franklin, Ph.D., a rehabilitation specialist at the Beaumont Rehabilitation and Health Center in Birmingham, Michigan, analyzed 13,000 men's and women's medical records and exercise practices. His conclusion: A 30-minute daily walk significantly improved their heart function and reduced their risk of heart attack.

Compared with no exercise at all, physical activity just one day a week also significantly reduces risk of diabetes. That's what Harvard researcher JoAnn Manson, M.D., associate professor of medicine at the university and director of women's health at Brigham and Women's Hospital in Boston, found after analyzing health and exercise data from the Nurses' Health Study, an ongoing investigation of the diet and lifestyle of more than 87,000 female nurses.

Low-intensity exercise also provides significant psychological benefits. James Rippe, M.D., director of the Exercise Physiology and Nutrition Laboratory at the University of Massachusetts Medical Center in Worcester, asked 36 volunteers to walk on a treadmill at slow, medium or fast speed. "No matter what speed they walked," Dr. Rippe explains, "everyone felt less tense and stressed afterward."

## Moving toward Nature's Way

These studies and many others have spurred the American College of Sports Medicine (ACSM) and the Centers for Disease Control and Prevention (CDC) in Atlanta to change their recommendations about exercise.

"We made a mistake telling everyone they had to engage in strenuous, 20-minute aerobic workouts at least three times a week to obtain health benefits," says Steven Blair, P.E.D., director of epidemiology at the Cooper Institute. "The crucial factor is the total amount of exercise." How much is enough? "About 30 minutes a day," Dr. Blair suggests. It doesn't even have to be a half-hour all at once. Any short-duration exercise that adds up to 30 minutes works just as well. However, the ACSM and CDC still recommend aerobic exercise for optimal conditioning of the cardiovascular system—the heart and blood vessels.

"Strenuous aerobic exercise is great if you're in decent shape and enjoy it," Dr. Duncan explains. "But it's not necessary. What counts is exercise regularity. If you become just a little more active in your daily life and stick with it, your health improves significantly."

This new understanding of exercise marks a return to a more natural, traditional view of physical activity. Our ancestors didn't set aside time to exercise. They simply led physically active lives. They walked a great deal. They chopped wood, pumped water, churned butter, raised their food and washed their clothes largely by hand. Some of these activities were aerobic, but most were not. The distinction didn't matter to our ancestors because they were exercising naturally and steadily, every day of their lives. Now the experts are urging all nonexercisers to do the same.

## A Little Exercise: Big Benefits

Regular low-level exercise confers important health benefits, both physical and emotional. On the physical side, here's what exercise physiologists say it does.

*Helps control weight.* In addition to burning extra calories while you're exercising, physical activity boosts basal metabolic rate—the rate at which the body burns calories while at rest. When you're physically active, you continue to burn extra calories even after you stop exercising. "You may not lose 20 pounds taking leisurely strolls," Dr. Duncan says, "but you'll be better able to maintain your current weight. With low-intensity exercise and a low-fat diet, you'll probably lose a few pounds."

*Enhances sexual pleasure.* James White, Ph.D., professor emeritus in the Department of Physical Education at the University of California at San Diego and director of the Human Performance Laboratory there, recruited 95 healthy but sedentary men, average age 47, into one of two exercise programs four days a week. One group engaged in low-intensity 60-minute walks. The other participated in an hour of more strenuous aerobic exercise. After nine months, both groups reported increased sexual desire and pleasure. The aerobics group registered greater gains, but the low-intensity exercisers also reported increased sexual desire and more orgasms.

*Reduces risk of heart disease.* Heart disease is the nation's leading cause of death. Low-intensity exercise helps prevent it by strengthening the heart, reducing blood pressure, lowering cholesterol and combating obesity and diabetes.

*Reduces risk of stroke.* Stroke is the nation's third leading cause of death. (Cancer is number two.) High blood pressure is a key risk factor, and regular low-intensity exercise helps reduce it.

*Helps preserve bone.* Regular, moderate, weight-bearing exercise (walking, gardening, dancing and so forth) helps maintain bone density and prevent bone-thinning osteoporosis—a major health problem for women over 50.

*Builds strength, flexibility and stamina.* As you exercise, your muscles become stronger, your joints become more supple, and you can remain active longer without tiring. In other words, the more you exercise, the more you can exercise, the less taxing it feels, and the more likely you are to enjoy it and stick with it.

*Improves reaction time.* Waneen Spirduso, Ed.D., professor of kinesiology and health education at the University of Texas in Austin, asked volunteers of all ages to push a button when they saw a light flash. Some were exercisers, others were not. In every age group, the exercisers had faster reaction times. "Exercisers' muscles work better," Dr. Spirduso explains. "So do their minds."

*Improves recall.* Do you ever have trouble remembering names? Kathleen Beckman Blomquist, Ph.D., a postdoctoral scholar at the Sanders-Brown Center on Aging at the University of Kentucky in Lexington, tested fitness and name-recall in 66 adults ages 18 to 48. Those in the best shape had the best memories. Then she encouraged all of the participants to increase their physical activity. After 12 weeks, those whose fitness improved showed enhanced ability to recall names.

*Improves resistance to colds.* Low- to moderate-intensity exercise boosts the immune system, according to David Nieman, D.H.Sc., professor of health promotions in the Department of Health, Leisure and Exercise Science at Appalachian State University in Boone, North Carolina. In a study at Loma Linda University in California, Dr. Nieman assigned 50 nonexercising women to two groups. One group continued their sedentary ways and the other took brisk walks for 45 minutes a day. After 15 weeks, the exercisers reported only half as many days with cold symptoms. (However, ultra-strenuous exercise impairs immune function. When Dr. Nieman compared colds in runners who logged 20 miles a week with those who ran an extremely strenuous 60 miles a week, he found that the ones who were putting in the greater mileage had twice as many upper respiratory infections.)

*Improves sleep and minimizes insomnia.* Exercise feels invigorating, but several hours later it helps the body wind down to sleep. Many sleep disorders experts recommend low- to moderate-intensity exercise to improve sleep and treat insomnia. Just don't exercise shortly before bed or you may wind up feeling more invigorated than sleepy.

*Helps manage arthritis.* Exercise moves the major joints through their full range of motion, which helps keep them pain-free. Exercise also releases endorphins, the body's pain-relieving chemicals.

Modest exercise also produces the following significant emotional benefits.

*Greater self-confidence.* Exercise provides feelings of accomplishment, which boost self-esteem.

*Less stress and anxiety.* People who exercise regularly say they feel better able to cope with stress and tension.

*Mood elevation.* In addition to relieving pain, endorphins released by exercise also have an antidepressant effect. Many mental health professionals encourage exercise as a natural complement to other treatments for depression.

## Just Say Yes

So what's stopping you? Given all the benefits, just about everyone *wants* to exercise, but too often, obstacles get in the way. Do any of these excuses sound familiar? If they do, perhaps some of these suggestions may prove helpful.

*"I'm too busy."* Of course you're busy. You lead a harried, stressful life. That's why you need to exercise—to build the stamina, strength, flexibility, confidence and self-esteem to cope with all the demands you face.

*"I hate exercise."* Don't do anything you dislike. Ask your-

self what kinds of physical activities you like and simply do them more often. You don't have to run, do sit-ups and use a stair-climbing machine. Bicycling, gardening, folk dancing, bowling, roller-skating and Ping-Pong can be great exercise. If you can't think of physical activities you enjoy, recall the ones you liked years ago. Chances are you'll still enjoy them.

*"I've never been active; I'm too old to start now."* You're never too old to start exercising. In one study, researchers at the University of Dundee in Scotland divided 49 residents of a nearby old-age home into two groups. One engaged in reminiscence sessions twice a week. The other spent the time doing low-intensity exercise. After seven months, the exercisers stood up faster, moved more easily, had greater grip strength and experienced less depression.

Maria Fiatarone, M.D., professor of medicine at Harvard Medical School, came to the same conclusion while working with frail elderly residents of the Hebrew Rehabilitation Center for the Aged in Boston. She recruited ten men and women, ages 85 to 96, into a weight-lifting program. After eight weeks, their strength, muscle mass and walking ability all showed significant improvement. "The physical deterioration we have traditionally associated with growing old has nothing to do with chronological age," Dr. Fiatarone says, "and everything to do with lack of exercise." No matter how long you've been out of shape, you can get back into shape. Just start now.

*"I don't have big blocks of time to exercise."* "You don't need them," Dr. Rippe says. "Sporadic exercise adds up. If you take just three 10-minute walks a day during breaks, you're exercising 30 minutes." What kinds of physical activities do you already engage in—shopping, housework, cooking, child care? Just walk a little more briskly while shopping. Stretch, bend and lift a little more during housework and cooking. And play more physically with your pet or your children.

*"I feel self-conscious; I hate looking ridiculous."* You won't look ridiculous. You'll look like a person who's taking positive steps toward better health. You'll look good. Soon, you'll look even better.

*"I never seem to improve."* Chances are you just don't notice. Keep track of your progress. Make a chart showing how many flights of stairs you can climb before you feel winded or how long it takes you to walk around the block—anything that's measurable. Plot your progress weekly, and pretty soon you'll be looking back at how far you've come.

*"I can't afford to join a gym or turn my home into one."* You don't have to. Housework is also good exercise. Just do it a little more vigorously. Or take a walk. Walking is great exercise outdoors or around the local mall, alone or with friends.

*"I never stick with it."* You're not alone. Half of those who start an exercise program quit within six months. To keep from being a quitter, it helps to be realistic. For every year you've been out of shape, it takes about a month to get back in shape. It takes about eight weeks to start feeling the physical and emotional benefits of exercise and longer to lose weight.

It also helps to start slowly and not overdo it. You should be able to carry on a conversation while exercising. If you become breathless, you're overdoing it. Find a buddy and exercise together. Support each other. Vary your activities so you don't get bored.

*"I read that before I start exercising, I should check with my physician. That's a hassle."* Most people don't have to visit a doctor before starting a modest exercise program. But if you're pregnant or over 50, or if you smoke, it's prudent to consult a physician first. Ditto if you have a personal or family history of heart disease, high blood pressure, diabetes, asthma, varicose veins or any other chronic medical condition.

*"Exercise hurts; whenever I exercise I feel awful the next day."* If any physical activity causes sharp pain, stop doing it. Pain is a message that something is wrong. If it persists, see a doctor. However, it's normal to feel some muscle soreness 12 to 48 hours after exercise, especially if you're not in great shape. Soreness feels like a dull ache. It's no cause for concern, though you might want to take aspirin, ibuprofen or acetaminophen to relieve it. Wait until your soreness has subsided, then continue exercising. Over time, as you get in shape, soreness stops—unless you increase the duration or intensity of your workout.

## Getting Physical in Daily Living

What if you'd really rather not exercise . . . at all? Then don't. You don't need to engage in that formal activity known as "exercise" to get the benefits. Just put a little more oomph behind the things you do anyway every day, find a few activities you enjoy and find ways to get your body moving a little more often.

**Take a walk.** Walking is wonderful exercise. As a weight-bearing exercise, it also helps prevent bone-thinning osteoporosis, which plagues older women.

**Take the stairs instead of the elevator.** If you're out of shape, start by walking down. When you feel ready, walk up partway and work up to climbing all the way. When climbing stairs no longer leaves you winded, climb a little faster.

**Park a few blocks farther away.** Walk the extra distance to work, the mall, the movies, church or friends' homes. As you gain stamina, park even farther away or walk more briskly.

**Take a walk before lunch.** In addition to getting exercise, you may find you eat less for lunch and suffer less from midafternoon blahs.

**Stash a pair of walking shoes at work.** Slip them on for walks at lunch and on breaks.

**Buy a backpack.** Instead of driving to all your errands, walk as much as possible and use your backpack to stash those little purchases.

**Cancel "food dates."** Instead of meeting friends for lunch, coffee or dessert, make dates to take walks, go dancing or go for bike rides. Or make a date to visit a health club. Most clubs allow free one-time visits to check out the facility. Try several.

**Walk your dog.** If you don't have one, consider getting one. Dogs are great exercise companions.

**Make breaks count.** During TV commercials or breaks at work, get up and stretch or walk around. Encourage your housemates and co-workers to join you.

**Get personal.** At home or at work, don't automatically use the phone. Walk to neighbors' homes or co-workers' desks.

**Make the most of phone time.** Don't sit while talking on the phone—pace. Invest in a longer handset cord so you can walk farther, or get a cordless phone. If you must stand in one spot, march in place, raising your knees high. Or rise to your tip-toes. Do this five times, then do five knee bends. When you feel ready, do ten.

Or keep a small three-pound weight or a canned food item nearby and do some weight-training curls and presses. (For curls: With your arm straight, hold the weight down by your hip. Then bend your elbow and bring the weight up to your shoulder. For presses: Start with your arm in the curled position, then straighten it over your head.) Do five of each. When you feel ready, do ten.

**Make the most of unpacking groceries.** Curl and press those cans a few times. When you feel ready, try it with six-packs.

**Clean out your attic, basement or garage.** They probably need it, and all that lifting and carrying is good exercise.

**Mow the lawn.** Pushing a power mower provides surprisingly good exercise. Or for a somewhat more strenuous workout, retire your power mower and invest in a push model. (You may even find that the lack of fumes and a quieter machine make this onerous task more pleasant.)

**Tend a garden.** Digging, weeding, raking, cutting and hauling build strength, flexibility and stamina.

**Sweep some snow.** Unless you're in reasonably good shape, stick to small accumulations of dry, powdery snow, the kind that can be swept with a broom. Snow shoveling can be very strenuous, and every winter people experience heart attacks from overexertion. If you're out of shape or have heart disease or significant risk factors for heart disease (family history, smoking, diabetes, obesity, elevated blood pressure or cholesterol), don't shovel heavy, wet snow or major accumulations.

**Play with children.** Kids love swings and merry-go-rounds, and pushing them provides great arm exercise. Join in older children's games. Play tag. Go roller skating. Jump rope. Climb a play structure. Take a swim or a bike ride or a rowboat outing on a lake. You'll have so much fun, you won't notice you're exercising.

## CHAPTER 11

# THE HEALING FOODS

## Eating for Better Health

**H**ippocrates, the father of Western medicine, once said, "Let your food be your medicine." These words are as wise today as they were more than 2,000 years ago—if you eat healthfully.

Nutritionists say that as long as your overall diet is low in fat, high in fiber and based on whole grains, legumes and fresh fruits and vegetables, individual foods don't matter. They counsel variety, and they're right. Broccoli is terrifically nutritious, but an all-broccoli diet is not as healthful as one based on a variety of fruits, vegetables, whole grains and legumes.

## The Winning Foods

However, given a diet based on a healthy variety of nutritious foods, some foods still stand out as particularly valuable for the prevention and treatment of specific conditions. Here's an overview of some of the best healing foods and the conditions they help.

179

## Apples: The One-a-Day Treat

Apples won't keep all doctors away, but eating one a day should reduce your need to consult gastroenterologists, cardiologists and oncologists. The core, as it were, of apples' healing value is the soluble fiber—pectin—in its pulp.

More than 2,000 years ago, India's Ayurvedic physicians prescribed apples to relieve diarrhea. In tenth-century Britain, people said, "To eat an apple before going to bed/Will make the doctor beg his bread." This evolved into our familiar "apple a day" couplet.

*Cancer.* Pectin fiber binds carcinogens in the colon, speeding their elimination from the body, according to medical researchers. In addition, substances known as polyphenols help prevent the cell damage that causes cancer.

*Constipation.* Physicians recommend diets high in insoluble fiber, such as bran, to add bulk to the stool. Bulk stimulates bowel contractions and relieves constipation. As a soluble fiber, pectin doesn't add much bulk to the stool, but it acts as a laxative stool softener. Hard stools can be painful to pass. Apples help keep things moving comfortably.

*Diabetes.* Physicians also recommend high-fiber diets to control diabetes. Medical researchers say that apple pectin helps control blood sugar (glucose) levels in people with diabetes.

*Diarrhea.* Pectin helps relieve diarrhea because intestinal bacteria transform it into a soothing, protective coating for the irritated intestinal lining. Applesauce is a physician-recommended diarrhea treatment, part of the BRATT diet: bananas, rice, applesauce, tea and toast. And pectin is the "pectate" in the over-the-counter diarrhea preparation Kaopectate.

Some diarrhea is caused by bacterial infection. Pectin is not an antibiotic, but it does help minimize the intestinal damage triggered by several microorganisms—*Salmonella, Escherichia coli* and *Staphylococcus aureus*—that may cause diarrhea.

*Heart disease.* Pectin helps reduce blood cholesterol, a key risk factor for heart disease. In the presence of pectin, the cholesterol in foods remains in the intestinal tract until it is eliminated. Eat an apple when you have meat or dairy products and enjoy some protection from their cholesterol.

Dutch researchers, looking at the connection between heart disease and diet, found that men who consume a lot of polyphenols have an unusually low risk of heart attack. Later diet surveys showed that people in Holland obtained 10 percent of their polyphenols from apples.

## Beans: Good for the Heart

You're probably familiar with the naughty children's rhyme: "Beans, beans, good for the heart/The more you eat, the more you . . . " The first part is true, and as for the second, well, it can now be cut by up to 70 percent.

Beans deserve their reputation for causing flatulence, according to Miami dietitian Sheah Rarback, R.D. Flatulence results when carbohydrates (starches and sugars) arrive in the colon incompletely digested and are fermented by the bacteria there. The fermentation process releases gas. Any incompletely digested carbohydrate—from bagels to pasta—can ferment in the colon and cause gas. "But," Rarback explains, "beans are the richest sources of two particular carbohydrates, raffinose and stachyose, that the body cannot digest because humans lack the enzyme to do it."

If gas is a problem for you, don't swear off beans. Instead, boil, rinse and soak them. Boil dried beans in a covered pot for three minutes, then let them stand for two hours. Next pour off the water, add enough new water to cover the beans, then replace this water after two hours and let the beans soak overnight. Rinse them once more before cooking. Tests by U.S. Department of Agriculture (USDA) researchers show that this method cuts bean-induced flatulence in half.

Or you can add Beano to bean dishes. It contains the missing enzyme that allows the body to digest raffinose and stachyose. Beano is available at health food stores and some pharmacies and supermarkets.

Why would you want to go to all this trouble just to eat beans? Because they're good for you.

*Diabetes.* Bean cuisine gives everyone protection from heart disease, but endocrinologist James Anderson, M.D., professor of medicine at the University of Kentucky College of Medicine in Lexington, says that people with diabetes enjoy special bean benefits. Diabetes greatly increases the risk of heart disease, which is an excellent reason for anyone with diabetes to boost their bean consumption. In addition, the soluble fiber in beans also helps keep blood sugar under control.

*Heart disease.* Beans are a staple of the Mediterranean diet that helps prevent heart disease. Studies by Dr. Anderson show that eating a half-cup of cooked beans a day for about a month reduces cholesterol an average of 10 percent. The type of bean doesn't matter—pinto, black, kidney, lentils, garbanzos, soybeans, red, navy, white, baked; they all cut cholesterol. Why? Because they are high in soluble fiber, which helps eliminate cholesterol from the body. Every 1 percent decrease in cholesterol results in a 2 percent decrease in heart attack risk, so one daily serving of beans reduces heart attack risk about 20 percent, especially if it takes the place of meat, cheese or other high-fat foods.

*Lung and pancreatic cancer.* All beans are high in folic acid, one of the B vitamins. Research at the University of Alabama suggests a connection between folic acid deficiency and lung cancer. The researchers found high levels of the B vitamin in the lung tissue of healthy men, but much lower levels in cancerous lungs. Folic acid can also be found in abundance in green vegetables such as spinach and broccoli.

Paul Mills, Ph.D., assistant professor of preventive medicine at Loma Linda University in California, found that compared with people who ate beans rarely or not at all, those who ate them at least once a week enjoyed significant protection from pancreatic cancer.

*Neural tube birth defects.* Beans' high folic acid content also helps prevent potentially fatal birth defects of the spine. Over the last decade, so many studies have shown that folic acid prevents neural tube defects that doctors now recommend folic acid supplements for pregnant women. Beans don't replace recommended folic acid supplementation, but every time a pregnant woman bites into a bean burrito, she's taking a step to prevent these tragic birth defects.

*Osteoporosis.* Studies done at the University of Texas at Austin show that manganese—an essential trace mineral—is important for bone strength. Animals deficient in manganese develop severe osteoporosis, and these studies show that women with osteoporosis tend to have low manganese levels. Beans are a rich sources of manganese. So are pineapples, oatmeal, nuts and tea.

## Carrots: Not Just for Bunnies

What's up for health, Doc? Big orange carrots, that's what. Carrots are rich in the antioxidant beta-carotene. They're especially valuable for parents whose young children turn up their noses at vegetables, and the "wascawwy wabbit" who has tormented Elmer Fudd in innumerable cartoons has helped keep carrots popular with kids. Carrots are one of the few vegetables that travel well raw for kids' (and grown-ups') lunches and snacks.

Ever wonder why Bugs Bunny has lived so long? It just might be the carrots.

*Cancer.* Beta-carotene consumption has been linked to reduced risk of several cancers, notably lung cancer. Researchers at Johns Hopkins University in Baltimore analyzed beta-carotene levels in a large group of volunteers who donated blood in 1974. By 1983, 99 had developed lung cancer. Who were they? The ones with the lowest levels of beta-carotene.

British researchers have corroborated these findings. They discovered that increasing beta-carotene consumption from 1.7 to 2.7 milligrams a day reduced lung cancer risk more than 40 percent. The average carrot contains about 3 milligrams of beta-carotene. Not all of that is absorbed into the bloodstream, but a good deal is.

*Heart attack.* At the Institute for Pharmacological Research in Milan, Italy, scientists analyzed the diets and health of 936 elderly women. Compared with those who ate the fewest carrots and least fruit, those who consumed the most had an astonishing 60 percent fewer heart attacks.

*Macular degeneration.* This common eye disease of the elderly impairs the macula, the part of the retina that produces the sharpest vision in the center of the visual field. But people who eat the most fruits and vegetables enjoy some protection, apparently because certain nutrients preserve the macula. At the University of Illinois in Chicago, researchers analyzed the diets of 3,000 elderly people. Compared with those who consumed the least beta-carotene, those who ate the most had a 40 percent lower risk of macular degeneration.

*Stroke.* Compared with eating carrots once a month or less, a carrot a day reduces stroke risk by a whopping 68 percent. That was what Harvard researcher JoAnn Manson, M.D., associate professor of medicine at the university and director of women's health at Brigham and Women's Hospital in Boston, discovered in an eight-year analysis of the Nurses' Health Study, an ongoing investigation of the diet and lifestyle of more than 87,000 female nurses. Dr. Manson is not certain what accounts for carrots' ability to protect the arteries in the brain, but she speculates that beta-carotene plays a role.

In Belgium, University of Brussels researchers have strengthened the case for a "carrot effect" on the brain. Shortly after 80 people had strokes, the scientists analyzed their blood. Those with the highest levels of beta-carotene had the best survival rate.

## Cranberry Juice: Zaps Bad Bacteria

Many women drink cranberry juice in the belief that it helps prevent urinary tract infections (UTIs). Dorothy Barbo, M.D., director of the Center for Women's Health at the University of New Mexico in Albuquerque, recommends it for prevention and as a complement to antibiotic treatment. "In my experience," she says, "cranberry juice seems to inhibit bacterial growth."

*Incontinence.* Because cranberry juice helps deodorize urine, a report published in the *Journal of Psychiatric Nursing* suggested incorporating it into the diet of anyone troubled by urinary incontinence to reduce the embarrassing odor of this problem.

*UTIs.* During the 1840s, German researchers discovered that the urine of people who ate cranberries contained a bacteria-fighting chemical (hippuric acid). Sixty years later, American researchers speculated that urine acidified by a steady diet of cranberries might prevent UTIs. Women adopted cranberry juice enthusiastically, and several studies endorsed it. But by the late 1960s, naysayers claimed the tart berries did not significantly acidify urine and therefore could not prevent UTIs.

However, the latest research endorses the treatment. One study showed 73 percent of people with recurrent UTIs reported "significant improvement" after three weeks of drinking a pint of commercial cranberry juice cocktail daily. The researchers concluded that urinary acidity had nothing to do with the berries' effectiveness. Instead, they acted by preventing UTI germs from adhering to the lining of the urinary tract, thus reducing the likelihood of infection.

## Coffee: The Breathe-Easy Beverage

Caffeine is the world's most widely used stimulant. Most Americans get their caffeine from coffee. More than 80 percent of American adults consume caffeine regularly, with an average daily dose of about 280 milligrams—the equivalent of two five-ounce cups of brewed coffee, two to three cups of instant coffee, six cups of tea or six 12-ounce cola drinks.

"On balance, there is no persuasive evidence that moderate amounts of caffeine—a cup or two of coffee a day—are harmful," says Nancy Clark, R.D., director of nutrition services at SportsMedicine Brookline in Massachusetts and a fellow of the American College of Sports Medicine. And there's plenty of evidence that coffee has some positive uses, she adds.

*Asthma.* Coffee's ability to open up bronchial passages—making it a bronchodilator—helps prevent and treat asthma attacks. A standard bronchodilating medication is theophylline, a close chemical relative of caffeine. Joe Graedon, co-author of *The People's Pharmacy* syndicated newspaper column, recalls, "We once got a thank-you note from a woman who forgot to pack her asthma medication on her Hawaiian honeymoon. She started wheezing and got panicky, but then she recalled a column that recommended caffeine as an emergency substitute. She had a few cups of coffee and was fine."

*Common cold congestion.* Because caffeine opens up the bronchial passages, it also can help relieve the chest congestion of colds. "If you'd rather not take Sudafed or some other pharmaceutical decongestant, have a cup or two of coffee. It produces a similar effect," says James Duke, Ph.D., a botanist at the USDA Research Station in Beltsville, Maryland.

*Fatigue.* To coffee lovers, the deep, rich brew tastes divine. But the reason people line up at the coffee machine every morning is that caffeine is a powerful central nervous system stimulant that gets the blood pumping.

Caffeine can even give you a performance edge. British researchers had 18 male runners race 1500 meters on nine different days after giving them one to two cups of either regular or decaffeinated coffee. With the help of caffeine, the runners ran 4.2 seconds faster. In a similar study, American researchers had distance runners run and cycle until they were winded. After a rest period during which they drank about five cups of coffee, the athletes repeated the workout. With the help of caffeine, their stamina improved 44 percent in the running test and 51 percent in the cycling test. International Olympic Committee standards are that an athlete's urine may contain no more than 12 micrograms of caffeine per milligram before events. To reach that level, an athlete would have to drink at least five cups of coffee shortly before an event.

*Pain.* Several studies have shown that compared with plain aspirin, a combination of aspirin and a small amount of caffeine (on the order of 60 milligrams) relieves pain more quickly and effectively. Scientists aren't sure why caffeine boosts the pain-relieving action of aspirin, but they speculate the lift caffeine provides may play a psychological role in pain relief. Next time you have a headache or any injury that makes you reach for aspirin, wash it down with a cup of coffee. Some pain medications—such as Midol or Vanquish—already have caffeine added, so make sure you read the label.

## Fish: Source of Healthy Fats

The chief villain in the American diet is fat. A high-fat diet has been persuasively linked to an increased risk of heart disease, cancer, diabetes and other serious conditions. Fat may be Diet Enemy Number One, but it's both unrealistic—and unhealthy—to eat none at all. According to Dean Ornish, M.D., director of the Preventive Medicine Research Institute in Sausalito, California, whose ultra-low-fat diet is part of the only regimen ever to successfully reverse heart disease, the body needs less than 10 percent of calories to come from fat. Among the most healthful fats are the omega-3 fatty acids found in coldwater, saltwater fish: salmon, tuna, mackerel, sardines, anchovies and herring. Moderate amounts of omega-3's can also be found in swordfish, shark, striped bass and rainbow trout.

A great deal of research shows that eating these fish once or twice a week confers so many health advantages that Jean Carper, author of *Food: Your Miracle Medicine*, calls many modern afflictions, particularly heart attack, "fish deficiency diseases."

*Heart disease.* Omega-3 fatty acids help prevent the formation of artery-clogging plaques. Danish researchers analyzed the arteries and fat tissue from 40 consecutive autopsies at Frederiksberg Hospital in Denmark, using the omega-3 content of the fat tissue as a reasonable gauge of lifetime fish consumption. The people with the most clogged arteries had the lowest levels of omega-3's in their fat.

Omega-3 fatty acids also help reduce blood pressure and prevent the blood clots that trigger heart attack.

*Rheumatoid arthritis.* This is not the most common form of joint disease, but it's the most crippling. At Albany Medical College in New York, Joel Kremer, M.D., associate professor of medicine, recruited 33 people with rheumatoid arthritis. He gave them fish oil capsules, and after 14 weeks, they reported 30 percent less joint pain, and less fatigue as well.

## Garlic: Powerful Protection

Garlic is one of the world's oldest medicines, and it's still among the best. "If the term *wonder drug* can be applied to any food," Dr. Duke says, "garlic deserves that distinction."

Garlic appeared prominently in the world's oldest surviving medical text, the *Ebers Papyrus*, written somewhere in the neighborhood of 1500 B.C. It was an ingredient in 22 remedies for headache, insect and scorpion bites, menstrual discomforts, intestinal worms, tumors and heart problems. Modern science has validated several of these ancient prescriptions.

*Cancer.* Tantalizing evidence suggests garlic plays a role in preventing and treating cancer. In one study researchers separated mouse tumor cells into two groups. One was left alone. The other was treated with allicin, a major component of garlic. Then both batches of tumor cells were injected into mice. Those who received the untreated cells quickly died, but in the garlic-treated group, there were no deaths. Since then, other animal studies have shown similar results.

Of course, animal findings don't necessarily apply to humans, but another study suggests that garlic helps prevent human stomach cancer. Researchers analyzed the diets of 1,800 Chinese, including 685 with stomach cancer. Those with the cancer ate considerably less garlic. The researchers concluded that a diet high in garlic "can significantly reduce risk of stomach cancer."

*Heart disease.* Garlic contains chemicals (allicin and ajoene) that reduce blood pressure and cholesterol, and they help prevent the blood clots that trigger heart attack.

Several studies dating back to the 1920s confirm garlic's ability to reduce blood pressure in animals and humans.

More than a dozen medical journal reports document garlic's ability to reduce cholesterol. In one experiment, British researchers had volunteers eat a meal containing about four ounces of butter, which raises cholesterol. Half the group also ate about nine cloves of garlic. After three hours, the average cholesterol level in the nongarlic group increased 7 percent. But in the garlic group, it decreased 7 percent. The researchers concluded that garlic has "a very significant protective action" against high cholesterol.

Dr. Duke calls garlic "as potent as aspirin," which is now widely used to prevent the blood clots that trigger heart attack. To prevent heart disease, he recommends eating at least one clove of fresh garlic a day.

*Infections.* During World War I, doctors treated infected battle wounds with garlic juice. They also prescribed garlic to prevent and treat dysentery. Shortly after the war, Swiss researchers isolated alliin (*ALL-ey-in*) from the bulb. By itself, alliin has no medicinal value, but when garlic is chewed, chopped, bruised or crushed, its alliin comes in contact with an enzyme (allinase) and becomes allicin, a powerful antibiotic.

Garlic kills the bacteria that cause tuberculosis, food poisoning and bladder infections and the fungi that cause athlete's foot and vaginal yeast infections.

For minor skin infections, garlic juice may prove sufficient, but unless you're an experienced herbalist, don't rely exclusively on garlic to treat infectious diseases. Instead, take it in addition to standard medication. You must chew the fresh cloves to transform alliin into allicin. One medium-size garlic clove packs the antibacterial punch of about 100,000 standard units of penicillin. Depending on the type of infection, oral penicillin doses typically range from 600,000 to 1.2 million units, or the equivalent of about 6 to 12 cloves.

*Lead poisoning.* European studies show that garlic helps eliminate lead and other toxic heavy metals from the body. Lead interferes with thinking and causes other serious health problems, and children are particularly susceptible to lead effects. Add garlic liberally to spaghetti and pizza sauces and other foods children enjoy.

The only downside to garlic is garlic breath. If this is a problem for you, check your health food store for deodorized garlic.

## Ginger: The Spice with a Punch

Gingerroot is best known in the West as a culinary spice, but throughout Asia it's been revered as a healer since the dawn of history. Science has confirmed many of ginger's traditional medical uses—and discovered several benefits the ancients never dreamed of.

*Cancer.* Certain chemicals in ginger help prevent the cell damage that eventually leads to cancer. Ginger may even help treat cancer: One laboratory animal study showed it shrinks liver tumors.

Heart disease and stroke. Medical research shows that ginger reduces cholesterol. It also lowers blood pressure and helps prevent the blood clots that trigger heart attacks and some strokes. Finally, it contains nutrients that help prevent the arterial damage that leads to heart disease.

*Indigestion.* Ancient Asian sailors chewed ginger to prevent seasickness. The early Greeks adopted it as a digestive aid. After big meals, they ate ginger wrapped in bread. Over time, they added the herb to sweetened bread and invented the world's first cookie, gingerbread.

Three centuries ago, British visitors to China returned singing the praises of ginger tea for stomach distress. Soon after, the English developed stomach-soothing ginger beer, the forerunner of today's ginger ale, which is still a popular home remedy for nausea and vomiting. Ginger relieves indigestion and abdominal cramping by soothing the gastrointestinal tract.

*Morning sickness.* The anti-nausea action of ginger helps prevent and treat the morning sickness of pregnancy.

*Motion sickness.* Ginger relieves motion sickness better than Dramamine, a standard drug treatment, according to a study by Daniel Mowrey, Ph.D., director of the American Phytotherapy (plant medicine) Research Laboratory in Salt Lake City. Dr. Mowrey recruited 36 volunteers with a history of motion sickness and gave them either 100 milligrams of Dramamine or 940 milligrams of ginger powder. Then they were seated in a computerized rocking chair programmed to trigger seasickness. The people were able to stop the chair when they began to feel nauseated. Those taking the ginger lasted 57 percent longer than those on Dramamine.

## Nuts: They're Good for You

Nuts derive 70 to 90 percent of their calories from fat. As a result, the crunchy, delicious morsels have been verboten for people on low-fat diets, especially those interested in preventing obesity, diabetes, heart disease and the fat-related cancers, particularly breast, colon and prostate cancer. But this view began to change in 1992, when a major study of diet and health showed that noshing nuts reduced heart disease risk dramatically.

*Heart disease.* The 18-year study, based on annual surveys of the diet and lifestyles of 31,200 Seventh-Day Adventists, was conducted by Gary Fraser, Ph.D., professor of medicine at the Center for Health Research at Loma Linda University in California. Seventh-Day Adventists are an unusually healthy group: They are well-educated vegetarians who typically abstain from cigarettes and alcohol. As a result, they provide a unique window into the subtle factors that make the healthy even healthier. Surprisingly, compared with Seventh-Day Adventists who ate nuts rarely, those who munched them once a week had 25 percent fewer heart attacks, and five-times-a-week nut noshers cut their risk almost in half. Peanuts, almonds and walnuts were the most heart-protective nuts.

Dr. Fraser's study did not prove that eating nuts caused the reduction in heart attack, only that the two were associated. To investigate the causality issue, the Loma Linda researchers divided 18 healthy men, average age 30, into two groups. Both ate the same diet, with 30 percent of calories from fat, but in one group, two-thirds of that fat came from walnuts (about 20 whole walnuts a day). After a month, cholesterol levels in the walnut group dropped 12 percent, demonstrating that nut munching caused the decrease in heart attack that was observed in the earlier study.

How could high-fat nuts be good for the heart? Simple: Nuts are like fatty fish. They are among the richest plant sources of heart-sparing omega-3 fatty acids. The rest of their fat is unsaturated—not the heart-hurting saturated variety found in meats, dairy products and coconut oil. Finally, nuts also contain a good deal of selenium and vitamin E, both nutrients that help prevent heart disease.

But bear in mind: The beneficial "nut effect" occurred in people who were already eating a low-fat diet. Most Americans add nuts to extremely high-fat foods: cookies, brownies and ice cream. Nuts do not cancel out the damage done by these foods. In addition, most of the nuts consumed in the United States are heavily salted, and all that salt increases risk of high blood pressure and heart disease.

That said, if you eat a low-fat diet, there's nothing wrong with adding a few nuts.

*Osteoporosis.* Nuts are also rich sources of the trace minerals manganese and boron. As mentioned in the beans section of this chapter, manganese is valuable in preserving bone health. As for boron, Forrest Neilsen, Ph.D., director of the USDA Human Nutrition Research Center in Grand Forks, North Dakota, has shown that women whose diets contain low levels of this nutrient lose unusually large amounts of calcium from their bones. Other good sources of boron include beans and fruits, especially apples.

## Oats: Cholesterol Cutter

In 1963, a little-noticed study described what happened when Dutch researchers substituted oatmeal for bread in the diets of 21 male volunteers. Within three weeks, their cholesterol had fallen 11 percent, thanks to a type of soluble fiber in oats, beta-glucans, that impairs intestinal absorption of cholesterol so more is eliminated. But it took another 20 years before oatmeal and oat bran became rallying points for cholesterol reduction. Better late than never.

*Heart disease.* In 1992 a research team led by Cynthia Ripsin, of the Department of Family Practice at the University of

Minnesota Medical Center in Minneapolis, analyzed 20 studies that had investigated the "oat effect" on blood cholesterol. Eating the equivalent of one large bowl of oat-bran cereal or three packets of instant oatmeal lowered cholesterol an average of 7 percent in those with total cholesterol of 229 or higher and about 3 percent in those with lower cholesterol. Every 1 percent decrease in cholesterol correlates with about a 2 percent reduction in heart attack risk, so if your cholesterol is high, oatmeal for breakfast can cut your heart attack risk by about 14 percent.

However, the studies that Ripsin analyzed used oat products whose beta-glucans content varied widely. Oat bran is a better cholesterol cutter than oatmeal. Unfortunately, some food manufacturers add a tiny amount of oat bran but promote it in big type on their packaging. Look for foods that list oat bran as the first or second ingredient on the label. If you prefer oatmeal, check labels for fiber content and select the one with the most.

Finally, oat foods help reduce cholesterol only in the context of a low-fat diet. A sprinkle of oat bran on a piece of cheesecake won't keep you out of coronary intensive care. And watch out for oat-bran muffins. They are often so high in fat that they do more harm than good.

## Olive Oil: Heart Protection

"There is strong epidemiological evidence that olive oil offers significant cardioprotective benefits," says Walter Willett, M.D., Dr.Ph., chair of the Department of Nutrition at Harvard University. In plain English, olive oil is good for the heart.

*Heart disease.* Like all vegetable oils, olive oil is 100 percent fat, and fat is a prime contributor to heart disease and cancer. So how could olive oil be good for the heart? The reason appears to be that it's neither saturated, like the fats in meats, butter and dairy products, nor polyunsaturated, like the fat in many other oils. It's monounsaturated. Greeks and Italians consume almost as much total fat as Americans do—most of it in the form of olive oil—but have heart disease rates considerably lower than ours.

Dr. Willett believes that Americans should eat like people in those Mediterranean countries. He and colleagues at the World Health Organization argue that we should junk the USDA's new Food Pyramid, which recommends meat and dairy products two or three times a day, and replace it with a Mediterranean Pyramid, which discourages meat and dairy foods and promotes a semi-vegetarian diet with olive oil as the major source of fat. Of course, like any fat, olive oil should be used sparingly in the context of a low-fat diet. But recent research suggests that this tasty oil is a real healer.

Olive oil, particularly extra-virgin, cold-pressed olive oil, is high in nutrients that help prevent the development of plaques that clog arteries and increase heart attack risk.

Olive oil also raises levels of high-density lipoproteins (HDL, the "good" cholesterol) and lowers levels of low-density lipoproteins (LDL, the "bad" cholesterol).

In addition, olive oil helps prevent the blood clots that trigger heart attack. Blood clots form when special blood cells, called platelets, clump together and stick to coronary artery walls. In one study, British researchers asked volunteers to take three-quarters of a tablespoon of olive oil twice a day in addition to their regular diet. By the end of eight weeks, blood tests showed that their platelets were significantly less likely to clump.

*Stroke.* Many studies show that olive oil also lowers blood pressure, a key risk factor not only for heart attack but also for stroke. A study by researchers at the University of Kentucky in Lexington showed that two-thirds of a tablespoon of olive oil a day lowered systolic blood pressure (the first number in the pair used to express blood pressure) by about nine points and diastolic blood pressure (the second number) by six points.

## Soy Foods: Cancer Fighters and More

Can tofu help prevent breast cancer? Increasingly, it looks that way. Soy foods—soybeans, tofu, miso, tempeh, soy milk, soy protein and textured vegetable protein (TVP), but not soy sauce—offer all the healing benefits of the other beans. In addi-

tion, they contain unusually large concentrations of chemicals—
isoflavones and phytosterols—with cancer-preventive value.
These chemicals may help account for the low rate of breast cancer among Asian women, who eat soy foods as staples.

*Breast cancer.* Soy isoflavones and phytosterols first came
to American scientific attention at a National Cancer Institute
conference in 1990. Isoflavones, also known as phytoestrogens
(literally, plant estrogens) show the most powerful anti-cancer
effects. They are structurally similar to the female sex hormone,
and they bind to the same receptor sites on breast cells. But unlike hormonal estrogen, isoflavones and phytosterols do not
spur the growth of breast tumors. When the soy chemicals bind
to estrogen receptors, they prevent hormonal estrogen from
doing so, which in turn prevents tumor growth. (Tamoxifen, a
drug widely used to prevent breast cancer recurrences, works in
a similar fashion.)

Soy foods' marked influence on estrogen metabolism was
demonstrated by Kenneth Setchell, Ph.D., professor of pediatrics
at Children's Hospital Medical Center in Cincinnati. Dr. Setchell
had six women in their twenties with regular menstrual cycles
add two ounces of TVP to their usual diets. Within a month,
their menstrual cycles were two to five days longer. Longer menstrual cycles mean less lifetime exposure to estrogen and, many
scientists believe, less risk of breast cancer. Dr. Setchell then substituted the same amount of miso, a fermented Asian soy food,
for the TVP and found an even greater effect.

In addition, one isoflavone, genistein, is unique to soy foods.
Genistein has been the subject of more than 200 scientific studies since the 1960s. It appears to regulate the enzymes that turn
normal cells into cancer cells. Some studies have even shown
that genistein can turn cancer cells back into normal cells. Genistein also helps block the formation of new blood vessels to developing tumors, in effect strangling them.

*High cholesterol.* As beans replace meat in the diet, choles-
terol levels decline. But at the First International Symposium on
Soy and Chronic Diseases in Phoenix in 1994, Cesare Sirtori,
M.D., Ph.D., professor of clinical pharmacology at the Univer-

sity of Milan, presented research showing that, compared with other beans, soy foods are more effective cholesterol cutters. He recruited volunteers whose average cholesterol levels were very high (353 mg/dl) and who were already on low-fat diets. Some continued eating as they had been, while the others' diets were modified to include generous amounts of soy. After four weeks, the ones whose diets were unchanged showed no change in cholesterol levels, but among the soy eaters, average cholesterol levels plummeted 27 percent, to 257 mg/dl.

*Hot flashes.* In Japanese, there is no word for "hot flashes," the uncomfortable feeling of heat that plagues many women during menopause. Herman Adlercreutz, M.D., Ph.D., professor of chemistry at the University of Helsinki in Finland, thinks he knows why—soy foods. Hot flashes develop as production of hormonal estrogen declines. Dr. Aldercreutz suggests that the estrogen-like chemicals in soy replace declining hormonal estrogen and prevent hot flashes.

Japanese who eat a traditional Japanese diet consume about 24 pounds of soy a year. Americans consume about 3 pounds annually, mostly because soy protein is added to many processed foods. "Eat as much soy as you can," advises Susan Potter, Ph.D., assistant professor of food and nutrition at the University of Illinois at Urbana-Champaign, "as long as your soy foods are low in fat."

*Prostate and colon cancer.* Tofu and its soy cousins may also help prevent prostate and colon cancer. A 1989 study of 8,000 Japanese-American men in Hawaii showed that those who ate the most tofu had the lowest rate of prostate cancer. And Harvard researcher Charles Poole, Ph.D., discovered that as soy food consumption rises, colon cancer risk falls. Scientists theorize that in addition to soy's direct anti-cancer effects, people tend to use it to replace meat in the diet. Meat's high fat content has been linked to both prostate and colon cancer.

## Tea: A Healthier Choice

Tea is the world's second most popular beverage (after water), but most Americans consider it a poor second to coffee as a caffeine-laced pick-me-up or after-meal beverage. Recently, however, tea has gained new popularity, in part because of its medicinal value.

A cup of tea contains only about half as much caffeine as a cup of brewed coffee, and many people prefer its taste and consider its buzz less jarring.

*Cancer.* Studies suggest that chemicals known as polyphenols in tea help prevent cancer. Researchers in Shanghai compared the diets of 900 people with esophageal cancer with those of 1,500 who didn't have the cancer. The people with cancer drank significantly less green tea. A Japanese follow-up study showed the same result—the more green tea, the less cancer. Subsequently, scientists at Rutgers University in New Brunswick, New Jersey, added green tea to the drinking water of experimental mice and then exposed them to chemicals known to cause a variety of tumors in rodents. The mice who drank the green-tea-laced water developed considerably fewer tumors than the mice who drank plain water.

These studies prompted headlines proclaiming "Green Tea Prevents Cancer." Unfortunately, few Americans drink green tea outside of Asian restaurants; most Americans drink black tea. But the latest study shows that black tea has a similar effect. Rutgers biologist Zhi Wang, Ph.D., isolated the specific cancer-fighting antioxidant chemical in green tea; it is also present in black teas.

*Colds, congestion and asthma.* As with coffee, the caffeine in tea eases breathing by opening the bronchial passages. Tea also contains another stimulant, theophylline. Physicians often prescribe pharmaceutical theophylline preparations to treat asthma.

*Diarrhea.* Tea contains astringent tannins. Ancient Chinese physicians valued tea's mild astringency for treatment of diarrhea. Today's doctors agree, since mild astringents are widely used to treat diarrhea. Leading home medical guides suggest treating diarrhea with the BRATT diet: bananas, rice, applesauce, toast and tea.

*Heart attack.* In 1993, Dutch researchers discovered that men whose diets are rich in polyphenols have an unusually low risk of heart attack. Subsequent diet surveys showed that the heart-healthy Hollanders obtained some of their polyphenols from apples and onions but got a whopping 61 percent from black tea.

*Osteoporosis.* Tea is a good source of manganese, an essential trace mineral that helps preserve bone.

*Tooth decay.* Tea is a good source of fluoride, which prevents tooth decay. Both green and black teas contain more fluoride than fluoridated water, according to a report published in the *University of California, Berkeley, Wellness Letter.* The tannins in tea also help fight the bacteria that cause tooth decay.

## Yogurt: Live-Action Therapy

Yogurt is much more than a fast, creamy snack. If it's made with live-culture bacteria, it can prevent yeast infections and boost health in other ways.

*Lactose intolerance.* This condition is an inability to digest the milk sugar found in all dairy products. Symptoms include stomach upset, diarrhea, gas and abdominal cramps. Most people with lactose intolerance can digest yogurt without difficulty.

*Yeast vaginitis.* A daily cup of live-culture yogurt substantially reduces the risk of recurrent vaginal yeast infections. In a study, Eileen Hilton, M.D., an infectious disease specialist at New York's Long Island Jewish Medical Center, recruited 11 women who'd had at least five yeast infections during the previous 12 months. For one year, they ate one cup a day of yogurt containing live *Lactobacillus acidophilus* culture. During the study's final six months, the women averaged less than one yeast infection.

But before you rush out to the supermarket, take note: Most national brands of yogurt do not contain live L. acidophilus culture, and some of those with the bacteria do not contain enough to have the yeast-preventive effect. You're more likely to find live-culture yogurt among the specialty brands at health food stores. Or, Dr. Hilton says, make your own, using acidophilus milk.

## CHAPTER 12
# HEALING HUMOR

*Those Who Laugh, Last*

*"Life is too serious to be taken too seriously."*
—Joel Goodman, Ed.D.

In 1976, Joel Goodman, Ed.D., learned that his father had been hospitalized in Texas with a coronary aneurysm, a form of heart disease that seriously threatened his life. Dr. Goodman, a corporate consultant in Saratoga Springs, New York, dropped everything and flew to Houston to be with his mother during his father's surgery, an operation the doctors said he might not survive.

Every morning, Dr. Goodman and his mother took a shuttle van from their hotel to the hospital. "The driver was named Alvin," Dr. Goodman recalls. "He was a comedian and a magician. My mother and I were rigid with fear, but on the five-minute drive to the hospital, Alvin told jokes and did magic tricks—and worked wonders for us. He made us laugh, and for a few moments, we could let go of our tension."

*"Once you find the humor in a situation, you can survive it."*
—Bill Cosby

In 1978, Allen Klein's wife, Ellen, lay dying of cancer in a San Francisco hospital. Somehow a copy of *Playgirl* magazine found its way to her bedside. On a whim, she pulled out the male nude centerfold and asked her husband to tape it to the wall. "Isn't it a bit risqué for a hospital?" asked Klein, a businessman who was 40 at the time.

"Nonsense," his wife replied. "Just take a leaf from that plant over there and cover up the genitals."

Klein did as his wife requested. The leaf worked for the first day and the second, but by the third it had begun to shrivel. Little by little, it revealed what it had been intended to conceal. "Every time we glanced at that dried-up leaf," Klein recalls, "we laughed. Our laughter lasted only a few seconds, but it brought us together. It revived us and made our troubles easier to bear."

*"The art of medicine consists of amusing the patient
while nature cures the disease."*
—Voltaire

In 1964, *Saturday Review* editor Norman Cousins was suddenly hospitalized with severe pain, paralysis and gravel-like nodules under his skin. Eventually his illness was diagnosed as ankylosing spondylitis, a serious form of arthritis. Cousins's doctor said his chance of recovery was 1 in 500. A specialist called that optimistic—he'd never seen anyone recover from the disease.

Cousins was no doctor, but he was not entirely medically naive. His magazine had published several articles on discoveries that were new at the time, discoveries showing that the emotions have a profound impact on health. Negative emotions impaired the body's ability to function and heal. (Today this field is called mind/body medicine.)

Cousins figured that if negative emotions hurt the body, perhaps a large dose of positive emotions might help him heal. Given his grim prognosis, he had nothing to lose.

He began his unorthodox self-treatment program by asking

his visitors to bring him joke books. Despite his pain and difficulty moving, he found himself laughing uproariously, particularly at E. B. and Katharine White's *Subtreasury of American
Humor* and *The Enjoyment of Laughter* by Max Eastman.

In short order, Cousins's lab results improved. He could
move more easily, and the quality of his sleep also improved. "I
made the joyous discovery that ten minutes of genuine belly
laughter had an anesthetic effect that gave me at least two hours
of pain-free sleep," he says.

Buoyed by his success and bothered by the noise, bad food
and general unpleasantness of hospital life, Cousins checked out
and moved into a luxurious hotel nearby, where he "could laugh
twice as hard at half the price."

He had a movie projector and screen set up in his room (this
was in the days before VCRs) and rented Marx Brothers movies
and Three Stooges comedies. In addition, his friend Allen Funt
donated copies of the television show he produced, *Candid
Camera*, which featured hidden-camera film of people doing
silly things. To the amazement of Cousins's doctors, the more
he laughed, the more he improved. Within a few months, he
could walk using metal leg braces, and he returned to work.
Eventually the braces came off. After a while, he recovered his
ability to type, and his only residual disability was sluggishness
in his fingers while playing difficult compositions on the organ.

> *"A sense of humor makes a person healthy,
> wealthy and wisecracking."*
> —Henny Youngman

As you may know, Cousins described his unique recovery
program in his book *Anatomy of an Illness*, a huge best-seller
that awakened millions to the healing power of humor. Dr.
Goodman and Klein have not become quite as famous, but they
don't care: They're too busy laughing.

> *"Humor is an affirmation of humanity's
> superiority to all that befalls us."*
> —Romain Gary

Dr. Goodman's father survived his heart surgery, and his son returned to his consulting work in organizational development—building teamwork, encouraging creative problem-solving and generally helping large institutions run more smoothly. He completely forgot about Alvin, the amusing van driver—until one evening when "I happened to tune into a radio talk show whose host asked: 'What makes you laugh?' The listeners told him, and I found myself riveted by their responses. I began thinking about Alvin, and how I'd used humor in my organizational-development work, but I realized I'd never been serious about it."

Dr. Goodman got serious about humor and launched the Humor Project, an organization that has helped more than 500,000 businesspeople, educators, managers and health-care providers cultivate lightness of spirit in the face of life's weighty matters.

"Humor fit right into my work. Organizations run better, and people solve problems more creatively when they don't take things too seriously," Dr. Goodman explains.

The Humor Project is not a school for comedians. "Personally, I'm not a good joke-teller," Dr. Goodman admits. "Instead the project encourages people to see the 'divine comedy' in life all around them. When you look for humor, you find it, and life becomes more enjoyable and productive."

*"God gave us humor to compensate for the law of gravity."*
—Henny Youngman

Allen Klein's wife died in 1978. "Her death was an incalculable loss for me," he recalls, "but as the months passed, I began reflecting on what Ellen had taught me. Her most important lesson was that we're here to have a good time. She turned every occasion into an opportunity to enjoy herself, and everyone she knew became her playmate."

Klein sold his business and went to work for a hospice, helping the terminally ill deal with their final passage. He was struck by the way the hospice residents appreciated humor and benefited from it—and by how guilty their visitors seemed to feel about laughing while the Grim Reaper hovered so near. Klein decided to encourage humor by becoming a self-proclaimed "jollytologist." Eventually he wrote *The Healing Power of Humor* and now lectures internationally about using mirth to cope with stress, loss and disappointment.

## The Emotional Benefits of Humor

Take a moment right now and smile. Not one of those tight-lipped, corners-of-the-mouth grins you might give your boss's wife when she insists you have a second helping of something you can't stand, but a big, toothy grin.

Now focus on how the smile makes you feel. Chances are you feel a little better than you did a few sentences ago. Why? Because mental health is a two-way street. Smiling is not just a result of happiness. It's also a cause.

"Smiling," explains health educator Robert Cooper, Ph.D., president of the Center for Health and Fitness Excellence in Bemidji, Minnesota, and author of *Health and Fitness Excellence: The Scientific Action Plan,* "resets the neurochemistry of the brain toward more positive emotions."

The big smiles that encourage positive emotions are popularly known as ear-to-ear grins. But according to research by Paul Ekman, Ph.D., professor of psychology at the University of California's San Francisco Medical Center Langley Porter Psychiatric Institute, they should be called eye-to-eye grins.

Dr. Ekman says that tight-lipped smiles do not improve mental health. For a smile to boost feelings of happiness, it must involve the entire face, particularly the muscles in the outer corners of the eyes.

> *"A person without a sense of humor is*
> *like a wagon without springs.*
> *It's jolted by every pebble on the road."*
> —Henry Ward Beecher

A sense of humor—smiling and the laughter that often follows it—not only enhances our self-perception of happiness, it also improves our emotional outlook. "Humor gives us the power to go on," Klein says.

Norman Cousins is not the only person to use mirth to gain power over an illness. Abraham Lincoln employed it to fight bouts of depression throughout his life. Once during a bleak period of the Civil War, Lincoln's Cabinet sat dumbfounded as the President read to them from a book of humorous stories. Lincoln laughed, but no one else did. "Gentlemen," he said, "why don't you laugh? If I did not laugh, I'd die."

> *"Humor acts to relieve fear.*
> *Rage is impossible when mirth prevails."*
> —William Fry, M.D.

"Humor helps us cope," Klein asserts. Levity provides perspective and helps us see problems in a larger framework. Once Klein found himself caught in a long, slow-moving supermarket checkout line. He caught himself growing increasingly annoyed, and in an effort to cope, he tried to see the humor in his predicament. He wound up thinking "This line is moving so slowly, the woman ahead of me just sprouted cobwebs." By the time he paid for his purchases, he felt fine.

Of course, humor can't heal all wounds or replace all losses, but it can help overcome them. To comedian Michael Pritchard, laughter is like changing a baby's diaper: "It doesn't get rid of the mess permanently, but it makes things okay for a while."

> *"A smile is a curve that sets everything straight."*
> —Phyllis Diller

"Humor keeps us balanced," Klein says. Humor offers a refuge from negative emotions before we become desperate. "Once we can see the comedy in our chaos, we are no longer so caught up in it, and our problems feel like less of a burden."

## The Physical Benefits of Humor

Laughter is Nature's form of ho-ho-holistic medicine.

Scientists are not exactly sure why we have a sense of humor, but smiling and laughter are innate and therefore presumably confer some evolutionary survival advantage.

In one study, researchers rated the dispositions of a group of medical students, then followed them for 25 years. By age 50, 14 percent of those rated "hostile" had died, but among those rated "easy-going," the death rate was only 2 percent.

Babies begin to smile when they're only a few weeks old, and they typically laugh by nine weeks. At four months of age, healthy, nonabused babies laugh several times an hour, and they keep it up well into their school years. But then our culture's "get serious" socialization kicks in, and laughter declines.

"Adults often go days or weeks without laughing," says Leslie Gibson, R.N., founder of the Comedy Carts program at Morton Plant Hospital in Clearwater, Florida. "Some people seem to lose the ability to laugh and need help relearning it."

> *"Laughter is an orgasm triggered by the*
> *intercourse of sense and nonsense."*
> —Anonymous

William Fry, M.D., professor emeritus of psychiatry at Stanford University and an expert on the physiology of mirth, notes that a hearty belly laugh exercises a surprisingly large number of muscles. He estimates that 100 laughs provide a workout equivalent to about ten minutes on a rowing machine. Dr. Fry recommends laughter to everyone as a kind of "inner jogging," but he notes that it's especially important for those who are bedridden or otherwise unable to get much exercise.

Laughter also stimulates respiration and heart rate. This increases the oxygen content of the blood, helping all body systems perform more efficiently. At the end of a hearty laugh, blood pressure falls and a wave of relaxation washes over the body.

Like other forms of exercise, laughter releases endorphins, the body's feel-good, pain-relieving brain chemicals. In one study, researchers at Allegheny College in Meadville, Pennsylvania, divided a group of volunteers into two groups and exposed them to increasingly painful electric shocks. One group watched a Bill Cosby comedy routine and the other watched a video on gardening. The participants were able to turn off the electric shocks when they became too painful. Guess which group could stand more discomfort.

## Warning: Humor May Be Hazardous to Your Illness

The latest research shows that humor also boosts the immune system's ability to fight disease. At Western New England College in Springfield, Massachusetts, Kathleen Dillon, Ph.D., professor of psychology, explored the effects of humor on production of salivary immunoglobulin A (IgA), an antibody in the mouth and throat that fights the common cold. She measured IgA in healthy volunteers before and after they viewed each of two videos, an instruction program about anxiety and the comedy, *Richard Pryor Live*.

After viewing the instruction video, the participants showed no change in IgA levels, but after *Richard Pryor Live*, their IgA levels increased markedly. Next time you feel a cold coming on, run down to your local video outlet and rent a few comedies. They may not prevent the cold, but who knows? They just might.

## The Healing Uses of Laughter

As a fourth-grader, Leslie Gibson had the misfortune to be fat and wear glasses. "I was on the receiving end of a lot of nasty humor," the now-trim 37-year-old nurse recalls.

To escape her tormentors on the way home from school, she used to duck into the shop of a shoemaker she knew. "He told me that if I could get the kids to laugh with me, they'd stop laughing at me." It worked. Gibson became the class clown, and the taunting ceased.

As a nurse, Gibson began teaching stress management skills to patients at Morton Plant Hospital. She used humor and eventually received a grant from Dr. Goodman's Humor Project to develop a Comedy Cart for the hospital. "It was a small audiovisual cart with a TV, VCR, comedy videos, games, gag items, humorous books and audiotapes," she says. "I wheeled it around the hospital as a free service to patients."

Gibson's Comedy Cart was an overnight sensation. Today her program includes ten carts for Morton Plant Hospital and two for its affiliated rehabilitation center. Volunteers wheel the carts around the hospital every weekday afternoon, and they've proved so popular that frequently patients must phone in reservations to guarantee a visit.

The Comedy Carts attracted media attention, and one day she got a call from the Ringling Brothers Clown College in Sarasota. Several clowns wanted to volunteer. Gibson now has 60 clowns who wheel Comedy Carts in full clown regalia: greasepaint, red noses, Bozo hair, clown costumes and oversized shoes. A few years ago, Ringling Brothers relocated its Clown College to Wisconsin, so Gibson opened her own.

"We take 20 people twice a year and they train for three hours five nights a week for eight weeks. Afterward we ask that they donate four hours a month to our program," she says.

*"The arrival of a good clown exercises more beneficial influence upon the health of a town than 20 donkeys laden with drugs."*
—Thomas Sydenham, seventeenth-century English physician

Clowning in hospitals has become a growth industry. At the Duke University Medical Center in Durham, North Carolina, Ruth Hamilton, founder of the Carolina Health and Humor Association (Carolina HA HA), set up the Laugh Mobile for cancer patients. Designed to look like an old-fashioned circus wagon, it contains an assortment of humorous materials, including practical joke items that patients are invited to use on the staff.

In New York, the Big Apple Circus launched the Clown Care Unit, whose initials, CCU, are a take-off on the coronary care units (CCUs) in many hospitals. "We specialize in the funny bone," says CCU staffer Dr. Loon (aka Kim Winslow). CCU members perform "clown rounds" three days a week for children at six New York hospitals.

These "doctors of delight" combine mime, juggling, slapstick, music and magic tricks for the amusement of the young patients and their families. CCU favorites include red nose transplants, a stethoscope that blows bubbles and "drawing blood"—with a sketch pad and a red marker pen.

> *"Seven days without humor makes one weak."*
> —Mort Walker

"Hi, this is Steve. You've reached my office. Leave a message and I'll get back to you. Please include the date and time of your call—and your shoe size."

This is not the typical family physician's phone message. But Steve Allen, Jr., M.D., assistant professor of family practice at the Binghamton clinical campus of the State University of New York Health Science Center in Syracuse, is not your typical family doctor. Dr. Allen is the son of the comedian and television personality of the same name.

Dr. Allen views humor as a way to counteract the stress associated with disease, literally dis-ease. While many physicians adopt an all-business, "professional" posture with their patients, Dr. Allen often mixes physical exams with juggling lessons and other forms of gentle silliness calculated to help his patients relax.

"Healing humor is not necessarily about telling jokes," explains Alison Crane, R.N., a psychiatric nurse in Skokie, Illinois, who founded the American Association of Therapeutic Humor in 1986. "I'm not very good at telling jokes and I stay away from them. Therapeutic humor is a way to build rapport and decrease people's anxiety about their illness and the health professionals they have to deal with. Humor humanizes caring, and when people feel they're relating to real human beings—not just automatons in white coats—they respond much better."

Instead of telling jokes, Crane often shares stories about her children. "Once I was having trouble getting through to an elderly woman," she recalls. "So I told her that my three-year-old daughter was in a quandary about what she wanted to be when she grew up. She couldn't decide between a garbage collector and a dolphin. The woman got a big kick out of that. She opened right up and started talking about her grandchildren."

*"Humor is the hole that lets the sawdust out of a stuffed shirt."*
—Henny Youngman

In 1974, San Francisco cardiologists Meyer Friedman, M.D., director of the Meyer Friedman Research Institute at Mount Zion Medical Center in San Francisco, and Ray Rosenman, M.D., published *Type-A Behavior and Your Heart,* about their studies showing that the belligerent, hard-driving, time-pressured behavior they termed *Type-A* substantially increased risk of heart attack. The book became a best-seller, and almost overnight *Type-A* became a household term. But critics said they would not be convinced until Dr. Friedman and Dr. Rosenman showed that changing Type-A's into more relaxed Type-Bs actually reduced their heart attack risk.

Dr. Friedman teamed up with Diane Ullmer, R.N., and they developed an intensive counseling program for Type-A heart attack survivors that was designed to help them mellow out and smell the roses. Among other exercises, participants were encouraged to use mirth. Whenever they felt the bile of hostility rising within them, they were taught to find humor in the situation and point it out instead of yelling about the problem. They were also instructed to laugh at themselves at least twice a day. After three years in the counseling program, 9 percent of the participants had had recurrent heart attacks. But in the group that did not receive counseling, the heart attack rate was 19 percent, a highly significant difference.

## How to Bring More Humor into Your Life

Why don't we laugh more often? Mainly because we've learned not to. Parents and teachers spend a good deal of time telling children "Wipe that smile off your face"; "Get serious"; "Stop smirking"; "Settle down"; and "Stop acting silly." In addition, laughter requires both spontaneity and surrender of control. As people become adults, they place a good deal of value on self-control and often feel ambivalent about spontaneity.

But a mature adult should also understand the need for levity now and then. When Steven Spielberg was filming the holocaust movie *Schindler's List,* he became so saddened by his subject that a few times a week while on location in Poland, he called comedian Robin Williams and asked him to run through some stand-up routines. If you have a particularly funny friend, you might do the same, but if not, tickle your funny bone with the help of these suggestions from Klein and Dr. Goodman.

**Know your audience.** Humor is individual. *Psychology Today* magazine once published 30 jokes and asked readers if they found them funny. More than 14,000 readers from all over the map replied. Every joke was rated "very funny" by some readers and "not at all funny" by others. In the words of comedian Henny Youngman, "Humor is a form of communication understood by some and misunderstood by most."

**Laugh at yourself.** "Those without a sense of humor," Youngman once quipped, "can be very funny." Of course, they don't mean to be, and when people begin laughing, those who are unintentionally funny may become embarrassed, self-conscious or insulted. If this happens to you, try to step outside yourself and see your gaffe the way your audience sees it. Laugh at yourself and people laugh with you, not at you.

**Keep it tasteful.** Don't poke fun at anyone's race, ethnic group, gender, weight, occupation or anything else that might be offensive. Also avoid sarcasm and ridicule. If there has to be a butt of the joke, target yourself or some inanimate object.

**Develop a humor first-aid kit.** Keep a funny book or tape close at hand and dip into it several times a day. Wear humorous buttons and post cartoons, amusing bumper stickers and other witty items where you live, work and play.

**Instead of flowers or food, give sick friends humorous gifts.** Try a joke book, a comedy video or a few gag items.

**Keep an eye out for the absurdities of everyday life.** Amusing quips and situations happen all the time. If you look for them, you'll find them.

**Encourage others to laugh.** Mirth is contagious.

## CHAPTER 13

# HEALTHY HABITS

### Making Changes That Last

**J**ean Antonello was one of the millions of Americans who ate too much, put on extra weight and then struggled desperately to lose it.

The New Brighton, Minnesota, nurse started dieting at age 13, and for the next 17 years she lived a nightmare, alternately starving herself and then bingeing on anything in sight. Her weight yo-yoed from 118 to 198. She felt depressed, out of control and filled with self-hatred. Like most compulsive dieters—or smokers, alcoholics, spendthrifts or other people with a habit they'd like to change—Antonello believed her main problem was a lack of "willpower."

Before her wedding, she lost 40 pounds, but within a year, she gained it all back, and then some. "I was always at war with myself. I hated it," Antonello recalls. Her postwedding weight gain triggered a personal crisis. She knew she couldn't go on as she had been, but she had no idea what to do.

If this sounds familiar, you're not alone. At some point in life, just about everyone wishes to break a bad habit and replace it with a good one. The good news is, it can be done. You can do it. Even if you've already tried and failed several times, you can break bad habits and replace them with good ones.

211

Millions of people with no more willpower than you possess have lost weight, quit smoking, turned their finances around, gotten in shape and made other major life changes. You can, too—not immediately, not all at once and not without considerable effort. But with introspection, preparation, help from loved ones and a new understanding of how habits change, you can do it.

## How "Bad" Is Your Habit?

Every January 1, millions of Americans vow to change by adopting New Year's resolutions. Fittingly, this burst of self-improvement energy comes hard on the heels of the holiday season, when too many people eat too much, drink too much and spend too much.

According to Anne Simons, M.D., assistant clinical professor of family and community medicine at the University of California's San Francisco Medical Center and author of *Before You Call the Doctor,* surveys of New Year's resolutions show that Americans want to lose weight, get more exercise, quit smoking, spend more time with loved ones and manage their finances more effectively.

These five goals concern different areas of life, but the steps involved in accomplishing them are similar. This chapter focuses mostly on weight loss because an estimated 70 million Americans—about one-third of the population—are dieting at any given moment. But weight-loss experts' recommendations can easily be adapted to help change any bad habit.

How can you tell if a habit is "bad"? Some habits—smoking, alcoholism, drug addiction and compulsive gambling—are clearly destructive. But others occupy a gray area. If you're 15 pounds overweight, that's not great, but it's not terrible. The same could be said for credit card debt or watching three hours of TV a night. How bad do things have to get before they should be changed?

"It's up to the individual," Dr. Simons says, "but if any habit feels bad, it probably is bad."

A habit becomes bad when it makes you feel out of control, when you keep doing it—or in the case of exercise, not doing it—despite the little voice inside you that says "Change this."

One problem, according to specialists in addictions, is that people with bad habits often vehemently deny having a problem: "I'm not hooked on cocaine. I can stop any time." Think about the habits in your life. If any of the following statements apply to you, it may be time for a change.

- I'm secretive about my habit.
- I feel ashamed and guilty about it.
- I lie about it.
- I do it to take my mind off other problems.
- Sometimes it interferes with things in my life I consider important.
- I used to enjoy it more than I do now.
- I do it even when it's not pleasurable.
- People I know have said they think I have a problem.
- I'd like to change it, but I don't know if I can.

If you agreed with any of these statements, congratulations. You've taken a giant step away from denial and realized that you have a habit you'd like to change.

## Getting Ready for Change

Once you've decided to change a habit, don't attempt to do it all at once. Some people do manage to quit smoking "cold turkey," but sudden life changes seldom stick. Before Jean Antonello lost 30 pounds once and for all, she prepared herself to make the change. It took her two years to escape the starve/binge mindset and another nine months to develop a personal weight-loss plan she could live with. Almost three years after she decided to lose weight for good, she finally felt ready to do it.

"I'd spent half my life wondering why my appetite was out of control," Antonello explains. "Luckily, by the time of my crisis,

I had some scientific training as a nurse. I decided to research my problem scientifically. Instead of focusing on what was wrong with me, I interviewed people who were naturally thin—who could eat anything and not gain weight—to learn what was right with them."

Antonello discovered that those who were naturally thin were not obsessed with food as she was. They ate when they felt hungry and stopped when they felt full. "I realized that willpower was not my problem. Dieting was," says Antonello. "If you periodically starve yourself, your body thinks you're living through a famine, and it takes steps to assure your survival. You become obsessed with eating, and when food becomes available again, your body stores fat to prepare for the next 'famine.' I needed to convince my body that the famine was over. I needed to learn how to eat."

That prospect panicked Antonello. She was scared to stop, scared to make the changes she should. She was also terrified of failing again. But this time she felt better prepared. An estimated 90 percent of dieters do not achieve permanent weight control, but Antonello did because she took the time to get ready.

Change takes time and personal commitment. But above all, it takes preparation. "Before you can break bad habits and establish good ones, you have to get ready," says psychologist Thomas Wadden, Ph.D., director of the Center for Health and Behavior at Syracuse University in New York. "Most people talk themselves out of the change they'd like to make. The challenge is to talk yourself into it."

If you're truly ready, terrific. Go for it. If you're not ready, analyze why not. "Then wait a month or so, and check in with yourself again," says weight-loss expert Kelly Brownell, Ph.D., professor of psychology at Yale University. "If you're not ready and you try anyway, you're setting yourself up for failure and disappointment."

Eleven years after she stopped dieting and lost weight once and for all, Antonello is justifiably proud of her achievement. She's especially proud of the almost three years she spent getting ready, because her main struggle, as she writes in her book,

# Smoking: The Greatest Challenge ━━━━

Which habit is harder to kick than heroin? Many experts say it's cigarettes. Obesity and alcoholism take a substantial toll on the nation's health, but cigarettes are worse, claiming more than 100,000 lives annually from lung cancer, heart disease and other smoking-related conditions.

Aspiring ex-smokers can adapt the suggestions in this chapter to their own situations, but here are some additional tips to help you quit.

*Travel light.* Never carry cigarettes with you.

*Occupy your mouth.* Whenever you want a cigarette, sip a glass of water instead. This way, you'll be replacing a bad habit with a good one.

*Move that body.* Whenever you want a cigarette, take a five-minute walk instead.

*Be stingy.* Stop buying cigarettes in cartons; buy only single packs instead.

*Finish the job.* Smoke the last cigarette in one pack before buying the next one.

*Beg a little.* Ask a friend to hold your cigarettes for you. That way you have to ask each time you want one.

*Focus on what you're doing.* When you smoke, do nothing else—no TV, no coffee, no reading, drinking or talking on the phone.

*Go to your corner.* Designate a "smoking place" in your home and smoke only there. Banish all ashtrays to your designated smoking place. Over time, move it to less and less comfortable locations, such as a corner of your basement. Then declare your home smoke-free and go outside to smoke.

*Be aware.* Record the number of cigarettes you smoke each day and display it prominently in your home.

*Distract yourself.* Recognize relapse temptations before they become crises. Instead of lighting up, call a friend, take a walk or a shower, chew gum or brush your teeth.

*Put it off.* Delay your first smoke of the day by 30 minutes. After a few months, add another half-hour. When you take a cigarette, delay lighting it for 10 minutes. After a few months, add another 10 minutes.

*How to Become Naturally Thin by Eating More,* was not against her weight but against her fears. Once she felt truly ready to lose weight, the pounds came off slowly but surely. "Looking back," she reflects, "I believe that if I hadn't taken the time to get ready for my change, I'd probably still be on the starve/binge, dieting roller coaster today."

The experts agree that careful preparation is crucial to habit-changing success. Here are some questions they recommend you ponder in preparation for permanent weight loss or any other significant life changes.

*How fed up are you with your bad habit?* Most people automatically say "Very." But often that's not the case. When psychologist Ronette L. Kolotkin, Ph.D., director of behavioral programs at the Duke University Diet and Fitness Center in Durham, North Carolina, asks people how their weight affects their daily lives, those who aren't ready to lose weight typically respond "Not much." The ones who are truly ready say, "I'm fed up, and I'm willing to do whatever it takes to change."

Being fed up means fed up, period. "People tell me, 'I know I should lose weight, but . . . ,' " says psychologist Diane Hanson, R.N., Ph.D., a lifestyle specialist at the Pritikin Longevity Center in Santa Monica, California. "That 'but' means they're not ready."

Dr. Hanson, 44, knows about weight-loss readiness from personal experience. Her mother added butter and cream to everything. Not surprisingly, by adulthood she was 30 pounds overweight. She yo-yo dieted for years, and then one day she realized she was truly fed up. No more "buts." She lost the 30 pounds in the early 1980s and has never regained them.

Steve Purser knew he was ready to lose weight when he too became truly fed up with his extra baggage. The 44-year-old San Francisco health official gained weight gradually from high school through college. "But it didn't bother me," he recalls. When he hit 30, his attitude changed. Once he felt committed to losing weight permanently, he dropped 20 pounds and has never regained more than 5 pounds.

*For whose benefit are you making this change?* "When

people tell me they want to lose weight for their high school reunion or because their doctor or mother-in-law has been nagging them, they usually gain it back," Dr. Kolotkin says. "External forces can help people start to lose weight, but any weight loss is rarely permanent. People who keep weight off lose it for themselves, because they're committed to doing it."

*What benefits do you expect?* Fairy tales end "happily ever after," but in real life, things are often messy—even for thin people. "It's amazing how unrealistic people can be about weight loss," says Dr. Kolotkin. "They think that slimming down will make everything wonderful. It doesn't."

Dr. Kolotkin contrasts unrealistic expectations about weight loss with the more realistic expectations most people have about job changes or second marriages. "People don't expect new jobs or marriages to be perfect. They know that to do so is a setup for disappointment. But when it comes to changing bad habits, many people have trouble getting past fairy-tale endings."

Be realistic. You probably won't become a movie star, but after you lose weight you'll be able to sit comfortably in a theater seat.

*What are you afraid of?* Consider the rewards of your bad habit—that's right, rewards. Being overweight might provide advantages that you'll have to sacrifice when you lose weight.

Some people build their social networks around friends who share their bad habit—people who are overweight, or smokers or race track regulars. Changing your life might cost you friends.

Other people use their bad habit as an excuse for not working on other problems. "They think, 'I have a lousy job or marriage because I'm fat,' " says Dr. Wadden. "If they lose weight, they lose their excuse for their other dissatisfactions. That can be scary."

Others believe their weight makes people take them more seriously. This idea is part of our language: A powerful person is a "heavy." A "lightweight" is a nitwit. "Several people have told me, 'When I'm heavy, people take more interest in what I say,' " says Dr. Kolotkin.

Some people fear a loss of friends or sexual attractiveness if

# Help Others Change Their Ways

Everyone wants to help those they love quit smoking, get fit, overcome obesity and substance abuse and make other health-oriented life changes. But too often, well-intentioned friends do more harm than good. Tom Ferguson, M.D., author of *The No-Nag, No-Guilt, Do-It-Your-Own-Way Guide to Quitting Smoking,* asked 200 smokers how friends could best help them quit. They speak not just for smokers but for people with other bad habits as well.

*Can the commentary.* Don't nag, insult or shame the person into changing.

*Don't judge.* Separate the person from the habit. Smokers are not bad people. They are good people with a bad habit.

*Be supportive.* Praise and support the person for even the smallest effort to change. When the person is in the throes of trying to overcome the bad habit, call regularly to offer support and be available 24 hours a day by phone to help the person deal with relapse crises.

*Think before you act.* Never offer cigarettes to a smoker, alcohol to an alcoholic or high-fat foods to someone who's trying to lose weight.

*Love a little.* Remember the hardest thing you've ever done. Recall your own struggle to accomplish it. Respect others who are on similar paths.

they lose weight. "Our culture says that thin is sexy," explains Maria Simonson, Ph.D., Sc.D., director of the Health, Weight and Stress Clinic at Johns Hopkins University in Baltimore, "but many men are sexually attracted to heavier women."

Others, especially women, fear increased sexual attractiveness if they lose weight. Why fear sexiness? Because it often means wolf whistles on the street and obnoxious approaches by neighbors, co-workers and friends' husbands. "Being thin," Dr. Kolotkin explains, "can be a real hassle."

A key part of preparing to change any bad habit involves

confronting your fears of success. If you've used your weight as an excuse for inaction on other problems, you won't be ready to lose until you've explored those issues. Once you do, weight loss can help build the self-esteem necessary to deal with them. And if you think your weight adds to your clout or sexiness, consider modifying your weight-loss goal. "Maybe you shouldn't lose 75 pounds," Dr. Kolotkin says. "Maybe you should stop at, say, 40."

As for fear of unwanted sexual advances, Dr. Kolotkin suggests losing weight slowly so you can learn to cope comfortably with new reactions to the new you. The best way to do it is to become more assertive. Practice saying things like "I'm flattered that you find me attractive now, but I never date people I work with." Or "I never fool around with married men, so forget it."

But perhaps the biggest inner fear that keeps people from breaking bad habits is fear of failure. "Every long-term dieter feels burned by all the diets that didn't work," Dr. Hanson says, "so they're skeptical about trying again." Dr. Hanson suggests viewing weight-loss attempts not as successes or failures but rather as experiments. "Think about what you've learned along the way," she says. "Analyze what you did right and what you need to do differently next time."

"I don't care what behavior pattern people are trying to change," Dr. Wadden says. "I never use the term failure. For most people, major life changes take several tries. It's frustrating to regain weight or return to smoking or to a destructive relationship, but that's usually a necessary step on the long and winding road to permanent change."

## Taking the Initial Steps

As you consider your emotional readiness for change, take some small but concrete steps in the right direction.

**Announce your intentions.** Tell your social support network that you're getting ready to make a major life change and ask for their support. This is not easy. It may be downright embarrassing.

"Going public" forces you to explain what you plan to do,

how you plan to do it and why this time will be different from your previous attempts. Going public might invite teasing ("But I thought you liked being fat.") or even ridicule ("*You?* Lose weight? Right. The day after hell freezes over.").

Going public is all part of a big process. When you make changes, the people around you must change, too—they must change how they think about you and their expectations of you. Some of your relationships may deteriorate, especially those based on shared indulgence in the habit you're trying to change. But other relationships will grow stronger, because it takes courage to change and people are attracted to those they consider courageous.

**Recruit buddies.** If you fear a loss of friends, try recruiting a buddy or two to help with your habit change—supportive, nonjudgmental friends you can turn to when you feel in danger of relapsing into your bad habit. (Buddies are a key component of Alcoholics Anonymous and other 12-step programs.)

**Keep a diary.** Your written record doesn't have to be elaborate or even contain complete sentences. Simply jot some notes about what you're doing, thinking and feeling whenever you indulge in your bad habit. Diaries help identify the triggers that prompt you to do what you'd rather not. Typical triggers include boredom, loneliness, rejection, frustration and difficult interpersonal encounters.

**Target your triggers.** Once you know what triggers the habit you're committed to breaking, plan ahead to minimize the likelihood of slipping into triggering situations. An overeater might decide to catch the bus farther from that seductive bakery. An alcoholic might decline offers to attend the office's weekly TGIF party. A smoker might commit to having a cup of herbal tea after meals instead of lighting up.

**Hold the line.** As you prepare to lose weight, quit smoking, eliminate credit card debt or make other changes, a good way to begin is to maintain your bad habit without allowing it to get worse.

If you're 40 pounds overweight, don't jump right into a weight-loss program. Instead, for a few months, maintain your current weight. If you smoke ten cigarettes a day, don't increase the number. Or if you owe $3,000 on your credit cards, maintain that level of debt. "Holding the line for six months is a real success," Dr. Wadden says. "It shows people that they have more control than they thought they had. That boosts their confidence as they move on to the next step, real change."

**Distinguish between ordinary and extraordinary stress.** People who aren't ready to change always find reasons not to try. But sometimes those who really feel fed up face major life problems that make changing difficult, if not impossible.

"Everyone has 'background obstacles,'" explains Dr. Brownell, "bills and hassles with kids and jobs. But if you're facing extraordinary problems—divorce, serious illness, a death in the family or job loss—then you may be too preoccupied to lose weight or make other changes."

How long should a person wait after a major problem before tackling a bad habit? "It depends on the individual," Dr. Wadden says. "But you should feel more or less back to normal and no longer preoccupied by the stressor."

Occasionally, however, serious life problems may spur change. "A woman who has just decided to leave a destructive marriage may be facing divorce," Dr. Brownell explains, "but if she feels excited about starting a new and better life, it might be a good time for her to lose weight."

**Use Nature's cures.** Bad habits reflect a loss of self-control. This book describes healing arts that help foster self-control and combat the feelings of stress and inner emptiness that lead to many bad habits. Incorporate a few of Nature's cures into your life. Try biofeedback, cognitive therapy, companionship, exercise, low-fat eating, meditation, sleep, tai chi and chi gong, vegetarianism, visualization, guided imagery and self-hypnosis, walking or yoga.

## Taking the Plunge

Okay, you're committed. You've gone public and recruited a few buddies. You know what triggers your binges, and you've devised ways to avoid them. You've successfully maintained your habit without allowing it to get worse. Now it's time to get serious about change. Here are some additional steps to take.

**Pick a meaningful start date.** When Steve Purser, the San Francisco health official who lost weight and kept it off, realized that he was prepared to forgo alcohol and substitute walks for desserts, he didn't plunge right in. "I waited until the first of the year. I'm not really sure why," he says. "It just felt right." Pick a start date that's personally meaningful to you: January 1, your birthday or the anniversary of some event that pushed you to make your change.

**Make some small changes.** "People who focus only on their weight usually regain what they lose," Dr. Kolotkin says. "Permanent weight loss means making small, manageable changes and sticking with them for life."

Of course, change is never easy. It often feels threatening, especially when it's "for life." That's why part of getting ready to lose weight or change any habit involves deciding which changes are small enough to feel manageable and nonthreatening. In other words, which changes are no big deal?

" 'Dieting' means making drastic short-term changes that never last," says fitness instructor Joan Price, author of *The Honest Truth about Losing Weight and Keeping It Off.* "To keep weight off, make small changes over time and incorporate them into your life for good. Be honest with yourself. Don't even consider a change you're unwilling to stick to."

To make your change, first list all the little things you're truly willing to do. Maybe you can't give up that cigarette after dinner, but you can live without the one after lunch. Perhaps you're repulsed by jogging, but it's no big deal to park one block farther from the mall and walk the extra distance. Or maybe you can't live without burgers, but you're willing to switch from cheeseburgers to plain hamburgers. These changes may sound insignificant, but they're not.

"It's the small changes that become permanent," Dr. Kolotkin says, "and permanence is crucial. I applaud switching from cheeseburgers to hamburgers—if it's for life."

Once you've listed all the changes you can live with, rank

them from easiest to hardest and make the easiest change—and no other. Within six months, it should become a permanent habit. Then make change number two and so on, one change every six months.

"It takes about six months for personal changes to become cemented as habits," Price says. "When you no longer have to struggle with one change, it's no big deal to make the next."

When Steve Purser felt ready to lose weight, he made only two changes. "I cut out alcohol, and instead of diving into sweets after dinner, I took a walk. If I still wanted dessert after my walk, I'd have it. But usually when I got home, I felt fine going without it."

**Be realistic; be patient.** "Tabloid headlines like 'Lose 15 Pounds in a Week' train people to be terribly impatient about weight loss," Dr. Kolotkin says. "Quick fixes never work. Weight doesn't come off quickly. If you're not ready to give it time, you're not ready to lose."

For those who want to become regular exercisers, here's a good rule of thumb: Calculate the number of years you've been out of shape. For every year, allow one to two months to get back into shape.

**Focus on benefits.** "Diets" are by definition temporary. "People never say, 'I'm going on this diet for the rest of my life,'" Dr. Kolotkin says. "They say, 'I'll try it for a while.' When they stop, they regain the weight."

Instead of dwelling on how much you're depriving yourself, remember why you're fed up with being heavy. "Mental preparation for weight loss," Dr. Wadden says, "involves refocusing your self-talk from 'I can't have this or that' to 'I'm going to look better, feel better, have more energy and wear the clothes I love.'"

After a few months of avoiding alcohol and taking his nightly walks, Purser was delighted to discover benefits he hadn't even imagined. "I had more stamina. I slept more soundly. And I felt less tired during the day," he says.

**Don't get trapped by perfectionism.** "Most people expect themselves to be perfect," says Susan Olson, Ph.D., a psychologist in Portland, Oregon. "When they make mistakes, they find it difficult to forgive themselves. Preparing for change means realizing that everyone makes mistakes. Learn to forgive yourself."

Think about how marriage works. When spouses fight, they don't immediately get divorced. After most marital mistakes, spouses forgive each other. That's part of any permanent relationship. Permanent habit control is similar. It means entering into a new, more forgiving relationship with yourself.

The quest for perfection leads to preoccupation with two other emotional demons—willpower and guilt. "When dieters realize they're not perfect," Antonello says, "they decide they have no willpower and feel guilty for being 'bad.' Of course, they're not bad. They're starving, and no matter how much willpower they muster, after a while they binge and feel guilty. But when people eat quality low-fat food normally, they lose weight without guilt and without the need for all that willpower."

**Don't compare yourself to others.** No matter how much weight you lose, there will always be people who look better than you do. No matter how well you budget your money, some people will have their finances more together than you do. It doesn't matter. To jettison bad habits and establish good ones, you don't have to be the best person in the world or even the best person on your block. You just have to change the person you are in the direction you want to go.

**Don't "exercise"; have more fun.** No one loses weight permanently by diet changes alone. Regular exercise is a must. Exercise also helps change other bad habits into good ones. It takes time that might otherwise be spent self-destructively, and it releases endorphins, the body's antidepressant chemicals, which contribute to feelings of well-being. Exercise is discussed in greater depth on page 169, but Price explains in a nutshell how to get off the sofa: "Don't 'exercise.' Just become a little more physically active in your daily life."

Price, 48, speaks from experience. As a child, she hated gym class and didn't learn how to swim or ride a bike until her midtwenties. "The only physical activity I enjoyed was dancing—but I had no idea it was 'exercise.'"

During her thirties, as part of a weight-loss effort, she tried bicycling and was amazed how much she enjoyed it. But she couldn't ride during the winter, so she regained lost weight. Casting about for a winter activity, she heard about an aerobic dance class at a local health club. "I'd never set foot inside a health club, and I felt terrified to enter. But my cycling had given me some confidence, and I'd always enjoyed dancing. I figured it was either try it or sit at home and eat."

At her first aerobics class, Price lasted all of five minutes. "I had no stamina," she recalls. But in the locker room, the other women were supportive. "Each one had a story about arriving for the first time thinking they were the only person who'd ever been out of shape," she says. Price stuck with the class and slimmed down permanently. Now she teaches aerobics.

"Half of those who start exercise programs stop within a few months," she explains, "and half of those who stop do so before their first session. They give up in advance because they force themselves to do things they don't enjoy."

To find a type of exercise you can live with, recall the activities you enjoyed when you were younger—bowling, Ping-Pong, tap dancing, whatever. Take up one of these activities again or try something that's close. Price's girlhood love of dancing led her to aerobics. "Find what works for you," she advises. "Two great activities that don't feel like exercise are gardening and walking."

Like other fitness authorities, Price recommends three or four half-hour workouts a week, but not immediately. "To start, try going just five minutes three times a week."

That was what Price did after collapsing five minutes into her first aerobics class. She gave herself permission to stop after five minutes. "That changed the experience," she recalls. "Instead of feeling defeated before I started, I felt more positive: 'Five minutes? I can do that.' " Soon her five minutes became ten, and within a year, she could last an entire class and was greeting shy, overweight women in the locker room with her own first-time story.

**Think positive.** Practice affirmations: "I am in charge of my life. I can change." Some people dismiss personal pep talks as

# Making Changes: One Day at a Time

It was a very unlikely success story that began quietly in Akron, Ohio, in 1935, shortly after the repeal of Prohibition. Two self-confessed "hopeless drunks," stockbroker William Wilson and surgeon Robert Smith, M.D., met and vowed to help each other quit drinking.

Each had tried and failed many times, but there in Akron something clicked. They both stopped drinking for good with the help of a seat-of-the-pants program that involved 12 steps—6 of which refer to faith in a Higher Power. Their success attracted a small group of fellow alcoholics, who formed Alcoholics Anonymous (AA) in 1939.

Today the organization operates in more than 100 countries, has more than one million active participants and has spun off similar "12-step groups" that deal with addictions to narcotics and gambling, overeating and other self-destructive habits.

Here are 4 of the 12 steps.

1. Acknowledge your powerlessness over the problem and the fact that your life has become unmanageable because of it.
2. Recognize that you cannot fight the problem alone, that you need help from other people and from a Higher Spiritual Authority.
3. Be honest with yourself and with others. (AA directly confronts the denial of many alcoholics by insisting that everyone who speaks at meetings begin with "My name is _____, and I'm an alcoholic.")
4. Take an honest inventory of your life. Acknowledge both the good and bad you've done. Commit to improving yourself and making restitution for the harm you've done.

silly, but they can be surprisingly effective. Remember the classic children's story, "The Little Engine That Could." The engine kept repeating, "I think I can. I think I can."

**Grieve the loss of your old self.** Once you've begun to trans-

AA members never vow not to drink again. Instead they follow the organization's 24-hour plan, which involves not drinking just for today. Hence the slogan "One day at a time." It's a small goal, but one by one, the days accumulate, and soon members have been sober for weeks, months and years.

Members also exchange telephone numbers. If they ever feel tempted to drink, they call each other and talk out their troubles until the urge to drink passes. Or they call emergency crisis hotlines or attend AA meetings. In many communities, there are several meetings a day. The meetings combine the intensive self-examination of an encounter group with intimate success stories, a sense of belonging and the spiritual release of a religious revival. (Some people have difficulty with AA's religious overtones. Several nonspiritual groups have spun off from AA; one is the Secular Organization for Sobriety, or SOS.)

Anonymity is a cornerstone of AA. In an age when celebrity endorsements can make or break the reputations of everything from health clubs to drug treatment programs, the personalities of well-known participants often overshadow the programs they endorse. Not so with AA. The program is everything, and participants—even movie stars—remain anonymous beyond first-name identification. In keeping with its doctrine of anonymity, AA has no formal membership list, no president and just a few paid staff members scattered around the country in major cities.

AA is listed under Alcoholics Anonymous in the White Pages of local phone books (or in the business White Pages in directories that separate business and residential listings). Other groups, such as Overeaters Anonymous and Gamblers Anonymous, are listed similarly.

form your bad habit into a good one, it's time to bid farewell to the old you. "Remember leaving home? You felt excited, but you knew you'd miss your family and friends," says Dr. Kolotkin. "Losing weight or making other life changes has the same bittersweet quality. Give yourself a chance to grieve over the loss of your old lifestyle—even though you know it was bad for you. It's easier to open a new chapter in life when the previous one is really closed."

**Sidestep the saboteurs.** Okay, you've started to lose weight, but at the family picnic, there's Aunt Susie handing you a slice of apple pie, saying, "I made it just for you." Or you've given up alcohol and your boss decides to celebrate a new sales record with champagne. What to do? Dr. Olson advises telling your aunt, "I appreciate how hard you worked on the pie, but I'm also working hard to lose weight. I know you'll understand when I decline." As for your boss, say, "The new sales record is great. Part of the reason we achieved it was that I stopped drinking. I know you'll understand if I toast our success with a glass of mineral water."

Also practice sidestepping the "thought police." A friend who knows you're losing weight might say, "Should you have that cookie?" Dr. Olson suggests replying, "I know you want to help me. So far I've made two permanent life changes: no late-night dish of ice cream and a walk every day at lunch. Eventually I plan to eliminate cookies, but not yet. I need you to support my progress and not make me feel guilty."

**Chart your progress.** At Alcoholics Anonymous meetings, participants introduce themselves, then declare how long they've been sober, whether it's been a few hours or many years. This ritual is one way to chart progress in the battle against the bottle.

In fitness programs, chart how many minutes you walk, how many flights of stairs you can climb without feeling winded or any other measure of progress that's personally meaningful. When charting weight loss, however, many people weigh themselves daily. That's a mistake. Weight comes off slowly. "For permanent weight control, losing a pound a week is plenty," Dr. Kolotkin explains. "You don't see progress if you weigh in daily. Weigh yourself every week or two."

**Give yourself credit.** Think of the best parents you know. They lavish praise on their children for every little accomplishment. Be that parent for yourself. "To make permanent changes," Dr. Wadden says, "you have to become your own cheerleader. Don't lament, 'I only lost half a pound this week.' Say, 'All right! Another half-pound! That makes seven pounds in ten weeks. I'm doing it.' "

**Reward yourself at every step.** Part of cheering your own progress involves rewarding yourself, not with a hot fudge sundae if you're trying to lose weight or a shopping spree if you're trying to reduce credit card debt, but with little treats that reinforce your change efforts: a new pair of walking shoes or a phone call to tell an old friend about your progress.

Pace your rewards so that you earn at least one a week. "Don't fall into the trap of saying, 'I'll do this or that after I've lost 30 pounds,' " Dr. Wadden says. "Buy some new clothes now. See the symphony next week. Take a vacation soon. You deserve it."

**Consider getting help.** If you follow these suggestions for a year and still feel at the mercy of your bad habit, ask your family doctor for a referral to a therapist who specializes in your problem or to a social worker who can put you in touch with a support group.

## CHAPTER 14

# HEAT AND COLD THERAPIES

### Modern Benefits from Ancient Healers

Ever since our ancestors discovered fire and ice, healers have used heat and cold therapeutically—and they've debated how to use them most effectively.

Sprained your wrist? Wrap it in an ice pack, some say. No, others insist, use a heating pad.

Feeling anxious, stressed out or depressed? Some recommend that you soak or bake your cares away in a hot tub or steamy sauna. No, others retort, what you *really* need to do is jump into an icy stream or a cold pool.

Finally, the debate is over. Modern scientific research has clarified exactly when to use heat and cold. It has also transformed many traditional ideas about these therapies. If you still think a cold shower cools sexual ardor, for example, read on.

## Some Like It Hot, Some Like It Cold

The use of extremes of temperature as healing therapy goes way, way back. The ancient Chinese packed people in hot sand. Early Russians fashioned primitive steam baths. And throughout the world, wherever natural hot springs exist, those who lived nearby treasured them for both their medicinal and spiritual uses. American Indian tribes from New England to California considered hot springs so sacred and medicinal that during intertribal wars, sworn enemies suspended hostilities so both sides could bathe their wounds simultaneously. Tribes without access to hot springs sought healing and ritual purification in steamy sweat lodges. (In modern times, some cultures still have special appreciation for the healing powers of heat. Finland is the home of the sauna, and in that cold country the dry-heat chambers actually outnumber cars.)

Cold therapy also got its share of attention in the ancient world. In ancient India, Ayurvedic physicians prescribed cold baths for invigoration. And in ancient Greek healing temples, the afflicted bathed in cool water while praying to the deities of medicine—Hygea, goddess of health (whose name gave us the term *hygiene*), and Panacea, goddess of cures (whose name now means *cure-all*).

Frequently, traditional cultures have mixed heat and cold. For centuries, the Finns have alternated baking in saunas with stepping out into cold Arctic air or rolling in snowbanks. Half a world away, the Japanese bathed in cold streams after soaking in hot springs, a custom that survives to this day in Japanese bathhouses, where a cold plunge pool is located adjacent to the hot bath.

## The Healing Bathtub

Today we take bathing for granted, so it may come as a shock that from the fall of Rome until well into the nineteenth century, bathing as we know it largely disappeared in the West. Lack of indoor plumbing and the problem of heating large amounts of water made extended full-body baths a luxury most people enjoyed only rarely.

It wasn't until around 1840 that bathing for health and healing caught on in the United States, thanks in part to overseas travelers, who came home with enthusiastic stories of Europe's luxurious spas. By the time of the Civil War, hundreds of "water-cure" establishments dotted the countryside from the Northeast to the Western frontier (which then was located at the Mississippi River).

Water-cure advocates were divided into two camps—hydrotherapists and resort developers. The hydrotherapists prescribed hot and cold baths, exercise, a vegetarian diet and abstinence from alcohol, coffee and tea to the emerging middle class. The resort developers, on the other hand, built luxury European-style spas around springs in places like Saratoga, New York. Aimed at the well-to-do, these resorts served all manner of food and drink.

By the 1850s, water-cure establishments offered group bathing, hot and cold sheet and blanket wraps and personal sitz baths—along with claims that hydrotherapy could cure everything from "female troubles" to opium addiction.

As time passed and indoor plumbing made hot-water bathing routine, naturopathic physicians adopted many hydrotherapy practices. Modern naturopaths often recommend hot or cold baths for such ailments as hemorrhoids, depression, rashes and circulatory problems.

Meanwhile, most of America's European-style luxury health spas fell from fashion around World War I, only to boom anew since the 1970s as relaxation retreats where many of Nature's cures can still be found. Noted spas include Hot Springs, Arkansas; Esalen Institute in Big Sur, California; and several establishments in Calistoga, California.

## Healing with Heat

Few activities feel more relaxing than an interlude in a hot bath, hot tub or sauna. Since 1969, when backyard inventor Roy Jacuzzi of Walnut Creek, California, added air jets to an old grape press and created the first Jacuzzi hot tub, bathing has emerged from the privacy of the bathroom and returned to what it was in ancient Rome—a way to combine relaxation with socializing. But hot baths do more than help us destress. According to an old Finnish proverb, "If the sauna can't cure it, nothing can." That's a bit of an overstatement, but recent studies show that heat treatments have many healing benefits.

**Arthritis.** The Arthritis Foundation recommends low-impact, weight-bearing forms of exercise—among them, walking and gardening—to help control joint pain and inflammation. Another way to gain the same benefit is to exercise—walk, run in place or swim—in warm water. The water's buoyancy helps cushion the joints from harmful impacts, and the relaxing warmth helps the joints move through their full range of motion.

**Eczema.** Japanese studies suggest that tooji—the traditional practice of bathing in hot springs—helps relieve eczema (also known as atopic dermatitis), a mysterious ailment that's often stress-related. It's not clear why hot baths help, but Andrew Weil, M.D., professor of preventive medicine at the University of Arizona College of Medicine in Tucson and author of *Natural Health, Natural Healing,* speculates that the hot water's stress-relieving effect may play a role.

In addition, tooji is a group practice in Japan. It's possible that companionship and group support may also play a role in relieving eczema. If you have eczema and a hot tub, it can't hurt to bathe with a friend.

**Hemorrhoids.** Some naturopathic physicians recommend sitz baths to treat hemorrhoids. A sitz bath consists of immersing just the lower body in warm water while elevating the legs.

**Insomnia.** The relaxation resulting from a hot bath or sauna helps many people let go of their daily cares and ease into sleep. "A hot bath within a few hours of bedtime definitely helps people fall asleep," says sleep expert Peter Hauri, Ph.D., director of the Insomnia Research and Treatment Program at the Mayo Clinic in Rochester, Minnesota, and co-author of *No More Sleepless Nights.* Taking a hot bath in the morning or afternoon would have no sleep-inducing effect, he adds.

**Muscle soreness.** Muscle aches often develop from minor overexertion. That's because the muscles involved have not been sufficiently conditioned to tolerate the extra demand placed on them, and the unexpected load damages some muscle cells. The damage triggers stiffness and the dull, aching soreness that begins within a few hours of the activity and may last for a day or two.

Heat can help relieve the discomfort in two ways. It opens superficial blood vessels, increasing circulation to stressed muscles. This extra blood carries oxygen and several components of the immune system's cellular repair kit that speed healing of injured cells. In addition, pain contributes to anxiety, which makes the pain worse. Heat's relaxing effect breaks this vicious cycle, soothing tensions and with them some of the discomfort. "I often recommend hot tubs or hot baths to soothe aching muscles," says fitness expert Suki Munsell, Ph.D., director of the Dynamic Walking Institute in Corte Madera, California.

**Premenstrual syndrome (PMS).** Hot baths help relieve the bloating and irritability of PMS, reports Israeli physician Shlomo Noy, M.D., co-author of *The Manual of Natural Therapy.*

There may also be some other, as-yet-unsubstantiated benefits. Spending time in a hot tub increases metabolism slightly, for example. So it could conceivably help control weight. (How's that for a pleasant weight-loss activity?) And at least one study suggests that heat's antimicrobial effect—similar to that produced by a fever—helps prevent colds.

There are some people, however, who would do well to stay out of hot tubs—pregnant women and men trying to conceive a child.

Hot tubs and saunas are not a good idea for pregnant women, according to Aubrey Milunsky, M.B.B.Ch. (a South African medical degree), director of the Center for Human Genetics at Boston University School of Medicine. In a 1993 study of 23,000 pregnant women, those who used hot tubs frequently during the first two months of pregnancy were almost three times more likely than nonusers to give birth to children with neural tube (brain and spinal cord) defects. Risk of neural tube defects was almost doubled for women who used saunas. (Dr. Milunsky found no increased risk from the use of electric blankets, which do not get as hot as saunas or hot tubs.)

There is also some evidence to suggest that extended use of hot tubs or saunas can depress men's sperm counts, since sperm

# Beware of Hot Tub Rash

Hot-tubbing feels great—but 8 to 48 hours after a steamy soak, you just might break out in an itchy rash. "Hot tub rash is nothing more than a minor annoyance," says Ray Breitenbach, M.D., associate clinical professor of family medicine at Wayne State University School of Medicine in Detroit. "It clears up by itself within a week. But it's a sign that the hot tub you used was not properly disinfected."

Hot tub rash is typically caused by bacteria that naturally live on the skin (*Pseudomonas aeruginosa*). Under normal conditions, these microorganisms pose no problems, but extended immersion in hot water stimulates them to reproduce rapidly, causing an itchy rash, most frequently on areas covered by bathing suits. Several factors increase risk of hot tub rash: higher temperatures, increasing numbers of bathers and water turbulence (through the use of Jacuzzi-type jets).

Since the first outbreak of "whirlpool dermatitis" was documented in 1975, thousands of cases have been reported. Showering beforehand does not prevent the rash, but bacterial overgrowth can be controlled by disinfecting the tub with chlorine. The Centers for Disease Control and Prevention in Atlanta encourage spa owners to maintain chlorine levels at one part per million (ppm) at all times. However, if unusually large numbers of people use the tub and keep the jets on, one ppm might not be sufficient. Extra disinfectant is a good idea before hot tub parties. Anything less would be, well, rash.

are heat-sensitive. Most urologists urge men in infertile couples not to take hot baths.

## Healing with Cold

Across the northern United States, members of "polar bear clubs" delight in swimming in frigid oceans, lakes and streams every winter. "There's no better way to start off a new year," says Judy Irving, a 47-year-old San Francisco filmmaker who swims year-round in the chilly waters of San Francisco Bay.

Since Irving became a Bay swimmer several years ago, she says she's "never felt healthier."

Most Americans, on the other hand, view voluntary immersion in cold water as odd, if not crazy. Well, score one for the polar bears. Cold baths can be quite therapeutic.

*Asthma.* For centuries, cold baths have been a mainstay of traditional Japanese medicine's treatment of asthma. In 1994, Toshio Katsunuma, M.D., a fellow in allergy medicine at the National Children's Hospital in Tokyo, discovered why. He asked 25 children with asthma to stop taking their asthma medication for 12 hours. He then poured about a half-gallon of near-freezing water over their bodies. Within five minutes, sophisticated instruments showed that they were breathing significantly more easily. Later, similar treatment with warm water did not ease the children's breathing. It's not clear why cold water opens the bronchial tubes, which constrict during an asthma attack, but Dr. Katsunuma believes that it produces subtle changes in circulating hormone levels that play a role in constriction.

*Fever.* Cool baths were once routinely recommended for treating fever in the days before aspirin and other fever-reducing medicines. They're still a standard medical recommendation for childhood fevers.

*Low sexual libido.* For more than a century, cold showers have been touted to cool the fire of men's sexual desire. Research, however, suggests they might do exactly the opposite. Libido-dampening cold showers were first recommended by Englishman Robert Baden-Powell, founder of the Boy Scouts, who insisted they would banish "impure thoughts" from adolescent minds. He had no scientific evidence, but his recommendation was generally accepted in the West—until 1993, when Vijay Kakkar, M.D., put it to the test.

Dr. Kakkar, director of the Thrombosis Research Institute of Chelsea in England, was skeptical of Baden-Powell's advice because in his native India, cold baths have been recommended for centuries to invigorate men and enhance their sexual abilities. He subjected volunteers to cold baths and measured their reactions. Icy immersion increased the flow of oxygen within their bodies, boosting their energy. It also elevated their mood and enhanced their immune function. Finally, it increased the levels of testosterone in their blood. Getting more of the male hormone testosterone does not boost the sexual ability of men who already have normal hormone levels, but the increased energy level and mood elevation Dr. Kakkar's study revealed certainly wouldn't *suppress* the male libido.

Dr. Kakkar cautions that anyone with heart disease, high blood pressure or other chronic condition should consult a physician before plunging into cold water.

**Low sperm count.** Because heat kills sperm, researchers wondered if cooling the scrotum might increase sperm quality. In one study, New York urologist Adrian Zorgniotti, M.D., fitted 64 infertile men with special underwear that kept their scrotums unusually cool. After 16 weeks, more than two-thirds showed improved semen quality. If your sperm count is low, or if you're dealing with infertility, cold baths might help.

**Muscle soreness and joint injuries.** Baseball pitchers do it. Basketball and football players do it. After they leave the game, they often slap a bag of ice on their arms, legs or major joints. Athletic trainers believe that icing helps prevent muscle soreness and joint injuries by controlling the swelling caused by minor damage to muscle cells and ligament and tendon fibers. If ice isn't available or doesn't seem to do the trick, trainers recommend a heat treatment.

## First Cold, Then Heat

For some conditions, heat and cold are best used in combination.

**Emotional blues.** For minor emotional blahs, Dr. Noy recommends alternating hot and cold showers twice a day.

**Itching.** For itchy rashes, Dr. Noy recommends alternating hot and cold showers. Some people experience greater relief from a long hot shower followed by a brief cold one. Others prefer a long cold shower followed by brief hot one. Experiment to find out which technique works best for you.

*Muscle and joint injuries.* One minute you're dancing, running, playing tennis or doing something else athletic, and you're feeling fine. The next minute, you feel sharp pain in a muscle or joint. This isn't simple soreness from minor overexertion. It's a more serious injury: a muscle strain or a sprain.

Muscle strains are tears in a significant number of muscle fibers—more than the number that cause muscle soreness but fewer than the number involved in a torn muscle. Sprains are minor tears in the ligaments that connect bone to bone. Standard treatment involves using ice for the first 24 to 48 hours, then heat for another day or two, followed by a cautious return to activity.

Ice is the I in RICE—the acronym for the rest, ice, compression and elevation that constitute first aid for muscle and joint injuries. "Icing a painful muscle or joint immediately after the injury has an anesthetic effect, and it helps minimize swelling," says Anne Simons, M.D., assistant clinical professor of family and community medicine at the University of California's San Francisco Medical Center and author of *Before You Call the Doctor.* You can use either ice cubes or a frozen hot/cold gel pack.

If you use ice cubes, first place them in a plastic bag to prevent messy dripping. Wrap either ice or a gel pack in a cloth and apply it to the injured area for 20 minutes, then remove it for 10 minutes before reapplying. Do not apply ice or ice substitutes directly to the skin, Dr. Simons warns. It can cause skin damage equivalent to frostbite. For the same reason, do not keep an ice pack on an injured area for more than 20 minutes at a time.

After about 24 hours, or as soon as the pain and swelling are under control, Dr. Simons advises substituting heat for the ice pack. "Heat opens the blood vessels in the area," she says, "increasing blood flow, which speeds healing." Use a heating pad or hot compresses or take hot baths. You could also put a hot/cold gel pack in a microwave.

## CHAPTER 15

# HERBAL HEALING

Using the "Roots" of Modern Medicine

It's amazing where you can run into herbal treatments these days.

Recently, a 39-year-old woman who'd just had surgery to remove a cancerous breast tumor met with radiation oncologist Jerold Green, M.D., at California Pacific Medical Center's gleaming, high-tech radiation oncology unit in San Francisco. Dr. Green explained how he planned to treat her breast with x-rays to kill any cancer cells the surgery had missed. He also explained that, unless she took precautions, the treatments would cause a radiation burn on her breast resembling a bad sunburn. His recommendation: Aloe vera gel, an herb that has been used to treat burns for more than 3,000 years. "Buy it at our pharmacy or at any health food store," Dr. Green said. "Just rub it on your breast before and after each treatment."

A decade ago, most physicians scoffed at medicinal herbs. Some still do. But today, medical journals are publishing more herb research than ever. Consumers, who are fascinated by herbal medicine, continually ask their doctors about it. And the threat of plant extinctions has spurred new scientific interest in the healing power of "botanicals." As a result, many mainstream doctors are now incorporating herbs into their practices.

Harvey Komet, M.D., a San Antonio ear, nose and throat specialist, for example, prescribes ginkgo to patients with chronic ringing in their ears (tinnitus)—a condition that's notoriously difficult to treat. "I've gotten good results with ginkgo," he says.

Anne Simons, M.D., assistant clinical professor of family and community medicine at the University of California's San Francisco Medical Center and author of *Before You Call the Doctor,* suggests echinacea for colds and flu. "Studies show it has an antiviral effect," she explains. "I use it myself."

And gynecologist Dorothy Barbo, M.D., director of the Center for Women's Health at the University of New Mexico in Albuquerque, recommends cranberry juice to prevent bladder infections and as a complement to antibiotics used to treat the infections. "Cranberry juice seems to inhibit bacterial growth," she explains.

Other physicians now tout feverfew to prevent migraine headache, garlic to control cholesterol, saw palmetto to treat prostate enlargement, willow bark to prevent heart attack and ginger to relieve nausea. Medicine is moving forward into its herbal past as consumers and doctors alike rediscover the "roots" of healing—not to mention its leaves, stems and flowers.

## Herbal Medicine: Ancient and Thoroughly Modern

The botanical roots of modern medicine are everywhere—if you know where to look. Five thousand years ago, Chinese physicians discovered that a tea made from the ma huang plant, Chinese ephedra, relieved asthma and chest congestion. Today ephedra, available at health food stores and herb shops and through mail-order herb catalogs, is still widely used to treat the chest congestion of colds, flu and allergies.

In fact, millions of people who have no idea they're taking a medicinal herb regularly use a chemical modeled after a constituent of ephedra. "One chemical in Chinese ephedra is the decongestant pseudoephedrine," explains Varro Tyler, Ph.D., professor of pharmacognosy at Purdue University in West Lafayette, Indiana, and author of *The New Honest Herbal.* Pharmaceutical companies now synthesize pseudoephedrine as the decongestant in Actifed, Allerest, Contac, Tylenol Cold and Flu, NyQuil, Formula 44 and other cold formulas and allergy products. One brand—Sudafed—even takes its name from pseudoephedrine.

Ancient India's traditional Ayurvedic medicine dates back 4,500 years to the ancient Hindu text, the *Rig Veda,* which mentions 67 medicinal herbs, including senna to treat constipation and cinnamon for stomach upsets. These herbs are still used medicinally.

"Senna contains anthraquinone glycosides, chemicals that have powerful laxative action," says James Duke, Ph.D., a botanist with the U.S. Department of Agriculture's Research Station in Beltsville, Maryland, and author of many herb guides, including *The Handbook of Medicinal Herbs.* Senna is an ingredient in many commercial laxatives, including Gentlax, Senokot, Fletcher's Castoria and Innerclean Herbal Laxative.

"Cinnamon helps relieve stomach distress because its oil has antimicrobial properties," says Daniel Mowrey, Ph.D., director of the American Phytotherapy (plant medicine) Research Laboratory in Salt Lake City and author of *The Scientific Validation of Herbal Medicine.* Today we have better treatments for intestinal infections, but cinnamon has been incorporated into several toothpastes, in part because it tastes good but also because its antibiotic action helps kill the bacteria that cause tooth decay and gum disease.

And so it goes. Untold numbers of herbs used in healing during ancient times are still in use today, many of them incorporated into common over-the-counter and prescription medications. And researchers are continually finding new uses for medicinal plants.

## Acceptance Grows

These days, ever-increasing numbers of people are returning to herbs—or learning about them for the first time. Herbal beverage teas line supermarket shelves, and most health food stores do a brisk business in medicinal herb teas and tinctures (the liquid form of the herb plus alcohol).

Recently a woman who was about to begin chemotherapy following surgery to remove a malignant colon tumor met with her oncologist, Barry Rosenbloom, M.D., at Cedars-Sinai Medical Center in Los Angeles. After describing his state-of-the-art, three-drug chemotherapy program, Dr. Rosenbloom mentioned the treatment's major side effect, nausea. But he assured the woman that he could prescribe medication to treat it. "Oh, no," the woman thought, "not another drug."

Anticipating nausea from chemotherapy, the woman had already decided she wanted to try a friend's herbal treatment, ginger tea. She expected her oncologist to oppose the idea, so her friend armed her with information about research on ginger. (A scientific study showed that ginger relieves the nausea of motion sickness better than a standard pharmaceutical treatment, Dramamine.) The woman told Dr. Rosenbloom that instead of the anti-nausea drug, she'd really rather use ginger—then she braced herself for an argument.

"Ginger?" Dr. Rosenbloom said, "Sure, why not? It's very good for nausea. Drink ginger ale or grind up the fresh root and make tea. You know, ginger has been used to treat nausea for thousands of years."

## Regulatory Limbo

If herbs are so great, why aren't they more widely known and used?

To claim that any herb or pharmaceutical has medicinal value, it must be either a traditional medicine specifically exempted from current Food and Drug Administration (FDA) regulations or it must win FDA approval by passing a series of rigorous scientific tests. In the early 1960s, when current FDA rules were drafted, herbal medicine was nowhere near as popular as it is today, so only a few herbs were grandfathered in. One was mint, which contains menthol, an approved treatment for nasal and chest congestion. But the vast majority of herbs were not exempted. They were ignored.

The FDA approval process costs a fortune—more than

$100 million per drug. Large pharmaceutical companies have these vast sums and are willing to invest them, because new drugs can be patented and sold, often at high prices, to recoup development and approval costs. "But no one is going to put up that kind of money to prove to the FDA that garlic lowers cholesterol," says Mark Blumenthal, executive director of the American Botanical Council in Austin, Texas, and editor of the medicinal herb research journal, *HerbalGram*. "Many studies show that it does, but the FDA can't grant anyone exclusive rights to garlic, so there's no way to recoup the approval costs. The same goes for literally hundreds of other herbal medicines. You can't patent plants, so under current FDA regulations, there's no incentive to get them approved for medicinal use."

As a result, most medicinal herbs exist in regulatory limbo. They are sold as foods, not as medicines. Blumenthal and other herb advocates are working to change this situation, but in an odd way, it reflects herbal medicine's place in the natural world. The cultures that gave us medicinal herbs drew no distinction between foods and drugs. Traditional healers around the world have always said, "Let your food be your medicine."

## Concerns about Safety

Many people—and their doctors—who want to try herbs approach the subject with caution. If herbs really have medicinal value, are they safe to use?

Herbal experts say that medical journals through the years have tended to overreport herb hazards and underreport their benefits. Journals have created the impression that using medicinal herbs is a fairly risky thing to do. Statistics compiled by the American Association of Poison Control Centers tell a different story. During two recent (and typical) years, pharmaceuticals caused 974 deaths and 6,978 major nonfatal poisonings. Plants caused just 2 deaths and 53 major poisonings. Herbal medicines caused virtually no problems. The most hazardous plants were not herbal medicines but ornamentals: jade, holly, poinsettia, schefflera, philodendron and dieffenbachia. The typical victim was a child under age five who ingested the plant by accident.

While the vast majority of herbal medicines present no danger to health, using them does require knowledge and proper caution. Too much of any good thing can cause harm, and studies show that a few herbs that were once considered safe for internal use are in fact hazardous. In large doses, comfrey—a traditional digestive remedy—can cause liver damage. So can coltsfoot, long used to treat cough. In addition, just about any herb might cause an allergic reaction.

For healthy individuals who are not pregnant, the herbs in this book are all considered safe in recommended amounts. However, pregnant women should consult their physicians before using any medicinal herbs (or pharmaceuticals). Most herbal medicines should not be given to children under age 2. Children under 16 and anyone over 65 should dilute herbal preparations to reduce the dose. And those with chronic medical conditions should consult their physicians before supplementing medical therapies with herbs.

## How Herbs Are Sold

Medicinal herbs are available at health food stores, herb shops, supplement outlets, some pharmacies and supermarkets and through mail-order catalogs (see Resources). They're marketed in so many different forms that many people become confused. Here's what's available.

*Bulk herbs.* Typically found in jars or bins at health food stores, bulk herbs are the raw, dried plant material. They're available loose and are usually sold by the ounce. Bulk herbs can be used in teas, soaked in vodka to make tinctures, powdered to make tablets or capsules or moistened and placed under bandages as poultices.

*Oils.* These superconcentrated herbal essences are used in aromatherapy (page 37) and are for external use only. Many herbs that are safe to use in teas ("infusions") are poisonous when highly concentrated into essential oils. One example is pennyroyal—a member of the mint family that is the natural insect repellent in most herbal flea collars. In infusions, pennyroyal helps settle the stomach and relieve cough and chest congestion. But as little as two tablespoons of pennyroyal oil can be fatal. Never ingest any kind of herbal oil.

*Tablets and capsules.* Today, the word pills suggests pharmaceuticals, but the modern pill was actually invented by early America's leading herbalists, the Shakers. This religious community is best known for crafting fine furniture, but in the 1830s the Shakers began selling medicinal herbs by mail, and they had trouble shipping bulk herbs and tinctures. Shaker woodworkers solved the problem by drilling peg holes into small wooden frames. The herbalists hammered powdered herbs into the holes and created the first pills. Like tinctures, herb tablets and capsules store easily and travel well.

*Teas.* Technically "hot-water extracts," there are three kinds of teas: beverage teas, infusions and decoctions. Beverage teas are typically steeped for a minute or two. Infusions are prepared like teas but are steeped for 10 to 20 minutes to extract more of the plant's healing constituents. Decoctions require simmering the plant material in boiling water for 10 to 20 minutes. Drink infusions and decoctions cool, or reheat them. If taste is a problem (many medicinal herbs are quite bitter), add honey or sugar and lemon or mix them with a beverage tea.

*Tinctures.* These "alcohol extracts" are highly concentrated. Tinctures come in small bottles with eyedropper caps, and a few drops often pack as much medicinal punch as a cup of strong infusion. You can take some tinctures, such as echinacea, straight from the bottle, but most go down easier when added to beverage teas. Tinctures stay potent longer than bulk herbs or tea bags, and their concentration makes them compact—good for travel or conserving shelf space in medicine cabinets.

## Getting the Right Dose

Those who use over-the-counter and prescription pharmaceuticals always know exactly how much medicine they're taking because FDA regulations require precision. People who use herbs face more of a challenge.

Some herb companies offer standardized doses in packaged herbal preparations. But when you're using bulk herbs, you can't be certain how much of the active constituents are in the herb. Herb potency depends on such things as plant genetics, growing conditions, maturity at harvest, time in storage and preparation method. Also, some of the more expensive herbs are sometimes adulterated by unscrupulous dealers.

Even with all this uncertainty, in controlled doses, herbs cause fewer side effects than pharmaceuticals. Pharmaceuticals are highly concentrated, and pills and capsules have little taste, factors that make it easy to overdose. The active constituents in herbs are typically less concentrated, and most taste quite bitter, which discourages taking too much. The dosages recommended in this book represent a consensus of the opinions found in both traditional references (herbals) and modern scientific sources. In the few cases where these sources disagree significantly, *Nature's Cures* recommends the smaller amount, in the belief that it's best to err on the side of caution.

## The Healing Herbs

Once you decide you want to use herbs, you're still left with some key questions. Which herbs? And how do you use them? Here is a list of common, safe and effective herbs to choose from, along with information about the conditions they treat and directions for their use.

## Aloe Vera

In ancient Egypt (1500 B.C.), the *Ebers Papyrus* recommended aloe vera for skin problems, and the world has been using this herb ever since. Chinese, Greek, Roman and Arab herbalists recommended it for wounds, burns, rashes and hemorrhoids. During the 1930s, radiologists discovered aloe vera's effectiveness in treating radiation burns. The latest scientific studies show that the herb has clear value in treating minor cuts, scrapes and burns.

*How-to:* "Keep a potted aloe in your kitchen, where most household burns occur," says Dr. Mowrey. "That way it's handy when you need it." Snip off a leaf, slit it open, scoop out the jelly-like material (gel) and apply it to the affected area. Aloe vera gel may also be purchased commercially, but fresh gel works best. (Snipping an occasional leaf doesn't harm the plant.)

## Chamomile

When Peter Rabbit ate himself sick in Mr. McGregor's garden and got chased out at the wrong end of a hoe, his mother gave him chamomile tea, a traditional remedy for indigestion, anxiety and wounds. Peter's mom was a wise woman . . . er, bunny. German herbalists once used chamomile so extensively, they called it *alles zutraut,* "capable of anything."

That's an exaggeration, but recent studies show that this popular beverage herb does indeed calm jangled nerves, relieve stomach distress, prevent ulcers and speed their healing and help fight infection by stimulating the immune system.

"Chamomile tea is an excellent home remedy for indigestion, heartburn and infant colic," says Dr. Duke. "It also has mild relaxant and sedative properties."

*How-to:* For an infusion, use two to three heaping teaspoons of dried or fresh flowers per cup of boiling water. Steep 10 to 20 minutes. Reheat if desired. Drink up to three cups a day. Dilute infusions may be given to infants for colic.

In a tincture, use ½ to 1 teaspoon up to three times a day.

When using commercial preparations, follow package directions.

For a relaxing herbal bath, fill a cloth bag with a few handfuls of dried or fresh flowers and let the water run over it.

## Comfrey

The ancient Greeks used powdered comfrey root poultices on wounds. Modern science has discovered that the plant contains a chemical—allantoin—that promotes the growth of new cells. Comfrey also has mild anti-inflammatory action, adding to its value in wound and burn treatment. Traditional herbalists revered comfrey for digestive problems, but recent studies have shown that it contains liver-damaging chemicals, so internal use is no longer recommended. But for wounds, comfrey is still a great healer.

*How-to:* Mix the powdered root with water to make a paste. Apply it to the injured area and cover with a clean bandage. Change the bandage and comfrey preparation daily. "I've seen complete healing of major skin wounds using this method," says Andrew Weil, M.D., professor of preventive medicine at the University of Arizona College of Medicine in Tucson and author of *Natural Health, Natural Healing*.

## Dill Seed

Dill is best known as the spice in pickles. Centuries before refrigeration, herbalists discovered that adding dill increased the shelf life of pickles. Today we know why: Dill inhibits the growth of food-spoiling microbes. That's also why dill can soothe an upset stomach. Our word *dill* comes from the Vikings' word *dilla*, "to soothe." Dill has been used as a digestive aid from Europe to China for more than 1,000 years, and dillwater—cooled dill infusion—continues to be used as a stomach soother around the world. "For infant colic, I often recommend a combination of dill and fennel," Dr. Duke says. "Both soothe the stomach and are gentle enough for babies."

*How-to:* For an infusion, use two teaspoons of bruised seeds per cup of boiling water. Steep ten minutes. Reheat if desired. Drink up to three cups a day. Dilute dill infusion may be given cautiously to infants for colic.

In a tincture, use ½ to 1 teaspoon up to three times a day.

## Echinacea

Echinacea root was the Plains Indians' herb of choice for wounds, infections and insect and snake bites. Early settlers adopted echinacea, including Dr. H. C. F. Meyer of Pawnee City, Nebraska, who used it in a patent medicine that he touted as a remedy for dozens of ailments, including rattlesnake bite. In 1885 he sent a sample to Cincinnati pharmacist John Lloyd, an early president of the American Pharmaceutical Association. Lloyd scoffed at echinacea. Outraged, Meyer offered to appear in Cincinnati with a live rattlesnake and allow himself to be bitten in Lloyd's presence to prove that his herbal medicine worked.

Lloyd declined, but he took another look at echinacea and became impressed with its antibiotic properties. His drug firm popularized echinacea as an infection fighter, and other drug companies followed with their own echinacea products. During the early twentieth century, millions of U.S. medicine cabinets contained tincture of echinacea. But in the 1930s, as modern antibiotics became widely available, Americans largely abandoned this herb. Fortunately, Europeans continued to use it—and study it. German research has shown that the beautiful daisylike plant stimulates the immune system against viruses, bacteria and fungi. "Try echinacea as a first treatment for colds and flu, or for treatment of bacterial infections before resorting to antibiotics," suggests Dr. Simons.

*How-to:* Most herbalists recommend using a tincture. Add one teaspoon to water, juice or a beverage tea. Use up to three times a day.

For a decoction, add two teaspoons of root material per cup of boiling water and simmer 15 minutes. Drink up to three cups a day.

When using commercial teas, follow package directions.

Shortly after ingestion, echinacea causes an odd numbing of the tongue that is temporary and harmless.

## Ephedra

In addition to its decongestant value, Chinese ephedra has a long history of use in Asia as a coffeelike stimulant. Recent studies have also shown that ephedra boosts metabolic rate—the speed at which the body burns calories. As a result, it has shown some benefit as a weight-loss aid, but only in those who are significantly overweight. Ephedra can also increase heart rate and blood pressure, so don't use it if you have high blood pressure, heart disease, diabetes or glaucoma.

You should also not take ephedra if you have thyroid problems. In fact, ephedra has been shown to be harmful when taken improperly and should not be used by anyone with health problems. If you want to take ephedra or any product containing ephedra, you should discuss it with your doctor.

*How-to:* For a decoction, use one teaspoon of twigs per cup of boiling water. Simmer 10 to 15 minutes. Reheat if desired. Drink up to two cups a day.

In a tincture, take up to ¼ teaspoon a day.

When using commercial preparations, follow package directions.

## Feverfew

Some herbalists claim that this healer got its name from traditional use as a fever remedy—a tempting assertion, but incorrect. *Feverfew* is actually a corruption of the Old English featherfew, a reference to the plant's feathery leaf borders. The ancient Greeks and Romans prescribed it for gynecological problems. In 1640, British botanist John Parkinson called feverfew "very effectual for paines in the head," and a century later, another English herbalist, John Hill, wrote that "in the worst headache, this herb exceeds whatever else is known." But their recommendations were largely forgotten.

Then about ten years ago, a happy accident occurred. The wife of a doctor with the British National Coal Board had migraines. A coal miner confided that he'd been cursed with the horrible headaches until he began chewing two feverfew leaves a day. The woman tried the herb and noticed immediate improvement—fewer and less severe migraines. Intrigued, her husband urged a London migraine specialist to test feverfew. Now several studies have shown it to be effective. Feverfew also calms the digestive tract and may help reduce blood pressure.

*How-to:* For migraine control, chew two fresh (or frozen) leaves a day or take a pill or capsule containing 85 milligrams of leaf material. Most people prefer pills or capsules to leaves, since feverfew is quite bitter.

For an infusion, use ½ to 1 teaspoon per cup of boiling water. Steep five to ten minutes. Reheat if desired. Drink up to two cups a day.

In a tincture, take up to one teaspoon a day.

When using commercial preparations, follow package directions. Don't give feverfew to children under the age of 2. For older children or people over age 65, start with low-strength preparations and increase strength if necessary.

## Garlic

After ephedra, garlic is considered the world's second oldest medicine (along with its close botanical relatives onions, scallions, leeks, chives and shallots). The oldest surviving garlic prescription, chiseled into a Sumerian clay tablet, dates from 3000 B.C. The ancient world revered garlic as a virtual panacea, but none loved it as deeply as the Egyptians, who consumed so much that the Greek historian Herodotus called them "the stinking ones." As the centuries passed, Europeans hung braided garlic plants from their doorposts to keep evil spirits at bay—a custom echoed today in the garlic braids that adorn many kitchens.

During World War I, army doctors used garlic juice quite effectively to treat wounds and dysentery. After the war, scientists discovered why it worked: When chewed or chopped, garlic is a potent natural antibiotic. In fact, ten medium cloves pack approximately the same antibiotic punch as a typical dose of penicillin. Garlic also has antiviral properties.

"Garlic is a very useful herb," Dr. Duke says. "Studies show that it helps protect against stomach cancer and reduces risk of heart disease by lowering blood pressure, reducing cholesterol and decreasing the likelihood of blood clots that can trigger heart attack."

*How-to:* In food, use as seasoning to taste. The cloves' papery skins peel easily if you smash them with the flat side of a cleaver.

For an infusion, use six chopped cloves per cup of cool water and steep six hours.

In a tincture, take up to three tablespoons a day.

## Ginger

Scientific research has shown that ginger fights nausea better than the over-the-counter anti-nausea drug Dramamine. This root herb does more than simply soothe the stomach, however. An ancient Indian proverb says, "Every good quality is contained in ginger." Well, not quite, but studies show that it also boosts the immune system's ability to fight infection. And like garlic, it lowers blood pressure and cholesterol and helps prevent the blood clots that trigger heart attack.

*How-to:* For motion sickness, take 1,500 milligrams 30 minutes before departure. Ginger capsules are usually most convenient, but a 12-ounce glass of ginger ale also provides the recommended amount—if it's made with real ginger, not artificial flavor.

For an infusion, use two teaspoons of powdered or grated root per cup of boiling water. Steep ten minutes. Drink up to three cups a day. Dilute ginger infusion may be used to treat infant colic. If you buy whole root, refrigerate it.

## Ginkgo

A relic of the dinosaur age, ginkgo is the oldest surviving tree on earth. Poetically, it helps the oldest people. China's first historically recognized herbalist, Shen Nung (c. 3000 B.C.), called ginkgo "good for the heart and lungs." And traditional Chinese physicians have used it for thousands of years to treat asthma.

India's traditional Ayurvedic physicians believed ginkgo enhanced longevity. It was introduced into the West as an ornamental in the 1700s, and today thousands of huge ginkgoes adorn streets and parks from Prague to Portland, Oregon. But this herb was not used medicinally in the West until the early 1970s, when scientists proved old Shen Nung correct. Ginkgo really is good for the heart, lungs and longevity.

Studies show that ginkgo helps prevent asthma attacks. But its effectiveness against many infirmities of old age is astonishing.

Ginkgo increases blood flow to the brain, speeding recovery from stroke and improving memory, and to the heart, so it may help prevent heart attack. It also increases blood flow into the penis and helps some men with erection impairment.

When cholesterol deposits narrow the arteries in the legs, the result is a painful condition called intermittent claudication. In one study, ginkgo produced "significantly greater pain relief than standard therapy." Finally, studies show ginkgo effective in the treatment of chronic ringing in the ears (tinnitus), one form of hearing loss (cochlear deafness) and age-related vision loss (macular degeneration).

*How-to:* Bulk ginkgo cannot be used because it takes a huge number of leaves to make a small amount of medicinal preparation. Many herb companies market ginkgo products. Follow package directions.

## Ginseng

Prized above gold for thousands of years, ginseng root has been Asia's most revered "tonic." It was viewed as an aphrodisiac that strengthens the body, enhances health and aids longevity. Early Jesuit missionaries in Canada discovered American ginseng in 1704 and made a fortune shipping it to China. The herb was eventually discovered growing as far south as Georgia, and it quickly became one of the American colonies' most valuable exports, until overcollection just about wiped it out. Today American ginseng is farmed in Wisconsin. Most of the crop is shipped to Asia.

Until recently, Western scientists scoffed at ginseng claims. But research evidence is mounting that the herb helps the body resist illness and damage from stress. Studies show that ginseng stimulates the immune system, helps reduce cholesterol levels, protects the liver from toxic substances and increases stamina and nutrient absorption from the intestines. Asian Olympic athletes take it regularly to boost their performance.

*How-to:* Herb companies market ginseng teas, capsules, tablets and tinctures. Follow package directions.

For a decoction, add ½ teaspoon of powdered root per cup of boiling water. Simmer ten minutes. Drink up to two cups a day.

## Goldenseal

A favorite Native American infection fighter, goldenseal was widely used to treat battle wounds during the Civil War and has been a popular folk antibiotic ever since. A survey of folk healing in Indiana showed that goldenseal is still used extensively to treat wounds and infections. No wonder: "Many studies show that it's a powerful antibiotic," Dr. Mowrey says. "It also has immune stimulant properties."

*How-to:* For an infusion, use 1/2 to 1 teaspoon of powdered root per cup of boiling water. Steep ten minutes. Drink up to two cups a day.

In a tincture, take ½ to 1 teaspoon up to twice a day.

When using commercial preparations, follow package directions.

## Mint

The ancient Egyptians relied on peppermint and spearmint to relax the digestive tract. Chinese and traditional Indian Ayurvedic physicians used them to treat colds, coughs and fever. European herbalists adopted all these uses.

American colonists brought the mints to these shores, where they discovered that Native Americans were already using American mints to aid digestion, relieve cold symptoms and treat chest congestion.

"Mints continue to be widely used as stomach soothers," says Dr. Tyler. Try a cup of mint tea after eating. In addition, mint oil (menthol) is an ingredient in several over-the-counter indigestion remedies, including milk of magnesia. Menthol is also an FDA-approved decongestant used in such cold formulas as Vicks Vaporub. Finally, menthol has anesthetic properties. It's an ingredient in several pain-relieving skin creams, including Solarcaine.

*How-to:* For an infusion, use one teaspoon of fresh herb or two teaspoons of dried leaves per cup of boiling water. Steep ten minutes. Reheat if desired. Drink up to three cups a day. Peppermint has a sharper taste than spearmint, and it feels cooler in the mouth.

In a tincture, take 1/4 to 1 teaspoon up to three times a day.

When using commercial preparations, follow package directions.

For a relaxing herbal bath, fill a cloth bag with a few handfuls of dried or fresh leaves and let the water run over it.

## Rosemary

Long before refrigeration was available, the ancients noticed that wrapping meat in crushed rosemary leaves preserved it and imparted a tasty flavor. To this day, the herb remains a favorite addition to meat dishes, and its preservative action led to its use in herbal medicine. Meats spoil in part because oxidation turns their fats rancid. Rosemary oil retards spoilage and compares favorably with the commercial preservatives BHA and BHT. Rosemary's preservative action may help prevent food poisoning at your next picnic. Mix the crushed herb into burger meat and tuna, pasta and potato salads. Rosemary also helps soothe the stomach.

*How-to:* For an infusion, use one teaspoon of crushed leaves per cup of boiling water. Steep 10 to 15 minutes. Drink up to three cups a day.

In a tincture, use 1/4 to 1/2 teaspoon up to three times a day.

## Saw Palmetto

This palm tree native to the southeastern United States produces a dark berry that was used by physicians a century ago to treat urinary problems. By the 1950s, it had been abandoned.

Recently, though, several studies have shown that extract of saw palmetto berries helps treat prostate enlargement, the urinary bane of men over the age of 50. The prostate grows larger with age and eventually pinches the tube through which urine exits the body (the urethra), making it difficult for older men to empty their bladders. In these studies, daily use of saw palmetto extract significantly increased urine output.

*How-to:* For relief of prostate symptoms, the recommended dose is 160 milligrams twice a day. It's impossible to obtain that dose from the plant material; it would require a half-pound of berries a day. A company called Phyto-Pharmica markets Saw Palmetto Complex capsules containing 80 milligrams of extract. Since the company sells only to licensed health professionals such as physicians, pharmacists, acupuncturists and chiropractors, ask a health professional to order saw palmetto for you from Phyto-Pharmica, P.O. Box 1358, Green Bay, WI 54305. Take two capsules twice a day.

## Slippery Elm Bark

The colonists found Native Americans using the inner portion of slippery elm bark as a food and as treatment for wounds, sore throat, cough—anything than needed soothing. Early Americans adopted the herb enthusiastically. In fact, no food or drug of today comes close to matching the place of honor slippery elm held in eighteenth- and nineteenth-century America. Great elm forests covered the East, and even in cities the versatile bark was always close at hand.

Coarsely ground and mixed with water, it became a spongy mass used to bandage wounds. Ground and mixed with milk, it turned into a soothing, nutritious food similar to oatmeal, which was used to soothe sore throats, coughs, upset stomachs and infant colic. And slippery elm sore throat lozenges were a fixture in home medicine chests.

Today, tragically, Dutch elm disease has decimated our elm forests, and our landscape and herbalism are poorer as a result. But the beneficial bark is still available in bulk and in herbal cough drops and sore throat lozenges.

*How-to:* For a poultice, mix the powdered bark with water to make a paste. Apply the paste to the affected area, then cover it with a bandage. Change the bandage and slippery elm preparation daily.

For a soothing decoction, use one to three teaspoons of powdered bark per cup of water. Blend a little water in first to prevent lumpiness. Bring to a boil and simmer for 15 minutes. Drink up to three cups a day.

## Valerian

In the thirteenth century, when the elders of Hamelin, Germany, refused to pay an itinerant flute player for ridding the town of rats, the Pied Piper charmed the town's children away with his hypnotic music. At least that's how the modern version goes. In the original, the Pied Piper used music and valerian root, which contains hypnotic chemicals similar to those in catnip.

Studies show that valerian has tranquilizing and sedative properties similar to Valium's, but it's nonaddictive. In Europe, dozens of valerian-based sleep aids are sold over the counter. "It works," says Dr. Mowrey, "and it's safer than most pharmaceutical sleeping pills."

*How-to:* Valerian is quite bitter. Commercial preparations and tinctures are usually more palatable than the infusion. Follow package directions.

If you'd like to try the infusion, use two teaspoons of powdered root per cup of boiling water. Steep 10 to 15 minutes. Add sugar, honey or lemon or mix it with a beverage tea. Drink one cup before bed.

In a tincture, take ½ to 1 teaspoon before bed. Don't give to children under 2. For older children and people over the age of

65, start with low-strength preparations and increase strength
if necessary.

## Witch Hazel

Native Americans used the plant to make bows, and many
tribes drank witch hazel tea to treat colds, fever, sore throat and
menstrual cramps. They also rubbed the tea on cuts, bruises, insect stings and sore muscles and joints. In the 1840s, an Oneida
medicine man introduced this herb's medicinal uses to a patent-
medicine entrepreneur. Witch hazel has been a medicine cabinet
mainstay ever since.

Even mainstream M.D.'s who are skeptical of herbs recommend this traditional treatment for cuts, bruises, hemorrhoids
and rashes. More than one million gallons of witch hazel water
are sold in the United States annually.

*How-to:* Commercial witch hazel water should be used ex-
ternally only. It is available at pharmacies and some supermarkets. Moisten a clean cloth and apply it to the affected area.

## CHAPTER 16

# HOMEOPATHY

## Tiny Treatments with a Big Payoff

There are few things that pain physicians more deeply than having to watch helplessly as their children endure illnesses that they are powerless to treat. Hayward, California, podiatrist Steven Subotnick, D.P.M., felt this special agony some years ago when his 14-year-old son, Mark, was plagued by chronic bronchitis. Every few months the boy would develop the chest infection, and three times it progressed to pneumonia.

Dr. Subotnick felt his therapeutic helplessness keenly because he wasn't just any physician. In the world of sports medicine, he was a celebrity, a medical visionary who'd almost single-handedly wedded podiatry and running, developing the biomechanical insights responsible for curing thousands of runners' foot, ankle, shin and knee problems. Physicians around the world called for his advice. On the wall of his office was an autographed photo of basketball great Bill Walton, inscribed, "To Steve: Thanks for the help."

But Walton's thanks rang hollow as Dr. Subotnick watched his son cough, choke and wheeze through yet another bout of bronchitis. His wife, Jan, shuttled Mark back and forth to their family doctor, who prescribed the standard therapy—antibiotics. Each time, the antibiotics helped, but almost as fast as you could say "erythromycin," Mark developed another chest infection. By this time the Subotnicks were at their wits' end.

## Oh, No, Not Homeopathy!

At the time, Jan Subotnick was a stained-glass artist who was involved in a career change to hypnotherapy. She and her husband had always had different ideas about health and healing. Dr. Subotnick viewed the body as a machine. When stress on the foot threw it out of whack, you either cushioned it or went in surgically to fix it. Jan had always gravitated toward Nature's cures: health foods, acupuncture, meditation and so forth.

As she watched her son suffer, she recalled a friend who'd had a chronic ear problem. Regular doctors couldn't help her, but a homeopath did. She decided to take Mark to a homeopath.

Dr. Subotnick had always tolerated his wife's offbeat notions about health, but as far as he was concerned, homeopathy was ridiculous. It was scientifically impossible. Its alleged medicines were so dilute that quite often they didn't contain even a single molecule of the active ingredient.

"Steve wasn't happy with my decision," Jan recalls. "But he knew that once I made up my mind about something, that was that."

Jan scheduled an appointment for Mark to see William Gray, M.D., at the Hahnemann Clinic in Berkeley. Dr. Gray is a Stanford-trained physician who, like Samuel Hahnemann, creator of homeopathy 200 years ago, revolted against what he viewed as the downside of mainstream ("allopathic" or "regular") medicine: drugs that worked against the body rather than with it and whose side effects were sometimes as debilitating as the diseases they cured. Among the nation's estimated 2,000 homeopaths (about half of them M.D.'s), Dr. Gray is considered one of the best.

In an hour-long interview, he asked Mark all sorts of questions, not just about his illness but about his life. Did he like his food bland or spicy? Did he prefer to be indoors or out? Did he go along with the crowd or was he a loner? Did he like salt?

Sweets? Was he often thirsty? Dr. Gray considered Mark's overall symptom picture and prescribed a superdilute dose of mercury.

When Dr. Subotnick heard the word mercury, he flipped. Mercury was poison. Superdilute or not, he insisted that Mark not take it. But it was too late. His son already had.

"Shortly after Mark took the mercury, he got much sicker," Jan, now a hypnotherapist in Oakland, recalls. "He fell into bed and just slept. We were pretty worried. But when he woke up the next morning, he wasn't coughing and had no chest congestion. He was cured."

"It was amazing," Dr. Subotnick recalls. "I'd never seen a recovery like that."

Over the next year, Mark had two more bouts of bronchitis. Both times, he took homeopathic mercury and the infection cleared up overnight. Today his chronic chest problem is a fading memory. His mother says, "He hasn't had bronchitis in years."

In spite of himself, Dr. Subotnick couldn't help feeling intrigued by homeopathy. It wasn't the first time he'd ventured beyond the medical mainstream.

## Breaking New Ground

Steve Subotnick hung out his podiatry shingle in 1970. Among his first patients was a pioneering distance runner named Joe Henderson, editor of a fledgling newsletter called *Runner's World*. "Distance running wasn't popular back then, but I was 30 pounds overweight and eager to find a way to get back in shape. Joe urged me to try running, and I enjoyed it. It was good exercise, and as a podiatrist, I liked a sport that was so focused on the feet."

By the mid-1970s, running had become all the rage—and many of its casualties were hobbling into Dr. Subotnick's office. "At the time, the conventional medical wisdom was that the feet had nothing to do with knee problems," he recalls. "But as a runner, it was clear to me the two were connected. All these runners were coming to me for foot problems, but they also had bad knees. I theorized that problems with foot plant explained an enormous number of runners' medical problems up and down their legs."

Dr. Subotnick promoted this novel idea as the medical columnist for *Runner's World,* by then a national magazine. He also talked it up as a clinical professor of biomechanics and surgery at the California College of Podiatric Medicine in San Francisco. "Initially my colleagues scoffed at me. Medicine is very conservative," he says. "But my approach—correcting the foot plant—proved very successful, and eventually the doubters changed their minds. Seeing is believing. Today foot-plant correction is the standard of care."

## A New Look at an Old Therapy

Seeing is believing. Or is it? Dr. Subotnick had seen his son's suffering. He'd seen antibiotics do little more than create brief pauses between flare-ups of bronchitis. And he'd seen homeopathy apparently effect a cure. Jan Subotnick was certain that homeopathic mercury had cured Mark. But her husband remained unconvinced.

As a scientist, Dr. Subotnick never drew conclusions from a single case, or even from several. Such "anecdotal evidence" was intriguing, but it could not be considered conclusive. Perhaps Mark's cure was a delayed effect of the antibiotics. Or maybe it was just luck.

Nonetheless, Dr. Subotnick couldn't get homeopathy out of his mind. He checked through the scientific literature. Oddly, there were very few studies. Then by chance, while attending a medical lecture, he met homeopath Dana Ullman of Berkeley, whose company, Homeopathic Educational Services, is a national leader in promoting the controversial healing art. They talked, and Ullman offered to sponsor an experiment in Dr. Subotnick's office.

"Dana gave me six homeopathic treatments for sports injuries," Dr. Subotnick explains, "and some books with basic instructions on how to use them. I didn't know what I was doing, but in about 40 percent of cases, I got good results using things like *Arnica* (extract of mountain daisy), which is a general remedy for sports injuries, and *Ruta grav,* (extract of rue), which is good for sore knees. I got my best results in the area of swelling control. After foot surgery, it can take quite a while for swelling to go down. I found that with homeopathic medicines, it subsided much faster."

Or did it? Dr. Subotnick knew that any scientist could poke huge holes through his informal study. Perhaps his own improving surgical skills accounted for his patients' rapid recovery. In addition, he had no control group who received only standard care without homeopathy, so he had no basis for comparison.

More important, Dr. Subotnick's informal study was open to charges of experimental bias. To be scientifically credible, experiments must be "placebo-controlled" and "double-blind." In a scientifically rigorous study, participants are divided into two groups. One group receives the test medication, while the other group is given a placebo—a look-alike dummy treatment that has no benefit. In addition, neither the researchers nor the participants know who is getting which treatment until the end of the experiment, when the codes are broken and the data are analyzed.

Dr. Subotnick's office test was neither placebo-controlled nor double-blind. Perhaps his subconscious desire to see the homeopathic medicines work affected his judgment. Perhaps his encouraging remarks about the homeopathic medicines affected his patients' perceptions about their postoperative swelling. Or perhaps the homeopathic medicines were merely placebos. A number of scientific studies have shown that if you give people anything and call it medicine, about one-third of them report improvement.

In fact, homeopathy's critics charge that it's nothing more than an elaborate system of placebos. Dr. Subotnick's 40 percent success rate was within the realm of what could be expected from placebos.

Dr. Subotnick knew his study wasn't serious science. But something seemed to be going on. Maybe homeopathy was impossible, but that's what Alexander Fleming thought in 1928 when some mold accidentally landed on a bacterial culture in his lab and wiped it out. That "impossibility" gave us penicillin. On the other hand, just because something is unorthodox doesn't mean that it works.

Then one day in 1988, a famous wilderness adventurer consulted Dr. Subotnick. "He'd led mountain-climbing expeditions all over the world," Dr. Subotnick recalls. "But he'd developed a neurological problem that had deformed his foot. He couldn't climb. He could barely walk. He said, 'Doc, I've tried everything. You're my last hope. I need a miracle.'

"After examining him, I knew podiatry had nothing to offer, so I asked if he'd like to take a chance on homeopathy. He said he had nothing to lose, so I gave him *Zincum* (zinc), not really expecting that it could help such a serious problem. But it worked. Everyone was amazed: the patient, his regular doctor and myself. Today his 'untreatable' foot is almost normal, and he has no functional limitations."

The man's recovery certainly had all the markings of a miracle. But in medicine, "miracles" are not all that rare. Every day someone somewhere walks away from a wheelchair or outlives the doctor who diagnosed 'terminal' cancer. Dr. Subotnick didn't know what to think. But the adventurer's foot cure persuaded him to train as a homeopath.

In early 1989, he enrolled at the Hahnemann Clinic's College of Homeopathy, a four-year, four-day-a-month training program for licensed health-care practitioners interested in using homeopathy in their practices. The school is one of only a dozen homeopathic training facilities in the United States today, a far cry from the 100 schools that flourished around the country a century ago.

## Finding a Gentle Alternative

During the early nineteenth century, physicians knew little about diseases or what cured them. They treated most illnesses with bleeding, violent laxatives (cathartics), drugs that caused vomiting (emetics) and mercury, which had been shown effective against syphilis 200 years earlier and had evolved into a treatment for just about everything. These medications were called "heroic measures," but today it's clear that the heroism was entirely the patient's.

Consider the fate of heroic patient George Washington. One day in 1799, the 67-year-old but healthy father of our country developed a sore throat with fever and chills. Chances are he had tonsillitis or a strep throat. He probably could have been treated with rest, hot liquids and the herbal antibiotics of the day, including garlic and goldenseal. Instead, Washington's physicians bled him of four pints of blood, leaving him anemic and weak, then gave him cathartics and large doses of mercury. He was dead within 24 hours.

Many physicians of that time decided quite correctly that heroic measures did more harm than good. One was a German doctor, Samuel Hahnemann. Disgusted with heroics, Dr. Hahnemann quit medicine and worked as a medical translator to better acquaint himself with healing arts around the world.

Dr. Hahnemann did not reject all heroic treatments. On the contrary, he was impressed with several. One was cinchona bark, discovered in the 1630s in Peru by Jesuit missionaries. It was the first effective treatment for malaria, a scourge that had plagued Europe since ancient times. It was later shown that cinchona contains the antimalaria drug, quinine. Another was Edward Jenner's method of preventing smallpox. Jenner made a small incision in the person's skin and introduced some material taken from the blisters (pox) of cattle infected with cowpox, a nonfatal bovine relative of the dreaded human disease.

In healthy people, both of these treatments produced low-level symptoms of the illnesses that they were used to prevent. Dr. Hahnemann called the phenomenon *homeopathy*, from the Greek for "treatment by similars."

On the theory that hundreds of substances might be used to treat diseases in this way, Dr. Hahnemann tested medicinal herbs, animal materials and natural chemical compounds like salt on himself and catalogued their effects. Eventually he returned to practicing medicine, using his homeopathic medicines. Dr. Hahnemann's approach was much less drastic than heroic medicine's. He had considerable success in Germany and attracted a large following among both patients and physicians who were fed up with standard heroics.

Homeopathy came to the United States in the 1830s and quickly won many supporters, including Daniel Webster, John D. Rockefeller, William James and Mark Twain, who wrote in an 1890 issue of *Harper's* magazine that homeopathy "forced the old school doctor to learn something of a rational nature about his business."

But homeopathy was controversial from the outset. In contrast to the regular medical view that diseases had physical causes, Dr. Hahnemann believed diseases were spiritual in nature, a view rather like the Chinese perspective that illness results from an imbalance of yin and yang energy forces in the body.

## Modern Science Rebels

The allopathic view received a tremendous boost in the mid-nineteenth century when Louis Pasteur demonstrated that bacteria could cause illness and developed his Germ Theory—the idea that microorganisms cause disease. Once the Germ Theory became accepted, the "regular" doctors attacked homeopathy as "spiritualistic."

But the homeopathic belief that galled the regulars most was Hahnemann's Law of Potentization—the idea that homeopathic medicines grow stronger as they became more dilute. Potentization violated a fundamental principle of pharmacology, the "dose-response relationship," which says that the bigger the dose, the greater the effect. Many medicines that homeopaths consider "extremely powerful" are so dilute that they contain none of the active ingredient. A ditty from 1848 summed up the scientific critique.

> The homeopathic system, sir, just suits me to a tittle,
> It proves that taking medicines, you cannot take too little.

If it be good in all complaints to take a dose so small,
It surely must be better still, to take no dose at all.

Largely because of the Law of Potentization, most scientists up until recently have tended to dismiss homeopathy as utter nonsense, if not downright quackery. "Homeopathy represents a totally ridiculous approach to pharmacology," says William Jarvis, Ph.D., professor of preventive medicine and public health at Loma Linda University Medical School in California and president of the National Coalition Against Health Fraud. "It's not science. I think the Food and Drug Administration should crack down on it as health fraud."

## Gaining a Toehold

Yet, despite the Germ Theory and the heretical nature of homeopathic dilutions, Dr. Hahnemann's system flourished throughout the United States because it appeared to offer the best treatment for the infectious disease epidemics that swept the nation throughout the nineteenth century. But did it really?

One disease that won legions of converts to homeopathy was cholera, an often-fatal bacterial infection that causes severe diarrhea and vomiting. One convert was William H. Holcombe, M.D., son of a New Orleans regular physician, whose medical school professors relentlessly derided Dr. Hahnemann's system and turned out students who felt the same way.

Upon graduation, Dr. Holcombe joined his father's practice shortly before a cholera epidemic struck the city in 1849. The father-son team tried standard heroics to no avail, and scores of their patients died. Then the younger Dr. Holcombe read a newspaper account of homeopathic success against the epidemic in Cincinnati. Against his better judgment, he gave the homeopathic cholera medicine to one patient—without the man's knowledge.

That night, guilt over what he'd done kept him from sleeping. "What right had I to dose that poor fellow with Hahnemann's medical moonshine?" he wrote in his diary. The next

## Decoding Homeopathic Medicines

The names are exotic, but the ingredients are not. Homeopathic medicines are known by their Latin names or by Latin abbreviations. Here are the names and meanings of some widely used homeopathic medicines.

| Latin Name | Common Name |
|---|---|
| Allium cepa | Onion |
| Apis | Crushed bee |
| Arnica | Mountain daisy |
| Belladonna | Deadly nightshade |
| Bellis perennis | Daisy |
| Berberis | Barberry |
| Bryonia | Wild hops |
| Calcarea carbonica | Calcium carbonate |
| Calendula | Marigold |
| Cantharis | Spanish fly |
| Caulophyllum | Blue cohosh |
| Chamomilla | Chamomile |
| Cimicifuga | Black snakeroot |
| Colocynthis | Bitter cucumber |

morning he called at his patient's home, expecting to find him dead. Instead he found him well on his way to recovery. Dr. Holcombe became a homeopath and later served as president of the American Institute of Homeopathy, which for much of the nineteenth century rivaled the American Medical Association (AMA) in prestige and power.

Cholera is a telling example because, on closer inspection, it supports the critique that homeopathic medicines are simply placebos. Cholera has a well-deserved terrible reputation that dates back to biblical times, but today we know that the waterborne infection is not always fatal. For some people, the diar-

| | |
|---|---|
| *Cuprum metallicum* | Copper |
| *Euphrasia* | Eyebright |
| *Ferrum phos* | Iron phosphate |
| *Gelsemium* | Yellow jasmine |
| *Hepar sulph* | Hahnemann's calcium sulphide |
| *Lachesis* | Venom of the bushmaster *snake* |
| *Ledum* | Marsh tea |
| *Magnesia phosphorica* (Mag phos) | Magnesium phosphate |
| *Mercurius* | Mercury |
| *Natrum mur* | Salt |
| *Nux vomica* | Poison nut |
| *Oscillococcinum* | Duck heart and liver |
| *Pulsatilla* | Windflower |
| *Rhus tox* | Poison ivy |
| *Sarsaparilla* | Wild licorice |
| *Sepia* | Cuttlefish |
| *Sulphur* | Sulphur |
| *Urtica urens* | Stinging nettle |
| *Zincum* | Zinc |

rhea resolves by itself in a few days. And even those who develop serious symptoms may survive simply by drinking uncontaminated water to replace the fluids lost through the diarrhea and vomiting.

Nineteenth-century heroic medicine clearly hastened the deaths of many people with cholera because its cathartics and emetics increased fluid loss, which led to serious dehydration, circulatory collapse, shock and death. Homeopathy, on the other hand, did nothing to aggravate fluid loss, and for many with cholera, the illness may simply have run its course, with the homeopathic medicines having no real effect.

Did homeopathic treatment produce better survival rates than a placebo would have? We'll never know because there were no double-blind studies. It's clear, however, that heroic treatments were lethal and that doing nothing would have been vastly more therapeutic. Maybe homeopathy helped, but quite possibly it was simply a placebo that did no harm.

## Homeopathy on the Wane

In the 1890s, an estimated 15 percent of American physicians used some homeopathic medicines in their practices, but after the turn of the century, Dr. Hahnemann's system fell from medical fashion. Homeopaths adapted fairly easily to the ascendancy of the Germ Theory by downplaying Dr. Hahnemann's spiritual view of disease and focusing on symptoms, but other changes in standard medical procedures almost did them in.

By 1900 regular physicians had stopped using bleeding, cathartics, emetics and mercury. As heroic measures disappeared, the medical opposition, organized and led by homeopaths, lost steam.

Another factor was the AMA's unrelenting hostility. The AMA was formed in 1846 (two years after the organization of the American Institute of Homeopathy), in part to stem the tide of defections by regular physicians to Dr. Hahnemann's medical system. Around the turn of the century, the AMA decreed that physicians caught using homeopathy would be thrown out of the organization and shunned by their regular colleagues. Several physicians were excommunicated, and most others dropped homeopathy.

Then in 1909, the Carnegie Foundation hired Abraham Flexner, an education consultant, and Nathan Colwell, of the AMA, to evaluate the nation's medical schools. Their 1910 Flexner Report praised Harvard and Johns Hopkins, citadels of allopathic medicine, and chastised most other medical training institutions, reserving particular scorn for homeopathy. State legislatures subsequently invested huge sums in reforming the nation's regular medical schools on the Harvard-Hopkins model. As time passed, homeopathic schools fell into comparative poverty, which limited their ability to attract students. The last homeopathic school in the United States closed in 1940.

Meanwhile, increasingly scientific regular medicine savaged the Law of Potentization, and as the modern pharmaceutical industry developed—especially after the discovery of penicillin in 1928—Americans lost confidence in homeopathy's vanishingly dilute medicines. Homeopathy simply didn't make scientific sense, and Dr. Hahnemann's healing art virtually disappeared in this country. In the early 1970s, there were fewer than 100 homeopaths in the country.

## On the Comeback Road

In Europe and Asia, however, homeopathy remained quite popular. Today the physician to the British royal family is a homeopath, and a 1986 survey showed that 42 percent of British doctors refer some patients to homeopaths. Of the 11 percent of the British public who have tried homeopathic treatments, 80 percent expressed satisfaction, while only 7 percent were dissatisfied. Across the English Channel, 39 percent of French family physicians use homeopathy in their practices. In the Netherlands, the figure is 45 percent and in Germany it's 20 percent. Homeopathy is also popular in India. Gandhi used it, and today India has 120 four-year homeopathic medical schools and more than 100,000 practicing homeopaths.

During the last 25 years, America has witnessed a modest homeopathic renaissance. Today about 1,000 physicians incorporate homeopathy into their practices, and several thousand other health professionals—dentists, podiatrists, veterinarians, nurses and chiropractors—use it as well. A 1990 study by Harvard researchers suggested that more than 2.5 million Americans have used homeopathy. The Food and Drug Administration reports that since the 1970s, sales of homeopathic medicines have increased more than 100-fold, thanks in part to the fact that they are now carried at major drugstore chains, including Kmart, Payless, Walgreens and Thrifty.

# Homeopathy for What Ails You

Homeopaths believe in treating the person, not just the illness. Two people with similar symptoms who would be given the same medicine by a mainstream physician might be given different medicines by a homeopath, depending on their temperaments and other personal attributes that mainstream physicians generally ignore, such as their sense of taste.

In addition, classical homeopaths give only one medicine at a time, while others give more than one. For quite a while, this belief regarding individual treatment with single medicines stopped homeopaths from publishing consumer guides to self-treatment for everyday conditions. But in the last decade, several self-treatment guides have appeared that pay their respects to individual treatment with single medicines and then recommend one or more homeopathic remedies for common complaints. Here is a selection. When using these medicines, follow package directions.

Allergies: *Allium cepa, Apis, Euphrasia, Urtica urens.*

Bladder infection: *Cantharis, Sarsaparilla, Mercurius, Nux vomica, Berberis, Pulsatilla.*

Colds: *Allium cepa, Euphrasia.*

## Looking at the Evidence

For all the controversy homeopathy has generated, it's amazing how few studies have investigated the effects of its medicines. Only about 100 little-noticed reports have appeared in conventional medical journals worldwide since the 1960s.

The main reason for this paucity of research has been pigheadedness on the part of both homeopaths and their critics. Homeopaths insist that they are satisfied with their medicines and don't need rigorous experiments to prove that they work.

Cuts, scrapes, minor burns: *Calendula*.

Earache or ear infection: *Belladonna, Chamomilla, Pulsatilla, Ferrum phos, Hepar sulph*.

Flu: *Oscillococcinum, Gelsemium, Rhus tox, Bryonia*.

Menopause symptoms: *Sepia, Natrum mur, Lachesis, Calcarea carbonica, Sulphur*.

Menstrual cramps: *Mag phos, Colocynthis*.

Muscle cramps: *Mag phos, Colocynthis, Cuprum metallicum*.

Muscle soreness and sports injuries: *Arnica* (either internally or in an ointment).

Premenstrual syndrome: *Belladonna, Mag phos, Colocynthis, Cimicifuga, Chamomilla, Caulophyllum, Pulsatilla, Lachesis, Sepia, Natrum mur*.

Sprains and strains: *Ledum, Bellis perennis, Arnica, Rhus tox, Bryonia, Zincum*.

Their attitude is "If doubters want double-blind, placebo-controlled studies, let them spend the money on them." Meanwhile, the medical establishment has replied: "Forget it. There's no way we're going to spend a dime testing drugs that aren't even there."

That's pretty much where matters stood until the mid-1980s, when mainstream medical journals began publishing an intriguing trickle of studies that support homeopathy. In 1986, allopathic Scottish researchers at the University of Glasgow gave a homeopathic hay fever remedy to 144 people with pollen allergy. The study was double-blind and placebo-controlled. Neither the participants nor the researchers knew which people took the homeopathic medicine and which took the look-alike but inactive placebo. Compared with those who took the placebo, the homeopathic group showed a significant reduction in symptoms, and their need for antihistamines plummeted 50 percent.

In 1988, French allergist Jacques Benveniste, M.D., a nonhomeopath, diluted an antibody solution 1:10 (one unit of antibody to ten units of water) and then rediluted the resulting solution in the same way 120 times, to the point where it was so dilute that most likely the final solution contained none of the antibody. But the final solution still had a noticeable effect on white blood cells.

To explain this revolutionary finding, the French researcher postulated that water must have some as-yet-undefined "memory" and speculated that "water memory" might explain how vanishingly dilute homeopathic remedies work. In 1989, nonhomeopath British researchers used a double-blind, placebo-controlled study to test the superdilute homeopathic flu medicine *Oscillococcinum* (*AH-sill-oh-cock-SINE-um*) on 487 people. After 48 hours, compared with the placebo, *Oscillococcinum* relieved twice as many flu symptoms.

In another double-blind, placebo-controlled 1989 study, British researchers showed that a homeopathic microdose of poison ivy (Rhus tox) provided significant relief from the pain of fibromyalgia, an arthritic condition.

A 1990 double-blind, placebo-controlled study in Germany tested a combination of eight homeopathic medicines on 61 people with varicose veins. People participating in the study took the homeopathic cocktail three times a day for 24 days. The researchers used a battery of medical tests and patient reports to gauge the severity of their symptoms. Among those who took the placebo, symptoms grew 18 percent worse. But among those who took the homeopathic medicines, symptoms improved 44 percent.

In 1991 in the *British Medical Journal*, nonhomeopath Dutch researchers from the Department of Epidemiology at the University of Maastricht published an analysis of 105 studies of homeopathic medicines performed from 1966 to 1990, most taken from French and German medical journals not usually translated into English. Of the 105 studies, 81 showed positive benefits for homeopathic treatment, while 24 showed no benefit. However, some of the studies involved few people, and most were not double-blind, meaning that researcher bias might have played a role in the results.

So the Dutch investigators selected the 21 most scientifically rigorous studies and analyzed their results. Fifteen showed significant benefits from homeopathic treatment. While many questions remain about how homeopathy works, they concluded: "The evidence presented in this review would probably be sufficient for establishing homeopathy as a regular treatment for certain conditions."

Finally, in 1994, the first study involving a homeopathic treatment appeared in an American medical journal, *Pediatrics*. Jennifer Jacobs, M.D., assistant clinical professor of epidemiology at the University of Washington School of Public Health in Seattle, recruited 81 Nicaraguan children under age five who had acute diarrhea, a common cause of dehydration and childhood death in the Third World. She gave half the group the standard mainstream treatment—rehydration fluid containing water, sugar and salt. The other half received the rehydration fluid plus a homeopathic medicine individualized to the child's specific symptoms and temperament. Among the children in the control group, the diarrhea lasted an average of 4 days. But in the homeopathy group, it lasted only 2½ days—a significantly faster recovery.

Homeopathic microdose medicines are actually used routinely in two branches of mainstream medicine. One is vaccination, where a tiny amount of deactivated microorganism is given to stimulate an immune response that protects people from the disease that is caused by larger amounts of the active germ. The other is allergy shots, where tiny amounts of allergy-triggering substances are given to allow recipients to tolerate larger exposures without ill effects. Still, science can't explain homeopathy. It looks as if the controversial healing art is destined to remain a medical hot potato until we understand how it works.

## Some Doctors Love It

Like most homeopaths, Dr. Subotnick is not all that concerned with how homeopathy works. He's satisfied that it does. After completing his homeopathic training, he transformed one room of his medical suite into a homeopathic dispensary, crammed with shelves full of little vials with odd-sounding names: *Kali sulphuricum* (potassium sulfate), *Aurum iod* (gold iodide), *Calc fluor* (calcium fluoride) and *Natrum carbonicum* (sodium carbonate).

He gives them to patients like Leland, a 68-year-old retired United Airlines mechanic whose severe leg and foot cramps did not respond to standard medication. His primary-care physician suspected a biomechanical problem and referred him to Dr. Subotnick.

"I couldn't find any podiatric problem to account for his cramps, so I did a homeopathic workup," Dr. Subotnick says. "From his symptom profile, it seemed to me he needed *Cuprum metalicum* (copper)."

"It was the damndest thing," Leland recalls. "He gave me these little pellets, and in a few minutes my pain was gone. Just like that. I'd never heard of homeopathy, but whatever that stuff was, it worked."

Do colleagues look cross-eyed at Dr. Subotnick now that he's come out as a homeopath? "Some do," he says, "But I'm used to it. Back when I was doing my foot-plant work, everyone thought I was nuts—until it turned out I was right. You just do what you've got to do. I don't really care what the nonbelievers think. I haven't thrown out all of medicine to practice homeopathy. I still use x-rays, surgery and pharmaceutical drugs when I believe they're appropriate. But I also offer homeopathy—and recommend yoga and meditation when I believe they might help.

## How to Find a Practitioner

You want to try homeopathy. Where to look?

You might think that walking your fingers through the Yellow Pages would do the trick. It might, but with only a couple of thousand physicians and other health professionals practicing this medical discipline, you'd be lucky to find one in your neighborhood.

If looking in your telephone directory doesn't turn one up, you might try contacting a national homeopathic organization. Homeopathic Educational Services and the National Center for Homeopathy both sell a directory of licensed health professionals around the United States who also practice homeopathy. The directory includes physicians (M.D.'s and D.O.'s), podiatrists, physician assistants, nurses, dentists, chiropractors, psychologists and others. However, it does not list every U.S. homeopath.

Contact Homeopathic Educational Services at 2124 Kittredge Street, Berkeley, CA 94704 and the National Center for Homeopathy at 801 North Fairfax #306, Alexandria, VA 22314.

You might also try asking friends or anyone who teaches or practices any of Nature's cures in your area.

"I think doctors need to be more open-minded. The skeptics say they can't explain homeopathy, therefore it can't work. I used to feel the same way. I thought homeopathy was crazy. But science can't explain everything. Take love: I can't explain it, but I know it can have powerful effects. I feel the same way about homeopathy. I've seen it work."

## A Guide to Homeopathic Medicines

Most homeopathic medicines come from plants used in traditional herbal medicine. A few come from animal sources, while others come from naturally occurring chemical compounds. Some homeopathic medicines, such as mercury or belladonna, would be poisonous in large doses. But in superdilute homeopathic doses, they are safe when used as recommended. All homeopathic medicines are sold over the counter in health food stores, and they rank among the safest medicines available. There have been very few reports of adverse reactions to them.

Homeopaths use two abbreviations to describe a medicine's strength or potency, the decimal, or x, system, and the centissimal, or c, system. The x system is more popular in the United States and the c system in Europe.

In both, potency is expressed as a number followed by an x or c, such as 6x or 12c. A potency of 1x means a 1:10 dilution of the original substance, or one-tenth strength; 2x means 1:100, 3x is 1:1000 and so on. The number before the x equals the number of zeros in the dilution, so 6x indicates a dilution of 1 part in 1,000,000. A potency of 1c means a 1:100 dilution. The number before the c equals half the number of zeros in the dilution, so 3c indicates a dilution of 1 part in 1,000,000.

Most homeopathic medicines sold for home use vary in potency from 3x to 30x. If you choose to try over-the-counter remedies, follow the manufacturer's directions for potency and dosage.

Homeopathic medicines are not simply diluted. They are also shaken vigorously, or "potentized." Homeopaths believe that shaking transfers the medicine's essence to the water used to dilute it. This concept is important because solutions diluted beyond 24x (or 12c) may not contain even a single molecule of the original solution. Critics charge that these superdilute solutions are nothing but water. Homeopaths believe that medicines become stronger as they become more dilute and that even when enormously diluted, the medicine's "essence" or "energy" remains.

Homeopathic medicines typically come as tiny beads, tablets, or granules onto which the dilute medicine has been placed. To work properly, they should be treated carefully. Ullman, author of several guides to homeopathy, offers these tips on how to use homeopathic remedies.

**Store carefully.** Keep bottles tightly capped, away from direct sunlight and at room temperature. Also keep bottles away from strong-smelling chemicals such as perfumes and household cleaners. Do not leave bottles open. After removing the medicines, recap the bottles quickly.

**Handle with care.** Homeopathic physicians recommend touching these medicines as little as possible. Wash your hands before handling them. Shake the recommended number of beads or tablets from the bottle into its cap and then pop them into your mouth without touching them.

## Chapter 17

# LIGHT THERAPY

### Brightening Up the Winter Blues

Plants always turn to face the sun. People tend to do the same. For thousands of years people the world over have revered the sun as a great healer; some ancient cultures even worshiped the solar disk.

These days sun worship is more likely to take the form of a midwinter Caribbean vacation. And despite the well-publicized threat of skin cancer, the sun is still viewed more as a healer than a hazard—even among doctors and medical researchers.

Researchers have found a whole host of benefits from regular, moderate exposure to sunlight—or to sunlike artificial lights. Such exposure can help relieve winter blues and treat other forms of depression; minimize jet lag; shorten abnormally long menstrual cycles and treat psoriasis, eating disorders and some forms of insomnia. It can possibly even help relieve some symptoms of lupus—a serious disease involving the immune system.

## Banishing Winter Blues

In the late 1970s, Neal Owens of Rockville, Maryland, was a petroleum salesman with an odd problem. "Every spring and summer," he recalls, "I was my company's top salesman. But come fall and winter, my sales fell to last place." Owens's boss accused him of goofing off around the holidays each year, but Owens insisted he wasn't. "I just seemed to lose my get-up-and-go during the winter," he explains.

"Maybe you're sick," his boss said, "get a checkup." Owens saw his doctor, who ran a battery of tests, but all the results were normal. Owens wound up seeing a psychiatrist, who diagnosed depression and prescribed various stimulants and antidepressants. "But the drugs didn't help, and their side effects left me feeling worse," says Owens.

Then one weekend during the fall of 1982, Owens happened to catch a television show about depression. It mentioned that researchers at the National Institute of Mental Health (NIMH) in nearby Bethesda had begun studying an odd, newly identified type of depression that struck some people like clockwork every winter and caused other symptoms, including winter weight gain. They called it the seasonal blues.

Hey, that's me, Owens thought. As his mood darkened each winter, his weight climbed by 20 pounds. And as his depression lifted each spring, he lost the weight. Owens contacted the NIMH researchers and volunteered for their study, which involved a therapy that struck him as bizarre—sitting beside bright lights for several hours a day.

"I was skeptical," Owens recalls. "The best antidepressants weren't helping me. How could I possibly get relief from something as ordinary as light? But I was desperate, so I signed on." Owens credits what is now known as light therapy with saving his sanity and possibly his life.

## Feeling SAD

Everyone recognizes "spring fever"—the giddiness that lifts the spirits as the short, dark days of winter become the longer, sunnier days of spring. Doctors first noticed its opposite number, annual winter depression, 150 years ago, but the condition remained a medical footnote until the early 1980s. Then researchers began linking the darkening of moods to the lack of sunlight from around November through March.

Winter blues, researchers have determined, varies in severity from mild "winter blahs" to moderate "winter doldrums" to severe winter depression. This severe form is now medically known as seasonal affective disorder, or, aptly enough, SAD.

People with the mildest winter blues function normally throughout winter, but by February they feel vaguely out of sorts, according to San Francisco psychiatrist Michael Freeman, M.D. "They typically develop the late-winter irritability popularly known as 'cabin fever,' followed by a welcome surge of spring fever energy as the days lengthen."

Those with moderate winter blues can function throughout winter, but not quite normally. "They feel more down," Dr. Freeman explains, "and suffer more noticeable cabin fever. They often feel an increased need for sleep, gain a few pounds and may have difficulty getting out of bed in the morning."

Like Owens, people with severe winter blues become seriously depressed each autumn and can't function normally until spring. SAD shares several symptoms with other forms of depression: lethargy, joylessness, hopelessness, anxiety and social withdrawal. In addition, people with SAD crave additional sleep, experience daytime drowsiness even if they get their sleep and gain a good deal of weight, often feeling irresistible cravings for sweets.

## Let There Be Bright Light

A decade ago, researchers noticed that some people with SAD regularly went south for winter vacations. After a few days of sun, they invariably felt better, and they continued to feel fine for a few weeks after their return. "The extra day length and greater light intensity temporarily relieved their depression," says SAD expert William Sonis, M.D., professor of psychiatry at the University of Pennsylvania in Philadelphia.

This observation led to another treatment that proved equally effective—daily exposure to high-intensity, artificial sunlight (full-spectrum light minus the ultraviolet rays, which cause sunburn and increase the risk of skin cancer). Among the scientists who proved the effectiveness of light therapy were the NIMH researchers contacted by Owens. In that early study, they loaned him a 70-pound box resembling a TV, with four fluorescent lights instead of a screen, and instructed him to sit in front of it for four hours a day, two hours before breakfast and two after work.

"The time investment was a major hassle," Owens recalls, "but after a week, I felt much better." Still, he felt skeptical. The lights might be helping, he thought, or perhaps his improvement was a delayed benefit of the new antidepressant he'd been taking. Then the NIMH researchers asked him to return the light box. "Within a few days, I felt awful again," Owens recalls. "I realized that the lights really helped."

By the mid-1980s, bright-light therapy (phototherapy) had become the treatment of choice for SAD, says Michael Terman, Ph.D., director of the Light Therapy Unit at Columbia Presbyterian Medical Center in New York City, "but at four hours a day, it took so long that for most people, it just wasn't feasible." Then Dr. Terman's additional studies showed that the evening session was unnecessary. Morning-only bright-light therapy cut treatment time in half. A few years later, Dr. Terman cut it further by brightening the lights.

Light intensity is measured in "lux" units. The typical home is illuminated at a level of about 250 lux. Early light boxes emitted 2,500 lux, which sounds like a lot but really isn't. "That's the brightness of outdoor light shortly after dawn," Dr. Terman explains. "At noon on a summer day, you can have 120,000 lux."

When Dr. Terman constructed a 10,000-lux light, he found that people with SAD obtained effective relief with daily exposure of just 30 minutes. "You put the unit on your kitchen table," he explains, "and by the time you've finished your morning coffee, you're protected for the day."

SAD symptoms typically begin to lift about a week after the start of phototherapy. But as Owens learned the hard way, they return shortly after discontinuing treatment. As a result, author-

(continued on page 286)

# Lag and Light

Does this sound familiar? After an overnight trans-Atlantic flight, you arrive at your Paris hotel at 4:00 A.M. French time. You're wiped out, but you can't fall asleep. Finally you doze off but you sleep fitfully. When you awaken a few hours later, you feel hung over, even though you had no alcohol on the plane. You stumble out to a charming cafe where everyone is enjoying breakfast croissants, but you're not hungry. You continue to feel out of sorts for several days.

Jet air travel has made the world much smaller and more accessible, but its downside is jet lag—an annoying combination of disorientation, nighttime insomnia, daytime fatigue, out-of-sync appetite, difficulty concentrating, decreased reaction time and general malaise. Here's the problem: Your body may be in Paris, but your internal clock is still back in Chicago.

Any travel across time zones can disrupt your body's natural rhythms, but most people don't experience noticeable jet lag unless they cross three or more. Jet lag typically becomes more pronounced with age and when flying east—the body has a harder time adjusting to a shorter day than a longer one.

Travel-disrupted body rhythms generally reset themselves within two to five days, but when you have only a week in Scandinavia and you want to be alert for that boat ride around the fjörds that's scheduled for the day you arrive, the natural recovery process takes too long. As early as 1958, scientists discovered that the internal clock is located in a group of cells along the track of the optic nerve. Recently, Al Lewy, M.D. professor of psychiatry at Oregon Health Sciences University in Portland and director of the Sleep and Mood Disorders Laboratory there, determined that carefully timed exposure to outdoor light can ease time-zone transitions.

Here are Dr. Lewy's techniques to beat jet lag.

If you have flown east across fewer than six time zones, spend some time outdoors in the sun during the morning at your destination. Later in the day, avoid light by staying indoors under low light.

If you've flown west across fewer than six time zones, get your sun in the late afternoon and early evening and avoid the bright outdoor light in the morning.

If you've flown east across 6 to 12 time zones, avoid sunlight in the morning at your destination. And if you've flown west across 6 to 12 time zones, avoid sunlight in the late afternoon and early evening. In both cases, spend time outdoors in the sun during midday, from about 10:00 a.m. to 2:00 p.m.

Follow these schedules for two or three days after arriving. They'll work even if the days aren't particularly sunny, according to Dr. Lewy. The outdoor light of a cloudy day is sufficient to reset internal clocks.

Other experts on jet-lag recovery—both medical researchers and frequent flyers—agree that other adjustments before, during, and after travel also help overcome jet lag. This is what they recommend.

**Alter your sleep pattern.** During the few days before your flight, adjust your sleep schedule according to the direction in which you plan to travel. Prior to flying east, wake up and go to sleep one hour earlier per day. Prior to flying west, rise and retire one hour later.

**Don't make it any harder than you have to.** Try to book a flight that doesn't require you to get up unusually early or stay up beyond your normal bedtime. Try to get a flight that lands in the early evening, destination time.

**Synchronize your watch.** When you board the plane, set your watch to your destination's time and begin adopting that schedule. Try to nap when it's night, destination time, and read, talk, eat and walk around when it's day there.

**Don't get too dry.** Drink plenty of fluids, but avoid both alcohol and caffeine.

**Do as the Romans do.** When you arrive, adopt your destination's schedule as much as possible while still observing Dr. Lewy's sun-exposure recommendations.

**Sleep when you should.** For help falling asleep, exercise early in the day and take a hot bath shortly before you wish to retire.

ities urge people with SAD to sit under bright light daily from
October through April.

Can prolonged daily exposure to 10,000 lux be harmful? No,
says Dr. Terman. Individual bright-light tolerance varies, however, and after a while, some people may start to feel uncomfortable. Overdose symptoms include queasiness and agitation,
but these symptoms disappear within a few hours of turning the
lights off.

"When people learn their limits and stay within them, they
don't have any problems," says Dr. Terman.

## Dawn's Earlier Light

Within just the last few years, scientists discovered that for
some people with winter blues, ultrabright light might not be
necessary. Dr. Terman was one of several researchers who confirmed that the light of simulated dawns also elevates depressed
mood.

Dr. Terman fashioned a simulated-dawn device using a night-
stand light fitted with a timer and a dimmer. At 4:00 A.M. the
light turned on, bathing the sleeping winter-blues sufferer in the
faint glow of artificial dawn. The light brightened over two or
three hours until the person awakened. In one early study, six
of eight people with SAD experienced substantial relief after two
weeks of awakening to simulated sunrises. Since then, other
studies have confirmed the effect.

## How to Brighten Your Mood

Bright-light boxes and dawn simulators may prove beneficial
for some people with seasonal blues. And experts in phototherapy offer other suggestions as well. Here's the scoop on how to
overcome everything from the winter blahs to a full-blown case
of SAD.

**Get more natural sunlight.** Trim the bushes around your
windows and keep your curtains and blinds open. Use bright
colors on walls and upholstery.

**Sit near windows whenever possible.** At school, at work, on public transportation and when dining out, head for the seat with the view. If you exercise indoors, work out near a window.

**Take a walk.** People with SAD often spend unusually little time outdoors in winter. A Swiss study showed that a one-hour walk in midday winter sunlight can significantly lift the spirits. For winter blahs and winter doldrums, a daily outdoor walk may be all that's necessary.

**Take a winter vacation in the sun.** "With a diagnosis of SAD," Dr. Freeman says, "it might even be tax-deductible."

**Try a dawn simulator.** These devices can be set like alarm clocks to produce an artificial dawn from one minute to three hours before the user awakens. A pocket-size SunUp unit costs about $200. Write to the SunBox Company, 19127 Orbit Drive, Gaithersburg, MD 20879.

**Try bright-light therapy.** To be of benefit, the light must enter the eyes, but you shouldn't look directly at bright-light appliances. Simply sit near them. Several companies now make bright-light boxes, among them the SunBox Company (address above) and Apollo Light Systems, 352 West 1060 South, Orem, UT 84058.

**Try a support group.** People with SAD have founded a nationwide support group, NOSAD, to help people with winter blues—and their families—cope with the condition. For free information, write to NOSAD, P.O. Box 40133, Washington, DC 20016.

**Educate yourself.** For more information on light therapy, send a self-addressed, stamped envelope to the Society for Light Treatment and Biological Rhythms, P.O. Box 478, Wilsonville, OR 97070.

## Light Therapy's Bright Future

Shakespeare called the eyes "the window to the soul." Increasingly, doctors are calling them a window to treating a remarkable variety of health problems with light. For years, sunlight has been a standard treatment for psoriasis, the poorly understood inflammatory condition that causes skin thickening and eruption of red, scaly patches. But recently, light therapy has been used successfully to treat several other ailments.

**Bulimia.** This binge/purge eating disorder typically develops in women during their teenage or early adult years. If bulimia remains untreated, it can cause serious physical and emotional problems. Some researchers have noted that bulimic episodes seem to occur most frequently in winter, leading to speculation that the illness might have a seasonal component. Raymond Lam, M.D., assistant professor of psychiatry at the University of British Columbia in Vancouver, asked 14 people with bulimia to spend 30 minutes each morning under either 500-lux lights (about twice as bright as typical indoor lighting) or 10,000-lux lights. Under 500-lux lights, bulimic episodes decreased 12 percent. But under the ultrabright lights, binge/purge eating plummeted 42 percent.

**Late-shift drowsiness.** There's a good reason why the work shift from midnight to 8:00 A.M. is called the graveyard shift. According to the National Commission of Sleep Disorders Research, people who work nights are two to five times more likely to fall asleep on the job and have accidents. Late-night sleepiness may impair the judgment of police, firefighters and ambulance drivers. In addition, a disturbing number of airline disasters have occurred in the wee hours.

Now phototherapy may come to the rescue. James Walsh, Ph.D., director of the Sleep Disorders Clinic at St. Luke's Medical Center in St. Louis, asked 30 graveyard-shift workers to perform a series of tasks every hour for one night. He also gauged their sleepiness using standard tests. The next night, he replaced their 500-lux lighting with 9,000-lux lights. After only one night under the bright light, the workers' accuracy improved dramatically, while their sleepiness decreased, Dr. Walsh explains. "One night's exposure to bright light seems to have shifted their biological clocks, enabling them to perform better on subsequent nights," he says.

**Lupus.** Lupus is an autoimmune disease—meaning that the immune system mistakes the body's own tissues for germs and attacks them. It strikes many more women than men and can cause a confusing array of symptoms, including fatigue, rashes, joint pains and kidney damage.

People with lupus are usually warned to avoid sunlight because it can aggravate their symptoms. But rheumatologist Hugh McGrath, Jr., M.D., associate professor of medicine at Louisiana State University in New Orleans, discovered that one type of ultraviolet sunlight, UVA-1, helps relieve lupus symptoms. He exposed ten women with lupus to a combination of UVA-1 and ordinary fluorescent light for ten minutes a day five days a week for three weeks. Nine of the ten women reported less joint pain, fatigue and other symptoms.

*Night-owl insomnia.* One type of insomnia involves a nightly inability to fall asleep until the wee hours—and often the abuse of alcohol and sleeping pills to bring on the sandman. It's called delayed sleep phase syndrome (DSPS), or night-owl insomnia, and it usually develops during the teen years. Researchers blame it on having a maladjusted biological rhythm that doesn't say "good-night" until several hours past a normal bedtime.

Bright-light therapy looks like the best bet for relief. In one study, a research team led by Norman E. Rosenthal, M.D., chief of environmental psychiatry at the psychobiology branch of the National Institute of Mental Health in Rockville, Maryland, arranged for 20 people with DSPS to spend two hours each morning under a bright-light appliance and then wear dark goggles for two hours before dusk. After a few weeks, participants fell asleep two hours earlier and woke up the next morning feeling more alert and refreshed. When contacted six months later, almost all the participants reported purchasing bright-light appliances.

*Nonseasonal depression.* The winter blues are just the tip of the depression iceberg. Some 10 to 15 million Americans are seriously depressed, and the condition's most tragic consequence—suicide—claims 30,000 lives a year. The success of light therapy in treating SAD has led to studies of its effectiveness for nonseasonal depression—with promising preliminary results.

In a study done at the University of California at San Diego, psychiatry professor Daniel F. Kripke, M.D., divided 50 men with severe nonseasonal depression into two groups. Half spent seven consecutive evenings in a room illuminated with 1,600 watts of bright light. The other half spent the time in a room with the lights turned low. Compared with symptoms in the dim-light group, symptoms in the bright-light group improved 18 percent.

*Prolonged menstrual cycles.* The typical menstrual cycle lasts about a month, but some women's extend up to twice as long. Long cycles might be an advantage for some women—less premenstrual syndrome, for example—but for women trying to have children, long cycles limit opportunities for conception. In a pilot study, Dr. Kripke normalized extended menstrual cycles by using an amazingly simple treatment—the women were exposed to the light of a 100-watt light bulb while they slept.

The women slept with the light on for five nights near the middle of their extended cycles, and the cycles became shorter. Dr. Kripke doesn't know why this treatment works, but he speculates that the light affects regulation of female sex hormones. If so, phototherapy might one day be used to treat some cases of infertility.

## Shedding Light on the Problem

These studies are all preliminary. Currently, light therapy is not an accepted treatment for nonseasonal depression, menstrual regulation, night-owl insomnia, bulimia or lupus. But if you have an abnormally long menstrual cycle, it can't hurt to try Dr. Kripke's therapy. If you have another of these conditions, discuss the possibility of light therapy with your physician.

## CHAPTER 18

# LOW-FAT EATING

*The Key to Health, Longevity and Weight Control*

Biochemist Ron Goor, Ph.D., of Bethesda, Maryland, had a family history of serious heart disease. His father had the first of three heart attacks in 1943 at age 31, when Ron was only 3. As a result, Dr. Goor grew up with parents who preached the gospel of low-cholesterol, low-fat eating. But their young son didn't listen. "I thought, 'Why should I?' " Dr. Goor, now 54, recalls. "My father was the one with heart disease, not me."

When Dr. Goor turned 31, he felt perfectly healthy, but the haunting memory of his father's first heart attack spurred him to have his cholesterol measured for the first time. It was 311 milligrams per deciliter of blood (mg/dl), considerably higher than the average level of people who have heart attacks (235 mg/dl). It was much higher than the 200 mg/dl the American Heart Association (AHA) recommends as the safe maximum and way above the 150 mg/dl level that heart disease experts suggest as the ideal level for health. Dr. Goor was at high risk for an early heart attack, just like his father's.

"My cholesterol scared the hell out of me," he says. "I was a heart attack waiting to happen."

Dr. Goor's heart attack risk spurred a change of career. He

quit his job at the National Science Foundation and returned to school, earning a Master's degree in public health. In 1976, he went to work for the National Heart, Lung and Blood Institute as the coordinator of the Coronary Primary Prevention Trial (CPPT), an experiment to determine if heart attack risk could be reduced by lowering cholesterol. The results of the seven-year study were impressive: Cutting cholesterol definitely reduced heart attack risk. For every 1 percent decrease in cholesterol level, heart attack risk dropped 2 percent. Many other studies have subsequently confirmed the CPPT's findings.

Participants in the CPPT cut their cholesterol with drugs or by reducing the cholesterol and saturated fat in their diets, or both. (Saturated fat is the type found in red meat, butter and whole-milk dairy foods). During the study, Dr. Goor went the exclusively dietary route and cut his cholesterol from 311 to 200—thanks to his wife, Nancy, an artist and children's book author, who loved to eat and refused to believe that dishes low in cholesterol and saturated fat had to be unappetizing.

For more than ten years, she tinkered with recipes and substituted ingredients, learning how to cook tasty, heart-healthy cuisine. The result in 1987 was *Eater's Choice: A Food Lover's Guide to Lower Cholesterol*, co-written by the Goors. It became a best-seller, and since then, the Goors have revised and expanded it several times.

As the 1980s turned into the 1990s, nutrition scientists learned that cholesterol and saturated fat were not the only villains in the American diet. They learned that all fats contribute to cancer, diabetes, arthritis, obesity and chronic high blood pressure (hypertension). Nancy Goor returned to her kitchen and discovered that low-fat cooking was not only possible and delicious, it also had an immediate payoff—weight loss. This led to the Goors' second book, *The Choose to Lose Diet: A Food Lover's Guide to Permanent Weight Loss*.

Dean Ornish, M.D., made the same discovery. (See Ornish Therapy on page 368 for more on his program for reversing heart disease.) His program participants, who ate an ultra-low-fat diet using recipes developed by some of the nation's leading chefs, also lost weight—an average of 22 pounds during the first year—with no restrictions on the total number of calories they consumed. Most ate more than they were used to eating and still lost weight because their fat consumption plummeted. Dr. Ornish's latest book is *Eat More, Weigh Less*.

Neither Dr. Goor nor Dr. Ornish is a "diet doctor." They're health educators with low-fat programs for losing weight and reducing risk of the diseases that cause more than half of the deaths in the United States.

## How High-Fat Diets Hurt

After smoking, a high-fat diet is the second most lethal habit. According to a report published in the *Journal of the American Medical Association*, smoking causes 400,000 deaths a year. High-fat diets cause 300,000. Several more highly publicized social evils are comparatively small problems: alcohol (100,000 deaths), guns (35,000), auto accidents (25,000) and drug abuse (20,000). These statistics in no way minimize the tragedies of alcoholism, murder or drug addiction. But they provide a perspective on what's *really* killing us.

Few people cringe when Aunt Mary serves up large slices of banana cream pie á la mode, but from a public health perspective, she might as well be offering heroin. If this sounds a bit extreme, consider the dangers of dietary fat and judge for yourself.

**Heart disease.** The nation's leading cause of death, heart disease kills 720,000 Americans a year, most as a result of heart attacks. About one American in four has some form of heart disease.

Heart disease results from a process called atherosclerosis, which is directly linked to dietary fat. Fatty foods are high in cholesterol and free radicals, which are oxygen molecules that have lost an electron and become highly reactive. As they circulate in the blood, they snatch electrons away from other molecules, sometimes grabbing them from the cells that line artery walls.

The microscopic injuries that free radicals inflict begin a decades-long process that eventually narrows the arteries with cholesterol-rich deposits called plaques. Sometimes plaques rupture, spilling their contents into the blood. If a plaque ruptures in one of the coronary arteries that nourish the heart, its debris can cause complete blockage. Without food and oxygen to nourish its hard-working cells, part of the heart dies. That's a heart attack.

Although heart disease generally strikes after 40 in men and after menopause in women, atherosclerotic arterial damage begins in childhood. A 1993 study coordinated by Jack Strong, M.D., chair of the pathology department at Louisiana State University Medical Center in New Orleans, analyzed autopsies of 1,532 teenagers who died in accidents. *One hundred percent* showed atherosclerotic plaques in the aorta, the body's largest artery.

*Stroke.* Stroke is the nation's third leading cause of death, claiming 144,000 lives a year. There are two major types of stroke, one caused by bleeding in the brain (hemorrhagic), the other by blockage of an artery there (ischemic). About 75 percent of strokes are ischemic, and the vast majority of ischemic strokes are caused by cerebral thrombosis—blockage of a brain artery by a process similar to heart attack, involving atherosclerosis and plaque rupture.

*Cancer.* A high-fat diet does not contribute to all cancers, but many studies have linked it to several types, notably colon and breast cancer, which together account for more than 100,000 deaths a year. Other studies suggest that a high-fat diet may play a role in causing cancer of the prostate (38,000 deaths annually) and pancreas (26,000), possibly lung cancer in nonsmokers (30,000) and malignant melanoma (6,900). For this reason, the American Cancer Society (ACS) urges everyone to eat less fat.

Dietary fat contributes to cancer risk because of free radicals. A high-fat diet increases the number of these molecules in the blood. If they don't snatch electrons from artery walls, causing heart attack or stroke, they may grab them from the chromosomes that contain our genes. Chromosomes can often repair themselves, but if they continue to sustain significant damage for many years, cellular repair mechanisms may become overwhelmed, resulting in cancer.

*Obesity.* Many people use *obese* as a synonym for fat, but it has a more precise medical definition—a weight 20 percent heavier than what's recommended for one's height and build. Anyone who is 35 percent overweight faces a risk of premature death 50 percent greater than average. Obesity is a risk factor for heart disease, several cancers, high blood pressure, diabetes and arthritis. It is a problem only in countries with a high-fat diet. In addition to being hazardous to health, obesity is also an economic handicap, since obese people earn less money than those who are slimmer.

**High blood pressure.** High blood pressure is a major risk factor for heart disease and stroke. A high-fat diet contributes to this condition because it adds extra pounds. As weight increases, the heart must work harder to pump blood through all the extra tissue. As the heart's effort increases, so does blood pressure.

*Diabetes.* Diabetes contributes to an estimated 250,000 deaths a year. It involves an inability to metabolize blood sugar because of problems with the pancreatic hormone, insulin. In Type I (insulin-dependent) diabetes, the pancreas stops producing insulin. In more common Type II (non-insulin-dependent) diabetes, typically associated with obesity, insulin production may be normal, but food intake overwhelms the body's ability to process it.

*Arthritis.* Dietary fat contributes to the most common form of arthritis, osteoarthritis, because excess weight subjects the major joints to extra wear and tear. A high-fat diet also appears to increase the risk of rheumatoid arthritis (RA), the most serious and potentially crippling form of joint disease. Several studies suggest that a low-fat diet relieves RA symptoms.

*Multiple sclerosis.* For the last 50 years, Roy Swank, M.D., Ph.D., professor emeritus of neurology at the Oregon Health Sciences University in Portland and author of *The Multiple Sclerosis Diet Book*, has amassed evidence that a high-fat diet is a key risk factor for multiple sclerosis (MS), which causes an enormous number of symptoms, from blurred vision to paralysis.

His studies show that a low-fat diet minimizes MS symptoms. (For a more detailed description of his work, see Elimination Diets on page 150.)

The list really does not end here. Almost weekly, it seems, new research adds to the overwhelming evidence that too much dietary fat is a major health hazard. And top doctors are increasingly vocal about what needs to be done. "Most Americans who have chronic health problems would not have them if they ate a low-fat diet," says William Castelli, M.D., long-time director of the Framingham Heart Study, the nation's oldest ongoing research program into the causes of heart disease.

## Bad-Guy Fat Facts

Millions of Americans grew up believing that carbohydrates (starches and sugars) were the major dietary villains. They viewed potatoes and cakes as fattening and thought weight loss involved limiting the total number of calories they ate. Until fairly recently, the centerpiece of any restaurant "diet plate" was a ground beef patty.

In the last 20 years, however, nutrition scientists have shown that there's really only one villain in the American diet—fat. Carbohydrates, including fruits, vegetables, beans and grains, provide most of the body's energy.

Even long-vilified sugar doesn't hurt most people when used in moderation (and provided they practice good dental hygiene). As far as weight control is concerned, if you limit fat calories, you don't have to worry much about your total calorie intake.

"It's not the potato that's fattening," Dr. Goor explains. "It's the butter, sour cream and bacon bits people put on it. The same goes for sugar. Cakes, pies and ice cream are fattening not because they contain sugar but because they're loaded with fat. It's people's 'fat tooth,' not their sweet tooth, that gets them into trouble."

How could this be? It's simple: All calories are not created equal. One gram of carbohydrate or protein contains only four calories, but one gram of fat contains nine. "Fat calories really

## Loose Label Lingo

Great! We now have nutritional labels—courtesy of federal government regulations—that are designed to help us eat healthy. That means we won't ever again be fooled by claims that a food is "fat-free," "low-fat," or "lite." Right?

Wrong!

Just because the Feds got involved doesn't mean you're protected from the tricks of the advertising trade. Here are a few things to be aware of.

Even if a label says a food is "light" or "lite," the food can still have as much as 50 percent of calories from fat. A food can be labeled "light" if it has half the fat or calories of the regular version, even if the regular version packs a double whammy.

Serving sizes vary from product to product, so one big cookie could be considered "low-fat" when compared to a three-cookie serving of another brand. Three grams of fat per serving is considered low-fat, so if a company decides that half a cookie is a "serving," they can use the low-fat claim on some pretty high-fat snacks.

Finally, milk is exempt from these labeling regulations. So even if it says "low-fat," 2 percent milk still has 38 percent of calories from fat.

---

sneak up on you," Dr. Goor says. "A few handfuls of potato chips have the same number of calories as two medium-size baked potatoes topped with nonfat yogurt and steamed vegetables."

Carbohydrates have a lot of bulk per calorie, so eating them triggers feelings of fullness. It's difficult to overeat if you base your diet on them. "If you reduce your fat consumption from the typical 35 to 40 percent of calories down to the 10 percent level of my program," Dr. Ornish explains, "you can eat one-third more food without increasing your total number of calories. You feel full and satisfied but still reduce your risk of heart disease and the other fat-related diseases—and you lose weight. That's why I called my book *Eat More, Weigh Less.*"

Your body also uses fats in a different way than it uses carbohydrates. Your body uses most carbohydrates quickly and can only store about one day's worth in the form of glycogen (a complex sugar) in the liver and in muscle tissue. "If you eat normal amounts," Dr. Goor says, "carbohydrates are never stored as fat."

Fats, on the other hand, are not used right away. Your body stores them as fat in adipose tissue, which has an almost unlimited capacity to bulge. Unlike carbohydrates, fat doesn't cause feelings of fullness, so you keep eating and eating, gaining weight and increasing your risk of all the fat-related diseases.

Everyone must consume some fats because they are necessary for the synthesis of essential fatty acids. But you need only about 10 percent of calories as fat to produce all the essential fatty acids your body needs to function optimally.

If high-fat diets contribute to a host of diseases, do low-fat diets help prevent them? Doctors answer that question with a resounding yes.

Dr. Ornish's findings that his ultra-low-fat diet reverses heart disease have been corroborated by several other studies that were recently summarized in a report co-sponsored by the AHA, the ACS and the Center for Science in the Public Interest, a Washington-based consumer nutrition organization. That report says that if Americans cut their fat consumption by about one-third (down to approximately 20 percent of calories from fat), heart disease and cancer would decline significantly, and the nation's health-care bill would plummet $17 billion a year.

## Forward into the Past

Nutrition experts have started saying that we should eat as people used to. They're referring not to the way we ate before microwave ovens but rather to the way our ancestors did 10,000 years ago. In those days, the main problem with food was not overconsumption, as it is today, but rather finding enough to prevent starvation. Our ancestors solved this problem by storing fat quickly and easily in their bodies to see them through periods of famine. "Back then," quips Dr. Ornish, "it was survival of the fattest."

Today we have essentially the same genetic makeup as our starvation-threatened ancestors, but the very fat-storage mechanism that saved them is killing us. According to anthropologists S. Eaton Boyd, Ph.D., Marjorie Shostak, Ph.D., and Melvin Konner, M.D., Ph.D., authors of *The Paleolithic Prescription*, we've become caught in a dietary time warp. Like Rip Van Winkle, we've awakened in a world of high-fat foods that our bodies are genetically incapable of thriving on. The results? All the fat-related chronic illnesses that have become our leading causes of death.

To avoid these degenerative diseases, we need to eat more like our Stone Age ancestors. Dr. Boyd is an expert on ancient diets, and Dr. Shostak and Dr. Konner lived for several years with the Kung tribe of the Kalahari Desert in southern Africa, one of the few remaining hunter-gatherer peoples on earth. Together they pieced together what early humans ate: primarily plants—nuts, fruits, beans, grains and roots—with some game meats. But those meats were much different from ours. They contained only about 5 percent fat by weight, much less than our domesticated meat animals (30 percent fat by weight). Overall, these experts contend, the human body evolved to consume no more than about 20 percent of calories from fat, about half of what most Americans eat today.

Throughout the vast majority of human history, even after the arrival of civilization, agriculture and industry, people continued to eat more or less as they were genetically programmed to do. In 1910, Americans ate a diet based on carbohydrates, with only about 20 percent of calories from fat.

"They consumed more total calories than we do today, but far fewer from fat. And heart disease, cancer, diabetes, hypertension and obesity were all rare," says Neil Barnard, M.D., author of *Food for Life* and president of the Physicians Committee for Responsible Medicine, a professional organization in Washington, D.C., that promotes preventive medicine through nutrition.

Today, according to a report by the National Center for Health Statistics, American fat consumption averages 34 percent of total calories. That average is down slightly from 1978, when the figure was 36 percent, but averages can be misleading. Some Americans have cut way back on fats, but millions still consume at least twice as much fat as their great-grandparents did. Compared with 1992, in 1993 U.S. sales of butter, ice cream, high-fat cookies and fast-food meals increased by almost $1 billion. It's clear Americans still have a long way to go to reduce their risks of fat-related health problems.

## Evolving Away from Fats

There are two ways to reduce the amount of fat in your diet—by evolution or revolution. If you already have a fat-related medical condition or major risk factors for one, consider the more revolutionary approach discussed under "Revolution to the Rescue" on page 305. If not, the evolutionary path can reduce your fat consumption enough to add years to your life and life to your years.

Evolving one's diet away from fats begins with reading food labels. The new nutritional label created by the Food and Drug Administration states the number of calories from fat in one serving of the item. As a general rule, select foods that contain no more than 20 percent of calories from fat per serving. Beware, though: Sometimes the serving size is too small, representing less than what you're likely to eat. That means that the actual fat content of a more realistic serving is higher.

And don't be fooled by the Daily Value (DV) listing. The DVs, displayed in bold type on the new nutrition labels, tell you how much of a day's worth of fat, cholesterol, sodium and so forth the food provides, based on a hypothetical 2,000-calorie-a-day diet. But they can lead to a misunderstanding of the amount of fat an item contains. A snack food might have a fat DV of 25 percent, which might seem acceptable to the unsuspecting consumer, but still contain 75 percent of calories (or more) from fat.

As far as unlabeled foods are concerned, here are some guidelines.

*Fruits, vegetables and beans.* They're low in fat and high in

# A Bonanza of Guilt-Free Snacks

Snacks are the downfall of many an aspiring low-fat enthusiast. Chips, cookies, most candies, commercial popcorn and most other snack foods are a one-way ticket to high-fat trouble. But today, low-fat eaters can choose dozens of convenient, tasty, creamy, crunchy, satisfying low-fat snacks.

- Fresh, stewed or canned fruit (steer clear of ultrasugary heavy syrup)
- Air-popped popcorn (instead of butter, add black pepper, oregano or a little sprinkle of grated parmesan cheese)
- Bagels, bread, nonfat crackers or rice cakes with jam or preserves
- Chilled vegetable salad (steam the veggies, then add soy sauce, balsamic vinegar, orange juice or some other low-fat marinade and refrigerate)
- Fat-free tortilla chips with salsa
- Fat-free, low-salt pretzels
- Cornflakes with nonfat milk or yogurt
- Frozen bananas (peel the bananas, insert ice-pop sticks and freeze)
- Nonfat yogurt (add fresh fruit, or for crunch, try Grape-Nuts cereal, which is fat-free)
- Nonfat cottage cheese
- Nonfat frozen yogurt

carbohydrates, just the ticket for a healthy diet. Just don't cancel out their low-fat benefits by smothering them in high-fat butter, margarine or cream.

*Pastas and grains.* Here's another food group that's low in fat and high in carbohydrates. Eat more pasta and grains, as long as you're careful about what you add to them.

*Breads.* Eat as much bread as you want, but beware of crackers, muffins, biscuits, croissants and other bread treats that are high in fat. In addition, be careful about what kind of spreads you use. Low-fat choices include jellies, jams, preserves, mashed bananas, bean dip, nonfat yogurt and nonfat or low-fat cream cheese and cottage cheese. Butter, margarine, peanut butter and cheeses are high in fat.

*Nuts and seeds.* Nuts and seeds are high in fat. If you eat them by the handful, you can consume a great deal of fat. Use nuts and seeds sparingly to top fruits, vegetables, beans, pastas or grains. If you're looking for a little crunch, substitute Grape-Nuts cereal (completely fat-free) or toasted bread crumbs, oats or cornmeal.

*Eggs.* Use commercial egg substitutes in cooking and baking. For scrambled eggs or omelets, mix one real egg into mashed tofu or two or three eggs' worth of substitute.

*Meats.* Of all the red meats, only venison contains less than 20 percent of calories from fat. Beef, veal, pork, lamb, duck, sausages and lunch meats are all high in fat. But you don't have to eliminate them from your diet; simply change how you use them. Instead of building your meals around them, choose recipes that use small amounts of meat to flavor dishes based on vegetables, beans or grains, the way Asian cuisines do. If you love BLTs, you can still have them, but instead of four strips of bacon and one slice each of lettuce and tomato, pile on the L and T and crumble one strip of bacon over them.

And if you love burgers, select lean cuts of ground beef—the leanest is fat-trimmed top round. Ask your butcher or supermarket to grind it for you. Then thin your burgers by adding oatmeal and grated carrots. When you pan-fry ground beef for spaghetti sauce, brown it first, then place it in a colander and rinse it thoroughly with hot water. This removes a great deal of the fat.

*Chicken.* Skinless white-meat chicken breasts are low in fat and can be used in a virtually limitless number of low-fat recipes. But watch out—chicken skin is high in fat. If you eat it, you lose chicken's benefits. The meat can absorb a great deal of skin fat during cooking, so strip the skin beforehand. Dark-meat chicken parts (thighs and drumsticks) are also high in fat. You can still eat dark meat; just use it sparingly in recipes in which the main ingredients are vegetables, beans or grains.

Also beware of chicken hot dogs. They're often as high in fat as their pork or beef counterparts because they're mostly skin and dark meat. Finally, be careful how you cook your skinless chicken breasts. Fried or batter-dipped, they drip with fat. And butter- or cream-based sauces add significant fat.

*Turkey.* It's not just for Thanksgiving anymore. Ounce for ounce, a skinless white-meat turkey breast is even lower in fat than a chicken breast. These days, supermarkets sell it whole, sliced or in cutlets. If you pound turkey cutlets and cook them like veal, it's hard to tell the difference. But be careful—turkey carries the same caveats as chicken: Trim the skin and cook the meat skinless. Steer clear of dark-meat turkey, turkey franks and ground turkey (which, unless it's labeled white meat, can contain the more fatty dark meat and even high-fat turkey skin), and don't fry or use high-fat sauces.

*Fish and seafood.* Most fish and seafood, including cod, flounder, lobster, scallops, shrimp, snapper and sole, are low in fat. But several fish—herring, mackerel and salmon—are fairly high in fat. To keep your fish low-fat, bake, broil, poach or grill it or pan-fry it in wine. Don't fry it in butter or margarine or cover it with butter- or cream-based sauces. If you enjoy high-fat fish, use small portions and combine them with vegetables, beans and grains. Canned tuna comes packed in either water or high-fat oil. Choose the water-packed type.

*Butter, margarine and oils.* They're all 100 percent fat. Butter is the most harmful because it's the highest in saturated fat, which raises cholesterol and contributes to heart disease. But margarine contains trans-fatty acids, substances that also increase risk of heart disease.

Olive oil, a monounsaturated fat, does not increase risk of heart disease nor, according to some studies, the risk of breast or colon cancer. But olive oil is still 100 percent fat. Use it sparingly. One good way is to use less than the amount recipes call for. If a recipe suggests two tablespoons of olive oil, try one or less.

You can also substitute vegetable broth or sherry or try an oil spray. Most people who cook with sprays, which are available at supermarkets, use less oil than they would if they simply poured liquid oil into their pans.

*Salad dressings.* One easy way to trim fat from your meals is to use fat-free dressings on salads. Pritikin and other brands are available at most supermarkets. Or try vinegar or lemon juice with just a splash of oil.

*"Low-fat" prepared foods.* The dishes sold by Weight Watchers, Lean Cuisine, Jenny Craig and other similar programs claim to be low in fat. They are lower in fat than those found in the typical American diet, but most still derive more than 20 percent of their calories from fat. And they are not low enough in fat to significantly reduce the risk of fat-related medical conditions. In addition, they use small portion size to reduce the total number of calories, so people who eat them often feel unsatisfied and risk bingeing on high-fat items.

*The new nonfat foods.* If reading this section has left you scratching your head and wondering what's left to eat, cheer up! Increasing consumer demand for nonfat items has filled supermarket shelves with all sorts of seemingly sinful yet fat-free foods. Do you love cream cheese? Now there's fat-free cream cheese made from skim milk. Does the word dessert make you salivate for ice cream? Try nonfat frozen yogurt or sorbet, which is made entirely from frozen pureed fruit.

Pretzels, chips, cookies, breakfast cereals, cheeses and sour cream all come in nonfat versions. Supermarkets now carry literally hundreds of nonfat items. The next time you go shopping, open your eyes to the new world of nonfat food alternatives. What you see—and taste—just might surprise you.

In addition to paying attention to the fat content of foods, here are a couple of other tips to help you evolve your diet into a more low-fat, healthy version.

*Eat mindfully.* While eating, don't do anything else. Don't read, work, do household chores or watch TV.

*Eat breakfast.* For most people it's easier to banish the fat from breakfast than from any other meal. Try toast with jam, apple butter or nonfat cream cheese; a nonfat cereal or oatmeal with skim milk or nonfat yogurt and fresh fruit; or a fruit salad with nonfat cottage cheese. "A good breakfast provides energy," Dr. Ornish explains, "and reduces midmorning food cravings that send people scurrying for Danishes and doughnuts."

## Revolution to the Rescue

An evolutionary approach may not trim enough fat from your diet to prevent health disaster if you already have any of the following conditions: heart disease, high blood pressure, diabetes, obesity, a fat-related cancer or a history of thrombotic stroke or its precursor, mini-strokes called transient ischemic attacks (TIAs).

You may need the kind of revolutionary diet changes Dr. Ornish has used to reverse heart disease. The Ornish diet is similar to the one Nathan Pritikin developed in the mid-1970s to combat heart disease. (Pritikin died in 1985, but several Pritikin Longevity Centers continue to promote his program, and most supermarket diet sections stock ultra-low-fat Pritikin items.) Both the Ornish and Pritikin diets derive only 10 percent of calories from fat.

Dr. Ornish's revolutionary diet is really quite straightforward. He divides foods into three groups.

*Anytime.* You may eat these foods whenever you feel hungry and until you feel full: fruits, vegetables (except high-fat avocados and olives), beans and grains.

*Sometimes.* You may eat these foods in moderation: nonfat dairy products (milk, yogurt, sour cream and cheeses); egg whites; nonfat or very low-fat commercially prepared foods (whole-grain cereals, nonfat salad dressings, egg substitutes, Pritikin soups, Entenmann's fat-free baked goods, Health Valley nonfat soups and chili and Life Choice frozen dinners, which use recipes from Dr. Ornish's program).

*Beware.* These foods should be avoided as much as possible: meats (including chicken and fish), oils (all kinds, including

margarine and most salad dressings), nuts and seeds, dairy products that are not nonfat, alcohol, sugar (which often comes in
treats that are laced with fat) and any commercially prepared
item with more than two grams of fat per serving.

The Ornish diet may sound rigorous, even impossible. But
just as some smokers quit cold turkey rather than slowly cutting back on cigarettes, many people prefer the Ornish method
to the evolutionary approach.

## Restaurant Dining the Low-Fat Way

Even if you eat a low-fat diet at home, it's often difficult to
pass up high-fat items when dining at restaurants. A generation
ago, this wasn't much of a problem. Eating out was a rare treat,
take-out was a rarity and only a few pizza places delivered.
Today, eating out is routine, many people couldn't survive without take-out, and all sorts of restaurants deliver.

If you go out for lunch every day at work and eat out or take
out a few other times each week, restaurants wind up as the
source of one-third of your meals—or more.

"Low-fat restaurant dining requires a few adjustments," says
Newton, Massachusetts, dietitian Hope S. Warshaw, R.D., author of *The Restaurant Companion,* a guide to healthful dining.
"But it's actually easier—and tastier—than it might seem. With
a little forethought and information, anyone can eat out without
bulging out."

Here are some tips from nutrition experts to help you find
your best restaurant bets.

**Know where fat lurks.** To fight fat, steer clear of anything
fried or sautéed and anything prepared creamed, breaded, Alfredo, Hollandaise, tempura, batter-dipped, au gratin, en croûte,
phyllo-wrapped, in puff pastry, in potpie, in a croissant or with
gravy. And avoid all of these sauces: béarnaise, béchamel, beurre
blanc and crème fraîche.

**Never say never.** Remember, restaurant dining should be
pleasurable. If you know a restaurant serves the world's most
heavenly chocolate cheesecake, enjoy it without feeling guilty.

Just make sure the rest of your meal—and your other meals that day—are low in fat.

**Know what's low in fat.** Feel free to enjoy most items that are served broiled, grilled, baked, boiled, roasted, poached or steamed. Savor fish, seafood, skinless poultry, lean red meats, salads, pasta with pesto or tomato sauce, fresh fruits and vegetables, whole-grain items and frozen ices, sorbets, sherbets and nonfat frozen yogurts.

**Know your ethnics.** Some ethnic cuisines—Chinese, Indian, Vietnamese, Cambodian, Middle Eastern and Japanese—tend to be low in fat. These cuisines generally do not deep-fry foods. Stir-fried foods are okay, but stay away from deep-fried Japanese tempura. Many dishes in these cuisines are prepared entirely without meats, sauces and dairy products. Enjoy the many poultry, fish, seafood, vegetable and noodle dishes. In Asian cuisines, the pork and beef dishes include relatively small servings of meat, which helps keep their fat content low.

On the other hand, some eating establishments—delis, steak houses, pizza places, barbecue and burger joints and French, German, Mexican, Cajun and Italian restaurants—tend to serve food that's high in fat. But even in these danger zones, it's not difficult to find tasty low-fat dishes.

**Watch those meats.** If you order meat, always trim off all visible fat. At delis, try a turkey sandwich and coleslaw or soup and a salad. At steak houses, stick to the leaner cuts: sirloin, tenderloin and flank steak. Prime cuts are high in fat, and one of the fattiest is prime rib.

**Make that pizza lean.** At pizza places, the high-fat toppings are the cheeses and meats. Ask for less cheese and more vegetable toppings. Or forgo the cheese altogether and order a pesto pizza. Steer clear of sausage, bacon, hamburger and pepperoni. If you must have a meat topping, the leanest is Canadian bacon.

**Watch those burgers.** Many hamburger joints now serve grilled skinless chicken breast sandwiches. If you can't resist a burger, order one topped with salsa or grilled onions and mushrooms, not bacon, cheese or sour cream.

**Get savvy in Italian restaurants.** It's hard to find low-fat lasagna, cannelloni, manicotti or saltimbocca. But chicken, fish and seafood dishes become problems only when they are served parmigiana or covered with other cheeses or cream sauces. Tomato-based marinara sauces are lower in fat than pesto, which is lower than meat sauces or cream-based white Alfredo or cheese sauces.

**Cruise that Continental menu.** At French, German and Continental restaurants, look for dishes that are grilled, broiled, steamed, roasted, marinated or en brochette. Broiled veal and rack of lamb may seem sinful, but they're relatively low-fat choices. Duck served with the skin on and with a cream sauce is very high in fat. But skinless duck breast slices with a fruit sauce or glaze is a fairly low-fat choice.

**Screen those beans.** The high-fat items at Mexican restaurants include the cheeses, sour cream, guacamole and refried beans, if they are prepared with lard. Ask for whole beans instead of refried and skip the toppings—or ask for nonfat yogurt instead.

**Enjoy Cajun carefully.** At Cajun restaurants, casseroles and dishes served breaded or under creamy sauces are high in fat. Blackened and grilled dishes are lower-fat choices.

**Pick your fish.** At seafood restaurants, grilled or broiled dishes are quite low in fat—unless they are served with a sauce containing butter, cheese or sour cream. Stay away from breaded or fried dishes and those served with high-fat sauces.

**Survive fast foods.** Even fast-food outlets now offer some low-fat choices: salad bars and grilled chicken breast sandwiches. If you opt for the salad bar, however, make sure you steer clear of those high-fat dressings and creamy pasta dishes.

**Don't sabotage your oatmeal.** Oatmeal is a great restaurant breakfast item. Just beware of high-fat toppings such as nuts, butter, whole milk, half-and-half or cream. Stick with skim milk and fruit.

**Love those baked potatoes.** Baked potatoes are tasty low-fat lunch and dinner items, but skip the cheese, bacon and sour cream toppings. Instead go with salsa, broccoli or nonfat yogurt.

**Shun cream soups.** At lunch, look for cup-of-soup-and-half-sandwich combinations—as long as the soup is not "cream of something." Combinations satisfy the need for variety. Vegetable and bean soups are nutritious, filling and usually low in fat. Soups with a chicken stock base are higher in fat, but they're still a better choice than a croissant ham-and-cheese sandwich.

Beware the high-fat sandwich. Mayonnaise and "special" sandwich sauces are high in fat. Stick to mustard, ketchup, salsa and barbecue sauce.

**Forget french fries.** Select rice, pasta or a baked potato instead.

**Plan ahead.** A little forethought is better than hours of self-recrimination for what you should have done. It's no big deal to plan for low-fat dining out. If you're happy at home with a simple breakfast of toast and coffee or a bowl of cereal with skim milk, don't even look at the menu. Just order your usual meal and don't get tempted by the Belgian waffles or bacon-and-sour-cream omelet. If you're happy with a salad for lunch or a baked potato and a steamed vegetable for dinner, don't look at the menu. Just order them.

**Think small.** Patronize restaurants that offer a large selection of appetizers, such as marinated vegetables, unusual salads and pasta dishes and exotic fish and seafood items. Try one or two appetizers instead of an entrée. But steer clear of pâtés, puff pastries and cheese plates (especially fried cheese).

**Consider portion size in advance.** Before you and your companion are seated, suggest splitting part or all of your meals. And beware of buffets, smorgasbords and all-you-can-eat specials. They're setups for overeating. In addition, the dishes are often high in fat.

**Nibble before dinner.** Never arrive at any restaurant feeling ravenous. You'll choose more wisely and feel better about yourself if you take the edge off your hunger beforehand with a healthy low-fat snack: an apple, a banana or pretzel or a cup of nonfat yogurt.

**Beware of booze.** Alcohol is surprisingly high in calories (more than 100 calories per ounce). If you drink beer, wine or cocktails with dinner, drink water or iced tea at the same time to quench your thirst and help you nurse your drink. If you enjoy wine with lunch or dinner, order it by the glass. That way you won't feel obligated to polish off a whole bottle.

**Become more assertive.** Restaurants are in the business of service, so speak up. Let the staff know what you want. They don't resent it. That's what they're there for.

**Ask for substitutions.** Does a breakfast restaurant offer jam and margarine or just butter? Instead of a three-egg omelet, can you order a one-egg omelet with some egg substitute? And can you get skim or low-fat milk for coffee instead of cream or half-and-half? Do lunch and dinner restaurants offer entrée salads?

**Clear off temptation.** As you're seated, ask that the bread and butter or chips be removed or served later with your meal. While you're waiting, sip water, club soda or herbal tea. If you do keep the bread basket, remember that breadsticks, rolls and French bread are lower in fat than croissants and most muffins.

**Come prepared.** If a restaurant doesn't serve healthful dressings and condiments, discreetly bring your own. Salsa makes an excellent bread spread, salad dressing and vegetable topping. Or prepare some herb-and-lemon-juice salad dressing and bring it in a small container.

**Get skinned.** When ordering chicken, insist on skinless parts and ask if the skin was removed before cooking.

**Ask questions.** Even such presumably healthful dishes as broiled or grilled fish or skinless chicken can be smothered in high-fat sauces. Ask how sauces are prepared; if they are high in fat, ask for no sauce or sauce on the side. Ask for salad dressing on the side as well. Then dip your fork into the dressing before you spear any salad. That way you get a little dressing—but not too much—with each bite.

**Divide and conquer.** If you can't resist a high-fat dessert, split it with your companion or take part of it home.

**Stand firm.** Don't let yourself be corrupted by your dining companion. Well-meaning friends sometimes sabotage low-fat dining plans by coaxing, "Come on, live a little."

If a friend has previously led you to restaurant ruin, announce your intentions to eat healthfully before you arrive at the restaurant and insist that your wishes be respected. (You may have to endure some teasing, but that's easier than letting your slacks out an inch.)

**Beware of salads.** Not all salads are low in fat. A good one to avoid is the chef's salad with its cheeses, eggs and high-fat lunch meats.

**Catch yourself in the act.** Finally, whenever you catch yourself thinking, "Oh, what the heck . . . ," stop a moment, close your eyes, take a few deep breaths and ask yourself if you *really* want that item.

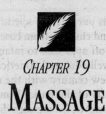

## CHAPTER 19
# MASSAGE

### Healing Hands, Touching Results

Touch is the only sense we cannot live without. People who are blind or deaf or have no sense of smell or taste can live to ripe old ages, but a century ago, Americans learned the hard way about the fatal consequences of touch deprivation and the life-saving benefits of massage.

A world-wide symbol of nurturance is the loving cuddling of babies. In many cultures, infants rarely spend any waking time out of an adult's arms until they crawl. Until the final years of the nineteenth century, American mothers also held their babies. But that changed abruptly when Luther Emmet Holt, M.D., published *The Care and Feeding of Children* in 1895.

Dr. Holt was a professor of pediatrics at the Columbia University School of Medicine in New York. He was also the "Dr. Spock" of his day. His book was a major best-seller and had enormous influence on turn-of-the-century child-rearing. Dr. Holt felt that in the new twentieth century, child care should break with its historical, "savage" roots. He railed against such traditional practices as cuddling and rocking babies in chairs or cradles. He believed that infants were "spoiled" by frequent handling and urged his legions of readers to put them down, feed them strictly by the clock and ignore them when they cried. Dr.

Holt believed that his purportedly scientific recommendations saved both parents and children from base "animal instincts."

Dr. Holt's hands-off approach to infant care was embraced by many affluent, well-educated Americans who were determined to greet the new century with the newest scientific wisdom and by the staffs of the nation's many orphanages and foundling homes. However, his message did not trickle down to poor, less educated women, who continued to hold, hug and cuddle their infants just as their ancestors always had.

By 1910, pediatricians were reporting a strange new early childhood disease that caused many healthy infants to withdraw, lose weight and die. They called it marasmus, from the Greek for "wasting away." At that time, the vast majority of early childhood diseases were associated with poverty, but marasmus was an odd exception. As the wealth of parents increased, so did their children's risk of the fatal illness.

Marasmus was especially epidemic at the nation's "best" foundling homes and orphanages. In a 1915 report that shocked the nation, New York City pediatrician Henry Dwight Chapin, M.D., detailed his tour of selected children's institutions, during which he discovered that few of the young residents survived to age two.

Curious about marasmus, an American pediatrician, Fritz Talbot, M.D., visited the Children's Clinic in Dusseldorf, Germany, where the wasting syndrome was rare. Dr. Talbot could not understand why, since German pediatric practices were virtually identical to American practices.

Then something caught Dr. Talbot's eye—an elderly nurse was working her way around the ward, cuddling and massaging each infant. The German doctors explained that without Old Anna's tender loving care, their best treatments didn't work, and many babies died.

Back in the United States, Dr. Talbot's experience fueled a rebellion against Dr. Holt's hands-off child-rearing theories. Anti-Holt forces also pointed to the thriving children of poor women who'd never heard of the Columbia professor and cuddled their kids like puppies.

Around 1920, New York's Bellevue Hospital pediatrics ward, once a bastion of Holtism, broke with the doctor and introduced "mothering," which encouraged frequent holding and rocking of the infants by staff and volunteers. Almost immediately, marasmus incidence plummeted and Dr. Holt's precepts fell from fashion. Today child development experts agree that infants cannot be cuddled too much.

## You Need to Be Touched

It turns out that frequent touching and cuddling, a spontaneous form of massage, not only helps infants thrive, it also contributes to adult happiness.

In the mid-1980s, while a visiting professor of psychology at Boston University, Carol Franz, Ph.D., unearthed a 1951 child-rearing questionnaire completed by the mothers of 400 Boston children who were then in kindergarten. Thirty-six years later, in 1987, Dr. Franz located 94 of the kindergarteners, then 41. Using a four-hour battery of surveys and interviews, she assessed their adult happiness—their enjoyment of their jobs, marriages, children and friends and their general zest for life.

Nothing that people typically consider prescriptions for happiness had anything to do with how fulfilled the participants felt. Their parents' wealth or poverty had no impact on their adult happiness. Neither did their parents' strictness or such childhood traumas as frequent moves, major injuries or even parents' divorces, alcoholism or death. Dr. Franz discovered only one clear predictor of later happiness—warm, affectionate mothers and fathers who cuddled their children and enjoyed spending time with them.

"I've always been affectionate with my children," says Dr. Franz. "That's just how I am. But the study suggests that parental warmth and affection—from fathers as well as mothers—equip children to create happy adult lives for themselves."

"Marasmus has never been documented after infancy," explains Stella Resnick, Ph.D., a clinical psychologist in private practice in Los Angeles, "but the fact that lack of touch can cause death shows just how important it is. We should think of touch as a nutrient transmitted through the skin. Just as we need a variety of nutrients, we also need many forms of touch: holding, cuddling, massage. Being held is one of life's primary pleasures. Cuddling is deeply nurturing. Massage is profoundly relaxing. We all have fears and anxieties. Warm human touch helps relieve them."

People in the United States are generally touch-phobic. When a crowd enters an elevator, the people distribute themselves so that no one touches anyone else. This observation had a profound impact on the late Sidney Jourard, professor of psychology at the University of Florida. He traveled around the world visiting coffee shops in hundreds of cities to count how often couples touched one another. In his home town of Gainesville, Florida, people touched just twice an hour, in Paris, they touched 110 times, and in San Juan, Puerto Rico, people touched 180 times an hour.

For most American adults, touching is reserved for lovemaking. A playful, massage-oriented love style is a key component of mutually fulfilling sex, but even out of bed, massage offers real pleasure and profound health benefits.

## Touching for Health

When a bruise or muscle strain causes pain, what's the first thing people do? Often before they even say "ouch," they grab the injured area and rub it.

Cave paintings discovered in the Pyrenees show that 15,000 years ago, our ancestors treated injuries with what looks like massage. Ancient Chinese and Ayurvedic physicians prescribed massage for many ailments as early as 3,000 years ago. During the fourth century B.C., Hippocrates, the father of Western medicine, said, "The physician must be experienced in many things, but most assuredly in rubbing."

In the New Testament, Jesus cured the blind by touching their eyes and the lame by touching their legs: "He laid his hands on every one of them and healed them" (Luke 4:40). As Christianity developed, priests laid their hands on the sick, and when the laying-on of hands fell from favor in the Church, the kings of France and England adopted the practice, using "the Royal Touch" to treat ailing supplicants.

"The benefits of massage," says Tiffany Field, Ph.D., professor of psychology, pediatrics and psychiatry at the University of Miami Medical School and director of the Touch Research Institute there, "include immune enhancement, insomnia relief, heightened alertness and relief from stress, anxiety and mild to moderate depression. Medicine is just beginning to rediscover the tremendous power of touch."

In the mid-1970s, Dr. Field recalls, "I'd never heard of marasmus, but my daughter, Tory, was born prematurely, and I became very interested in the medical care given preemies."

Concern about these frail babies' susceptibility to diseases spread by human contact led to the standard practice of keeping them in special isolation cribs called Isolettes. As a psychologist, Dr. Field was familiar with monkey research showing growth retardation and other problems in animals deprived of maternal contact. She became concerned that lack of human contact might retard her daughter's development. She launched a study to find out.

For 15 minutes three times a day, one group of preemies received gentle massage. The results were dramatic. Compared with untouched babies, those that were massaged gained 47 percent more weight and were sent home six days earlier. "Everyone benefits from touching preemies," Dr. Field explains. "The children are healthier, and the hospitals save a fortune." Since her first study, Dr. Field has conducted similar experiments on children born with congenital cocaine addiction. "Frequent touch helped them withdraw more easily and gain weight more quickly," she says.

Massage triggers the release of chemicals in the brain, such as serotonin, that enhance our sense of well-being. "We don't fully understand the biochemistry of touch, but it's very clear that human beings need it," Dr. Field explains.

Research compiled by the American Massage Therapy

# When Not to Massage

People with dozens of medical conditions and psychological problems can use massage to relax and gain all the other health benefits discussed in this chapter. But because massage affects so many body systems, some people should not use it.

Do not have a massage or provide massage—especially deep pressure styles—if the recipient is pregnant, acutely ill or feverish. Be cautious about giving a back massage to anyone with a back problem. Check with a physician before massaging anyone with a serious medical condition, such as cancer or heart disease. Finally, don't massage:

- The abdomen within two hours after eating.
- The abdomen in anyone with a hernia.
- Any area that's swollen, inflamed, infected or bruised.
- Any suspected broken bone or sprain.
- Arthritic joints.
- Rashes or other skin eruptions, including acne.
- Varicose veins.
- Thrombophlebitis (painful blood clots in the veins).
- Any area with a surgical incision.
- Areas known to contain tumors.

Association (AMTA) shows that in addition to releasing serotonin, massage has many other physiological effects on the body. Different massage styles have different effects, but from gentle rhythmic stroking of the entire body surface to sustained deep pressure applied on specific points, here's a sampling of effects.

- Massage feels enjoyable, reduces stress, calms nervous irritability, clears the mind and helps improve posture.
- Massage increases local circulation. Rubbing of the soft tissues opens blood vessels (vasodilation). This in turn speeds deliv-

ery of nutrients and elimination of cellular wastes, which spur healing of injured tissues.

- Massage produces general relaxation—reduction of pulse and blood pressure, deepening of breathing and relief of muscle spasms and cramping and the pain they cause.
- Massage speeds muscle recovery from exertion.
- Massage stretches connective tissue, which helps reduce pain and increase range of motion.
- Massage stimulates the release of serotonin, endorphins and other brain chemicals (neurotransmitters) that elevate mood and enhance feelings of well-being.
- Massage stimulates lymphatic circulation, which can help decrease swelling (edema).

Medical literature contains dozens of studies demonstrating the benefits of these effects. Here are some summaries of recent reports.

*Anxiety and depression.* Dr. Field divided 72 adolescent residents of a psychiatric hospital into two groups. One group of 20 viewed relaxing videos, while the 52 others received a 30-minute back massage every day for five days. Based on staff evaluations, the massaged group showed less depression and anxiety and more normal sleep patterns. In addition, their saliva and urine showed lower levels of stress hormones.

*Athletic performance.* Swedish researchers assessed the leg strength of eight competitive cyclists who pedaled to exhaustion on two different occasions. After one session, the men rested for ten minutes. After the other, they received a ten-minute leg massage. The researchers then measured the cyclists' leg strength and found it to be 11 percent greater after the massage. A similar 1994 study showed that a 30-minute postworkout massage significantly reduced the incidence of muscle soreness.

*Cancer pain.* At the University of South Carolina in Columbia, Sally Weinrich, R.N., Ph.D., associate professor of nursing, and Martin Weinrich, Ph.D., associate professor of epidemiology and biostatistics, divided 28 hospitalized cancer patients into two groups. One received a ten-minute visit, the other a ten-minute massage. Pain levels were then assessed using standard psychological tests. After just one ten-minute massage, pain levels decreased.

Norwegian researchers have shown why. They measured blood levels of endorphins, the body's pain-relieving chemicals, in a dozen volunteers before and after a 30-minute massage. The massage produced a 16 percent increase in endorphins, and the effect lasted for about an hour.

*Chronic pain.* Michael Weintraub, M.D., chief of neurology at Phelps Memorial Hospital in New York City, felt perplexed. Some of his chronic back pain patients did not respond well to anything mainstream medicine could provide. He offered them acupuncture, which helped quite a few, but some people had a fear of needles and wouldn't try it. So in 1989, Dr. Weintraub asked 63 of his patients to try two shiatsu-style acupressure massages a week in his office. The massages provided significant pain relief in 86 percent. Dr. Weintraub now works closely with several massage therapists.

*The common cold.* Boston researchers divided 32 elderly people into two groups. Members of one group lay on a massage table for ten minutes but did not receive a massage. People in the other group got a ten-minute back rub. Both groups provided saliva samples before and after. The elderly people who were not massaged showed no change in secretory IgA, a protein produced by the immune system that acts as the body's first line of defense against the common cold. But in those who received the massage, IgA increased significantly.

*Eating disorders.* Dr. Field says she has obtained "excellent results" from including massage in a comprehensive treatment program for women with anorexia nervosa and bulimia. "Women with eating disorders are so mentally divorced from the reality of their own bodies that they can't see what they look like. Massage helps them *feel* it."

*HIV infection.* Dr. Field's colleague, Gail Ironson, M.D., professor of psychology at the University of Miami, arranged for 40 HIV-positive men to have a 45-minute massage once a day, five days a week for one month. They all felt better, due at least

(continued on page 322)

# Therapeutic Touch:
# Massage without Touching

In Cinderella, the fairy godmother waves her magic wand over the young scullery maid and transforms her rags into a gown. Dolores Krieger, R.N., Ph.D., professor of nursing at New York University and author of *Accepting Your Power to Heal: The Personal Practice of Therapeutic Touch,* dispenses with the wand yet claims to heal many ailments with a few waves of her hands.

Dr. Krieger has popularized therapeutic touch, a massagelike healing art. Ironically, its practitioners, mostly nurses who call themselves "Krieger's Krazies," rarely touch their "healees." Instead they channel healing energy through their hands and into healees by rearranging the "energy field" that surrounds healees' bodies an inch or two away from their skin.

Dr. Krieger readily acknowledges the metaphysical nature of therapeutic touch as well as mainstream medicine's skepticism (even derision) about it. But she insists that it can reduce pain, anxiety and depression in adults, reduce stress in premature infants, accelerate wound healing, relieve premenstrual syndrome and boost metabolism by increasing the amount of oxygen carried in the blood.

Therapeutic touch is a contemporary version of the ancient practice of laying-on of hands. Dr. Krieger learned it from Dora Kunz, a traditional laying-hands practitioner. The roots of laying-on of hands stretch back to before the dawn of history, but Dr. Krieger says therapeutic touch also draws on traditional Chinese and Ayurvedic medical concepts, as well as modern physics.

In Chinese and Ayurvedic medicine, all living things possess life energy, *chi* or *prana,* that flows around the body along various pathways. According to these traditional practices, when the energy flow is disrupted, illness results. However, healers can transfer their own life energy to those who are ill if they consciously intend to do so. The energy transfer helps the sick person get well.

Meanwhile, modern physics views matter and energy as interchangeable manifestations of the same thing. Dr. Krieger says that therapeutic touch works on the healee's "energy body," and through it, helps heal the physical body.

Therapeutic touch begins with "centering." The healer enters a meditative state of deep relaxation and single-minded focus on the healee. Then the healer "assesses" the healee's ailments by circling his or her body at a distance of a few inches, "tuning in" to any perceived energy disturbances or temperature changes. Finally, the healer "rebalances" the healee's energy by using the hands to "unruffle" or "smooth out" any perceived energy disturbances. Typically, the process takes 10 to 20 minutes.

Dr. Krieger's book abounds with anecdotal reports of success using therapeutic touch, but the scientific literature on it is scant, with a few studies showing no significant benefits. However, several studies have shown benefits. Researchers at Healing Sciences International in Orinda, California, inflicted small, superficial experimental wounds on the arms of college-student volunteers, who extended their injured arms through a hole in a wall so they could not see what was happening on the other side. Some of the arms received therapeutic touch; others did not. The group treated with therapeutic touch experienced significantly faster wound healing.

"Therapeutic touch," says Michael Lerner, Ph.D., former Yale psychology professor and co-founder of the Commonweal Cancer Help Program in Bolinas, California, "makes assumptions about the nature of reality that are not universally shared in our culture. But at the Cancer Help Program, participants have the opportunity to give a therapeutic touch experience to someone and to receive one hemselves. For the vast majority of participants, the experience of both giving and receiving this form of simple touch with intent to heal is profoundly positive. Today's science cannot account for it, but something seems to be happening that medicine should attend to."

partly to a significant increase in their serotonin levels. They also showed an increase in natural killer (NK) cells, a key component of the immune system. This was the first time anyone ever boosted NK cells without drugs.

*Hospitalization stress.* Hospital treatment can help heal, but hospitalization can be an alienating, stress-provoking experience. Marian Williams, R.N., runs a six-month training program for nurses interested in learning massage at the California Pacific Medical Center in San Francisco. "It's very clear," she says, "that patients receiving massages require less pain medication and suffer less insomnia."

*Productivity.* Dr. Field gave a math test to a group of office workers. Then she arranged for them to receive brief massages twice a week for one month. The office workers subsequently finished a similar math test more quickly and with fewer errors.

## Types of Massage

There are almost as many styles of massage as there are practitioners. Most people who become massage therapists develop a personal style—"a little of this, a little of that"—just as master chefs tend to draw on elements of several cuisines.

In the United States, there are two basic massage styles, Swedish and shiatsu, with dozens of offshoots whose different names obscure the fact that many have a good deal in common. Esalen massage, laying-on of hands and therapeutic touch, among others, derive from Swedish massage. Acupressure massage, do-in (*doe-een*), polarity therapy and reflexology are just some of the styles that have roots in shiatsu.

In addition, some schools of hands-on healing combine massage with posture training, movement re-education or deep tissue manipulation.

## The Gift from Sweden

For most of the more than one million Americans who enjoy massage each year, massage typically means some variation of

Swedish massage, which was developed about 150 years ago by Peter Ling of Sweden, who integrated ancient Asian massage arts with a Western understanding of anatomy and physiology. Swedish massage came to the United States 100 years ago and has been a massage touchstone, as it were, ever since.

Depending on the preferences of the massage provider and recipient, Swedish massage varies in pressure. Some people prefer light, feathery strokes that push gently on the major muscle groups. Others enjoy deeper strokes with firm, rolling pressure that resembles the kneading of bread.

There are five basic Swedish massage strokes.

*Effleurage (EF-flur-ahj).* French for "touching," effleurage is the introductory stroke, the first one used on every part of the body. In addition to feeling great, it prepares the area for the other strokes. Effleurage involves long, gliding strokes—from the buttocks to the base of the neck, for example, or from the ankle to the thigh. The practitioner typically uses the whole hand, both palm and fingers, but for variety, effleurage strokes can be administered with the fingertips, the heel of the hand or even the knuckles.

*Petrissage (PET-ris-ahj).* This stroke involves grasping the muscle groups and lifting them, stretching them away from the bones and then kneading, pressing or rolling them.

*Thumb work.* More localized than either effleurage or petrissage, thumb work involves using the fingers and palms to anchor the hands in place, then using the thumbs to press on small areas and moving in a circular motion around them.

*Vibration.* This stroke involves placing the hands on a muscle group and moving them back and forth quickly in a shaking motion.

*Percussion.* This stroke uses the fleshy side of the hands to tap or chop.

## Shiatsu: Touching in Japanese

In Japanese, *shi* means "finger" and *atsu* means "pressure." Shiatsu massage is the Japanese adaptation of acupressure, which in turn is derived from Chinese acupuncture. Like acupuncture, shiatsu is based on the idea that life energy (*chi* in Chinese and *ki* in Japanese) runs up, down and around the body along pathways called meridians. Free flow of this energy produces health, and any blockages cause illness. Blockages occur at specific points, called *tsubo* in Japanese. Finger pressure on the points associated with each disease releases blocked energy, re-establishing healthy flow.

The meridians are nonanatomical. Practitioners of Asian medicine insist they exist, while Western researchers are equally convinced that they do not. Western scientists say that the meridians are actually the major nerve lines and that pressure on the approximately 75 most active points releases not blocked energy but rather neurotransmitters, chemical messengers between nerve cells that play a key role in many physiological actions, such as pain relief.

No matter which explanation one accepts, a good deal of laboratory evidence shows that finger pressure on the tsubo can help relieve pain, anxiety and stress and generally enhance feelings of well-being.

Shiatsu practitioners must learn two things: where the points are located and how to stimulate them. Charts and practice teach the former. When pressed, the points announce themselves with tenderness, tingling or mild discomfort (but not pain). Point massage involves a circular boring movement with the thumb or forefinger for about 30 seconds.

## How to Get or Give a Good Massage

If you want a good massage, *don't* go to a massage parlor in the sleazy part of town. At these fronts for prostitution, about the only thing you can't get is a good massage.

If you want a good therapeutic massage, get a recommendation from a friend or contact the AMTA at 820 Davis Street, Suite 100, Evanston, IL 60201.

It's possible—but not ideal—to learn massage from a book. A better way to learn is to take a class or view a video. For referrals to classes near you, contact the AMTA. Many massage videos are also available. Two of the best are listed in Resources on page 526.

Professional certification in massage therapy requires a good deal of training. But you don't need much instruction to give a wonderfully soothing massage. Here's what massage therapist Rebecca Klinger, the instructor in the *Massage Your Mate* video (see Resources) recommends.

- The recipient should shower beforehand and remove jewelry, glasses or contact lenses.
- The provider should have clean, short, smooth fingernails and wear loose clothing that does not restrict movement.
- The massage should take place in warm, quiet room (no phones).
- Soft, soothing music helps establish a relaxing atmosphere.
- If you don't have a massage table, place a sheet on a rug-covered floor. Do not use a bed, because beds absorb too much pressure when the provider presses. If you use the floor, a small foam kneeling pad often adds to the provider's comfort.
- Respect the recipient's privacy by covering him or her up to the neck with a sheet or large towel. Expose only the area being massaged: the back, leg and so forth.
- Oil is a must. Massage works best when strokes are lubricated. Any vegetable oil will do, but scented massage oils add an extra dimension of relaxation and sensuality.
- Massage oils can be messy. Have a towel close at hand to blot up any excess.
- Have some small pillows or rolled-up towels on hand to place under the recipient's ankles, neck or other places that need support as the massage proceeds.
- As the massage begins, both provider and recipient should breathe deeply for relaxation.
- The provider should pour a little oil into his or her hands and rub them together to warm them and focus healing energy in them. Don't pour the oil over the recipient. Accidental spills are jarring.

- The provider should begin with light strokes and proceed to deeper pressure only after the muscles in an area have relaxed and warmed up.
- The recipient should tell the provider if any strokes feel uncomfortable: too light, too deep or on a tender spot.
- The provider should never place pressure directly on the spinal column, just on the muscles on either side of it. The provider should also avoid the eyes and neck.
- The best massage comes from the provider's whole body, not just the arms. Giving a massage is like dancing. The whole body should be involved.
- If the provider has any doubts about what stroke to use, return to effleurage.

Even if you don't go in for formal massage, its health benefits can be yours simply by touching those you love more frequently—and being touched by them in return. Hug your children. Embrace your friends. Cuddle with your honey while watching TV. You'll feel calmer and better able to cope with stress. As the bumper sticker says, "Hugs Are Better than Drugs."

CHAPTER 20

# MEDITATION

*Portable Safe Harbor in a Stress-Filled World*

**M**ention "meditation," and what springs to mind? For many, it's an image of the Beatles studying transcendental meditation (TM) in India with its originator, Maharishi Mahesh Yogi. TM is one form of meditation, but there are many others. Some, like TM, are Asian spiritual disciplines focused on the breath or on a word or phrase (a mantra). Asian meditative disciplines have been widely practiced in America for only about 30 years.

Throughout history, Western culture has also been rich with meditative approaches to life's stresses and strains. Think of the worshiper praying, Henry David Thoreau sitting peacefully by the shores of Walden Pond, the woman on the bus quietly knitting or the fisherman perched on a rock overlooking a stream, intently watching his line.

Meditation is not just for yoga masters sitting cross-legged on mountaintops in the Himalayas. It's a flexible approach to coping with stress, anxiety, many medical conditions and the day-to-day "static" that robs us of inner peace. It's for anyone who ever thinks "I wish I felt less frazzled."

Today, Asian-style meditation has become as Americanized as flying to Thanksgiving family reunions. Perhaps that's why the new Pittsburgh International Airport boasts a large meditation room featuring a quiet ambiance, comfortable furniture and paintings of clouds. What better place than one of the nation's largest, busiest airports for a refuge from all the hustle and bustle?

## Medicine Discovers Mind Power

Asians have meditated for thousands of years. After the European powers colonized India and China, a handful of Westerners studied yoga, Buddhism, Hinduism and other meditative disciplines, but for the vast majority of Americans, the formal practice of meditation remained esoteric.

Then during the 1930s, two scientists, one European and the other American, independently stumbled on meditation as a form of therapy. Both developed thought-controlled techniques that produced deep relaxation. Johannes Schultz, M.D., a German psychiatrist and neurologist, was inspired by hypnosis to develop autogenic training—a set of visualization exercises that involve images of the limbs becoming heavy and relaxed. (To get all the details on autogenic training, see Visualization, Guided Imagery and Self-Hypnosis on page 443.)

Around the same time, Edmund Jacobson, M.D., a Harvard physician and physiologist, developed "progressive muscle relaxation"—conscious serial relaxation of the body's major muscle groups. Both techniques required a quiet room, deep breathing and a passive, observing attitude. Both relieved anxiety. And both remained obscure medical curiosities—until the 1970s, when, quite by accident, Harvard cardiologist Herbert Benson, M.D., brought meditation to the masses.

## Thinking Blood Pressure Down

The year was 1968, and Dr. Benson was using biofeedback to study monkeys with chronic high blood pressure, which is potentially life-threatening if the condition is not controlled. Some devotees of TM learned of his research and asked Dr. Benson to study them. They claimed that they could lower their blood pressure substantially simply by meditating, without fancy biofeedback equipment.

Initially Dr. Benson turned them down. "Why investigate anything as far out as TM?" he wondered. But the TM enthusiasts persisted, and eventually Dr. Benson relented. Much to his surprise, he discovered that TM did indeed reduce blood pressure. It also lowered the body's metabolic rate and oxygen consumption to levels that were unheard of except in animal hibernation or in the deepest stage of human sleep.

Dr. Benson became fascinated by Asian meditative disciplines, particularly TM, which is among the easiest to learn. When you learn TM, an instructor gives you a word or phrase—your personal mantra—which you promise not to divulge. You are told to sit quietly with your eyes closed and repeat the mantra over and over again for 20 minutes at a time once or twice a day.

The mantra functions to focus your mind on a single idea, representing the "oneness" of the universe. You're instructed to assume a passive, accepting attitude while repeating your mantra. When distracting thoughts intrude, you're instructed to simply observe them, accept them and gently return your mental focus to repeating your mantra.

As Dr. Benson's studies continued, he realized that the physiological changes caused by TM were not unique to it. They could be achieved by every deeply relaxing technique he investigated: Zen, yoga, hypnosis, autogenic training and progressive muscle relaxation.

The meditation-induced state of profound calm was, in fact, a natural human reaction, the physiological opposite of the well-known fight-or-flight reflex—the response to danger that prepares your body to defend itself or flee. The fight-or-flight reflex increases blood pressure, heart rate, breathing, metabolism and blood flow to the muscles.

The response triggered by all the relaxing disciplines did the opposite. It lowered blood pressure and slowed heart rate, breathing, metabolism and blood flow. Dr. Benson called the meditative reaction the relaxation response.

In 1975, Dr. Benson's book, *The Relaxation Response,* became a runaway best-seller. No matter where you stood on "spirituality," it had an important message to offer. For the scientifically inclined, it stripped meditation of its spiritual baggage and presented a powerful physiological case for deep relaxation that was palatable to Western rationalistic sensibilities. Meanwhile, for those with a more spiritual frame of mind, it demonstrated the real physiological value of religious meditative practices.

Dr. Benson presented meditation as one of Nature's cures—a physiological gift that anyone can use to calm down, cope with stress and, for those with spiritual inclinations, feel at one with God or the universe. Soon after *The Relaxation Response* appeared, people who would never have been caught dead in an ashram were meditating—and loving it.

Meditation had finally arrived in America, and quite by accident, Dr. Benson, now associate professor of medicine at Harvard Medical School and president of the Mind/Body Medical Institute at New England Deaconess Hospital in Boston, helped launch the field of mind/body medicine.

## Healing with Mind Power

During the two decades since *The Relaxation Response* first appeared, meditation has gone mainstream. Most people who practice it do so to reduce stress, anxiety, anger and other negative emotions. But increasingly, physicians prescribe meditation as part of the treatment for a large and growing number of medical conditions.

*Cancer.* "Cancer is very scary," notes Michael Lerner, Ph.D., former Yale psychology professor and co-founder of the Commonweal Cancer Help Program in Bolinas, California. "Meditation and other approaches to deep relaxation help center people so they can figure out how they'd like to handle the illness and proceed with life."

*Depression.* Feelings of helplessness, hopelessness and isolation are hallmarks of depression—the nation's most prevalent mental health problem. Meditation increases self-confidence and feelings of connection to others. "Many studies," Dr. Benson says, "have shown mood elevation in depressed people who regularly elicit the relaxation response."

**Heart disease.** Meditation is a key component of Ornish therapy, the only treatment scientifically proven to reverse heart disease. (To learn more, see Ornish Therapy on page 368.)

**High blood pressure.** As soon as Dr. Benson learned that TM reliably reduced blood pressure in meditators, he taught the relaxation response to 36 people with moderately elevated blood pressure. After several weeks of practice, their average blood pressure declined significantly, reducing their risk of stroke and heart attack.

**Infertility.** Couples dealing with infertility may become depressed, anxious and angry. To help them cope, Alice D. Domar, Ph.D., a psychologist at the Mind/Body Medical Institute, taught the relaxation response to one group of infertile couples. Compared with a similar group of infertile couples who did not learn deep relaxation, the meditators experienced less distress—and were more likely to get pregnant.

**Pain management.** Anxiety decreases the threshold for pain, Dr. Benson notes, and pain causes anxiety. The result is a vicious cycle: Compared with people who feel relaxed, those under stress experience pain more intensely and become even more stressed, which aggravates their pain. Meditation breaks this cycle.

Childbirth preparation classes routinely teach pregnant women deep breathing exercises to minimize the pain and anxiety of labor. Few call it breath meditation, but that's what it is.

Meditative techniques are also a key element in the Arthritis Self-Help Course at Stanford University. More than 100,000 people with arthritis have taken the 12-hour course and learned meditation-style relaxation exercises as part of a comprehensive self-care program. Graduates report a 15 to 20 percent reduction in pain.

Meditation may not eliminate pain, but it helps people cope more effectively. In a recent study at the Mind/Body Medical

# When Meditation Isn't Calming

By now everyone knows that meditation is always good for you, right? Wrong.

Adverse effects from meditation are not all that uncommon. In a 1992 study, Dean Shapiro, Ph.D., associate professor of psychiatry and human behavior at the University of California at Irvine, followed 27 people who attended a two-week meditation retreat. During meditation, 17 (62 percent) reported at least one adverse effect: fear, anxiety, confusion, depression or self-doubt.

Several other studies have shown similar findings, and in most it was the experienced meditators, not the beginners, who reported the most problems.

How could something that reportedly minimizes negative emotions cause them? Meditation experts point to several possible explanations.

First, some people have felt so stressed for so long that they are unfamiliar with deep relaxation and therefore feel threatened by it. Second, meditators are taught to accept nonjudgmentally whatever thoughts enter their minds. But sometimes extremely upsetting thoughts well up, and meditators are unable to remain nonjudgmen-

Institute, after people with chronic pain learned the relaxation response, their pain-related physician visits decreased 36 percent.

*Panic attacks.* Sometimes anxiety becomes paralyzing and people feel (wrongly) that they are about to suffer some horrible fate. Panic attacks are often treated with drugs, but studies by Jon Kabat-Zinn, Ph.D., associate professor of medicine at the University of Massachusetts Medical Center in Worcester and director of the medical center's Stress Reduction Clinic, show that if people who are prone to panic attacks begin focused, meditative breathing the instant they feel the first signs of an episode, they are less likely to have a full-blown panic attack.

tal. Third, meditation helps propel personal growth and deepen insight. But sometimes growth can be a painful thing. And finally, some people are temperamentally unsuited to meditation—they might not be able to sit still—and trying to do something they're incapable of causes problems.

Meditators are most likely to experience the downside of this relaxation technique during the first ten minutes of a meditation session, when they're unwinding into a state of deep relaxation, according to meditation researcher Patricia Carrington, Ph.D., clinical associate professor of psychiatry at the University of Medicine and Dentistry of New Jersey/Robert Wood Johnson Medical School in Piscataway and author of *Freedom in Meditation*. The unwinding process is not always smooth, she notes. Sometimes jarring thoughts or feelings pop up.

Occasional "side effects" of meditation are no reason to stop doing it, Dr. Carrington says. But if you begin to feel that meditation's costs outweigh its benefits, switch to another stress management activity, such as bodywork, walking, tai chi or yoga.

*Psoriasis.* This disease causes scaly red patches on the skin. A pilot study at Dr. Kabat-Zinn's clinic suggests that compared with the skin patches of people with psoriasis who receive only standard medical therapy, the skin patches of those who also meditate clear up more quickly.

*Respiratory crises.* Asthma, emphysema and chronic obstructive pulmonary disease (COPD) all restrict breathing and raise fears of suffocation, which in turn makes breathing even more difficult. Studies at Dr. Kabat-Zinn's clinic show that when people with these respiratory conditions learn breath meditation, they have fewer respiratory crises.

*Illness in general.* "It doesn't seem to matter what type of medical condition brings people to the Stress Reduction Clinic,"

Dr. Kabat-Zinn observes. "Over the eight-week program, they usually report a reduction in symptoms."

Many of Nature's cures—acupressure, aromatherapy, biofeedback, exercise, heat and cold therapies, massage, music therapy, tai chi and chi gong, visualization, guided imagery and self-hypnosis and yoga—incorporate elements of meditation.

## Learning the Relaxation Response

Of all the forms of meditation, the relaxation response is one of the easiest to learn.

Here's how to bring forth the relaxation response: Find a quiet place with a comfortable chair and sit with your eyes closed. Select a single word or phrase—"one," "peace," "ice cream," "God help me" or whatever suits you.

Silently repeat this phrase to yourself over and over again for an extended period of time once or twice a day. Begin with a minute or two and work up to 20 minutes or a half-hour. While doing so, try to empty your mind of all other thoughts.

While meditating, assume a passive, accepting, nonjudgmental attitude. When distracting thoughts enter your mind—and they're inevitable—notice them and accept them (no matter how bizarre they might be), then let them go as you return to focusing on your word or phrase.

In another type of meditation, practitioners focus on their breath. Instead of a word or phrase, they concentrate on the process of inhaling and exhaling deeply. The other steps remain the same.

After a while, in addition to deep relaxation, the relaxation response (or any classical meditative or prayer discipline) produces something extra—a feeling of well-being or wholeness that lingers long after you resume your normal activities. Religious meditators describe this effect as "feeling the Divine presence" or "feeling closer to God."

Mind/body physicians suggest that meditation's residual effects—improved stress-coping abilities—function metaphorically as a kind of emotional vaccine that "immunizes" against anxiety and distress. Scientists believe this effect may be part of the reason that people who worship regularly stay healthier than those who are not religiously observant.

In 1992, Kenneth Ferraro, Ph.D., professor of sociology at Purdue University in West Lafayette, Indiana, confirmed this observation in using a survey that asked 1,500 Americans about their health and religious affiliation. Compared with regular religious "practicers," the "nonpracticers" were more than twice as likely to say they were in generally poor health (9 percent versus 4 percent.)

## Mindfulness: Living in the Moment

In mantra and breath meditation, you focus on a word or your breath and try to empty your mind of everything else. This mental clearing is what most people mean when they refer to meditation.

But there's another kind of meditation, a practice Buddhists call *vipassana,* or insight meditation. Dr. Kabat-Zinn calls it mindfulness—the art of becoming deeply aware of the present instant. Mindfulness helps you turn down all the noise in your head—the guilt, anger, doubts, uncertainties and "shoulds" that upset us moment to moment. Mindfulness is a technique that encourages you to stop and smell the roses.

"The key to mindfulness," Dr. Kabat-Zinn explains, "is not so much *what* you focus on but *how* you do it, the quality of the awareness you bring to each moment." That awareness, he says, should be meditative in the sense of being a silent witness, accepting and nonjudgmental. However, mindfulness does not imply resignation to abuse or injustice. It teaches *acknowledgment* of the moment-to-moment reality and prepares those who use the technique to respond to that reality less impulsively and more effectively.

To teach mindfulness in his clinic, Dr. Kabat-Zinn hands each of his students a single raisin and asks them to eat it. Ordinarily people would simply pop the raisin in their mouths, chew a few times and swallow, largely unconsciously. But mindful, meditative raisin eating is much different. It begins with looking intently at the raisin, considering its shape, weight, color and texture. Next comes placing the raisin in the mouth, focusing on how it feels on the tongue as the mouth welcomes it with salivation. Then the mindful raisin-eater chews the raisin slowly and thoroughly, focusing on its taste and texture. Finally, swallowing the raisin involves following it all the way down to the stomach.

There are two kinds of mindful meditation—formal and informal. Yoga is a good example of the formal type. In a yoga class, participants focus intently on their breathing and the postures, moving slowly from one position to the next, exquisitely aware of their feelings during the process. Tai chi offers a similar dimension of mindfulness. Informal mindfulness involves turning the headlong rush of daily living into a collection of discrete moments of experience, each savored fully.

Of course, it's impossible to live life entirely mindfully. But try committing yourself to some mindful meditative moments every day, and chances are you'll feel less anxious and more self-confident.

One way to do this is to hang up the phone mindfully. Instead of jumping from call to call or from the phone to other chores, enter a mindful moment the instant you say good-bye. Hang up slowly. Let the receiver descend into its cradle like a feather falling in a light breeze. Ruminate on your connection to the person with whom you just spoke. Take a few deep breaths, then proceed with your life.

Once you commit to a mindfulness trigger—if not hanging up the phone, then perhaps sipping a cup of tea or eating fruit snacks, starting the car or petting your dog—it's not difficult to work a dozen mindful moments into each day.

## Body Scan Meditation

If you'd like to try a more formal type of mindfulness without attending a yoga or tai chi class, Dr. Kabat-Zinn recommends the Body Scan.

1. Lie on your back with your legs uncrossed, your arms at your sides, palms up, and your eyes open or closed, as you wish.

2. Focus on your breathing, how the air moves in and out of your body.

3. After several deep breaths, as you begin to feel comfortable and relaxed, direct your attention to the toes of your left foot. Tune into any sensations in that part of your body while remaining aware of your breathing. It often helps to imagine each breath flowing to the spot where you're directing your attention. Focus on your left toes for one to two minutes.

4. Then move your focus to the sole of your left foot and hold it there for a minute or two while continuing to pay attention to your breathing.

5. Follow the same procedure as you move to your left ankle, calf, knee, thigh, hip and so on all around the body.

6. Pay particular attention to any areas that cause pain or are the focus of any medical condition (for asthma, the lungs; for diabetes, the pancreas).

7. Pay particular attention to the head: the jaw, chin, lips, tongue, roof of the mouth, nostrils, throat, cheeks, eyelids, eyes, eyebrows, forehead, temples and scalp.

8. Finally, focus on the very top of your hair, the uppermost part of your body. Then let go of the body altogether, and in your mind, hover above yourself as your breath reaches beyond you and touches the universe.

## The Instant Calming Sequence

Meditation and mindfulness are great when you have enough control over your time to enjoy them. But what happens when a crisis requires immediate action?

There's no time to plop down in an easy chair for a 30-minute mantra meditation. "Not to worry," says Robert Cooper, Ph.D., president of the Institute for Health and Fitness Excellence in Bemidji, Minnesota, and author of *Health and Fitness Excellence: The Scientific Action Plan.* "If you take a few specific steps as soon as stress strikes, you can often stay calm, or at least minimize your distress."

Using scientific findings in the physiology of relaxation, Dr.

Cooper has developed a six-step program that minimizes the negative effects of stress the moment the body begins to feel stressed. He calls it the Instant Calming Sequence.

**Step 1: Practice uninterrupted breathing.** When stress strikes, immediately focus on your breath and continue breathing smoothly, deeply and evenly.

**Step 2: Put on a positive face.** Smile a grin that you can feel in the corners of your eyes. "The conventional wisdom is that happiness triggers smiling," Dr. Cooper explains. "But recent studies suggest that this process is a two-way street. Smiling can contribute to feelings of happiness, and in a stressful situation, it can help keep you calm." Try this simple test: Smile a broad grin right now. Don't you feel better?

**Step 3: Balance your posture.** People under stress often look hunched-over, hence the oft-repeated phrase "They have the weight of the world on their shoulders."

"Maintaining good posture works like smiling," Dr. Cooper says. "Physical balance contributes to emotional balance." Keep your head up, chin in, chest high, pelvis and hips level, back comfortably straight and abdomen free of tension. Imagine a skyhook lifting your body from a point at the center of the top of your head.

**Step 4: Bathe in a wave of relaxation.** Consciously sweep a wave of relaxation through your body. "Imagine you're standing under a waterfall that washes away all your tension," Dr. Cooper says.

**Step 5: Acknowledge reality.** Face your stressor head-on. Don't try to deny it or wish that it hadn't happened. Think: "This is real. I can handle it. I'm finding the best possible way to cope right now."

**Step 6: Reassert control.** Instead of fretting about how the stressor has robbed you of control, focus on what you *can* control and take appropriate action. Also, think clear-headed, honest thoughts instead of distorted ones. (For some hints on how to clear your thinking, see Cognitive Therapy on page 65.)

## CHAPTER 21

# MIND/BODY HEALING

### The Missing Link in Mainstream Medicine

Mention birthdays and most people think of gifts, cakes with candles and gatherings of friends and relatives. But birthdays also provide a unique window into the frontier of mind/body medicine, thanks to the "birthday effect"—the observation that birth date has a startling influence on death date.

This isn't astrology. It's what David P. Phillips, Ph.D., discovered in a study dealing with the birth and death records of 440,000 Californians. The professor of sociology at the University of California at San Diego wanted to know if deeply held cultural beliefs could influence the survival of people with major illnesses such as cancer, emphysema and heart disease, among others.

He focused on immigrants from China whose enduring commitment to traditional Chinese culture he inferred from three aspects of their lives: birth in China, residence in a city with a large traditional Chinese population (Los Angeles or San Francisco) and no autopsy at death, a procedure shunned by traditional Chinese culture.

Dr. Phillips found records for 28,169 traditional Chinese who'd died from 1969 to 1990 and sorted them by birth year and cause of death. Traditional Chinese believe that combinations of certain birth years and diseases bring bad luck. Those born in "fire" years, those ending in a six or a seven, such as 1937, are supposed to fare worse than others if they develop heart disease. People born in "earth" years, ending in eight or nine, have bad luck if they get cancer. Those born in "metal" years, ending in zero or one, have difficulty with respiratory conditions.

## Thinking Makes It So

Dr. Phillips compared every traditional Chinese person in his study with 20 individuals—the controls in his study—who did not share the Chinese view of bad luck but who matched the traditional Chinese subjects in sex and cause of death. His conclusion? A belief in bad luck can be fatal. Compared with the control population, Chinese who had ill-fated pairings died an average of three years sooner.

For a subgroup of people, Dr. Phillips found employment, religious and other information that suggested an even deeper commitment to traditional Chinese values. As commitment to traditional values increased, so did the birthday effect. Compared with other individuals, deeply committed traditional Chinese women with emphysema who were born in a year of respiratory bad luck died an average of eight years sooner.

"You'd have to conclude," Dr. Phillips says, "that values and beliefs, creations of the mind, play a significant role in health and longevity."

Western medicine's prescientific forebears would have agreed. They believed that the mind and body were inextricably linked and that whatever affected one had an impact on the other. "The soul's passions," Aristotle said, "seem to be linked with the body, as the body undergoes modifications in their presence."

## The Great Mind/Body Split

But by the seventeenth century, as the Age of Enlightenment launched modern medicine, early scientists rebelled against what they considered the superstitious spirituality of folk medicine and the spiritual dogmatism of religious medicine. They decreed that the mind and body were separate and distinct and rarely affected one another. Belief in mind/body dualism reached its zenith during the early twentieth century, after Louis Pasteur's Germ Theory of Illness became the foundation of scientific medicine. The Germ Theory held that microorganisms, not the vagaries of the mind, caused the vast majority of diseases.

Of course, mental illness was still possible, and within scientific medicine, psychiatry developed to deal with it. Psychiatrists knew that disturbances in the mind could cause "psychosomatic" symptoms in the body, such as chest pain and shortness of breath in those having panic attacks. In addition, a mind/body undercurrent continued to trickle through mainstream medicine.

At the turn of the century, noted medical educator Sir William Osler, M.D., a Canadian physician whose medical textbooks earned him knighthood in England and a distinguished professorship at Johns Hopkins University School of Medicine in Baltimore, said that the treatment of tuberculosis depended as much on patients' heads as their chests. And in the 1960s, Stanford psychiatrist George Solomon, M.D., observed that depression seemed to aggravate rheumatoid arthritis. He speculated that emotions played a role in the immune system's response to disease. In 1964, he proposed a new scientific field—psychoneuroimmunology (PNI)—to investigate how the mind (*psycho-*) and the nervous system (*neuro-*) affected the immune system.

Initially, Dr. Solomon's theory fell on deaf ears. If they couldn't identify a germ, doctors dismissed most complaints—especially those that were vague, chronic and reported by women— as existing "all in the head."

According to mind-separate-from-body medicine, the birthday effect should not exist. Assuming that everyone receives reasonably competent medical care, people with the same diseases should fare, on average, about the same. Only they don't.

Dr. Phillips discovered another culturally influenced birthday effect—this one among white Americans. In a 1992 report, he analyzed the birth and death records of 2,745,149 people and came up with some strange findings. Women's statistically expected death rate dipped well below average during the several weeks before their birthdays and then rose to a peak well above average during the weeks immediately after their birthdays. Men's death rate was significantly higher than average shortly before their birthdays but returned to normal soon afterward.

Like the case of the traditional Chinese, Germ Theory–based medicine cannot explain these odd patterns. But if we re-embrace the ancient view that the mind and body are actually one entity, the "bodymind," then the ups and downs of this birthday effect become not only understandable but enlightening. For seriously ill white Americans, birthdays are either lifelines or deadlines.

## Mind Matters

"Birthdays typically involve taking stock and comparing one's ambitions with one's accomplishments," explains David Sobel, M.D., regional director of patient education, director of the regional education department at Kaiser Permanente Medical Care Program of Northern California and co-editor (with Robert Ornstein, Ph.D.) of the *Mental Medicine Update* newsletter.

American men traditionally base their self-esteem on career performance, an area fraught with unrealistic ambitions. Not everyone can be chairman of the board. For men whose attainments fall short of their ambitions, an approaching birthday looms as a dreaded, depressing deadline. Those who are seriously ill and also disappointed in themselves in effect give up, throw in the towel and die before their birthday deadlines. Those who make it over the psychological birthday hump quickly return to the average death rate.

On the other hand, women have traditionally placed more value on relationships than careers. For seriously ill women, birthdays mean extra attention from family and friends. The fact that women's death rate dips before their birthdays suggests that anticipation of a celebration with family and friends acts as a lifeline. But afterward, when the party is over and the mailman brings no more cards, a letdown can set in, and women's death rate rises to a level well above average.

In addition to suggesting that we give the men in our lives extra support before their birthdays and the women extra support afterward, this study shows that symbolic occasions that are "all in our heads" can have a profound impact on our health, even hastening or postponing our deaths.

Welcome to the fascinating world of mind/body healing, a field that currently defines the shifting boundary between mainstream medicine and Nature's cures. Mind/body interactions are fundamental to natural healing and play significant roles in more than half the chapters of Nature's Cures: acupuncture and acupressure, aromatherapy, biofeedback, complementary cancer therapies, cognitive therapy, companionship, dreams, exercise, healing humor, healthy habits, massage therapy, meditation, music therapy, Ornish therapy, tai chi and chi gong, vision therapy, visualization, guided imagery and self-hypnosis and yoga.

## The Immune System Link

Mainstream medicine's mind/body Wall of Jericho first began cracking in the late 1960s and early 1970s at laboratories in New York City and Cambridge, Massachusetts. Curious about Indian yogis' ability to control physiological functions that at the time were considered beyond conscious reach, Neal Miller, Ph.D., then head of the Laboratory of Physiological Psychology at Rockefeller University in New York City, used simple reward-and-punishment training to teach rats to raise and lower their heart rates.

Meanwhile, in Cambridge, some practitioners of transcendental meditation showed cardiologist Herbert Benson, M.D., who is now associate professor of medicine at Harvard Medical School and president of the Mind/Body Medical Institute at New England Deaconess Hospital in Boston, that they could lower their blood pressure by sitting quietly, breathing deeply and mentally reciting a brief phrase, or mantra.

Dr. Miller and Dr. Benson demonstrated convincingly that the mind affected the body's stress reactions, either heightening or minimizing the harm stress can cause. But they never showed how the mind/body link worked, and in Western medicine, discoveries rarely become established until scientists understand their "mechanism of action." Until someone did, mind/body effects would be shunted off to the fringes.

Enter Robert Ader, M.D., Ph.D., director of the Division of Behavioral and Psychosocial Medicine in the Department of Psychiatry at the University of Rochester School of Medicine and Dentistry in New York. In 1974, when Dr. Ader was a professor of psychology, he was teaching rats to avoid sugar water. Each time they drank, he injected them with a drug that produced nausea. Unexpectedly, the rats did more than throw up. They sickened and died.

At first Dr. Ader thought his drug, which was not poisonous, might have been contaminated with something that was. But it turned out to be pure. Besides, the rat deaths were related not to how much of the drug they received but rather to how much sugar water they drank.

Dr. Ader read up on his drug and discovered studies showing that in addition to producing nausea, it also impaired immune function. He deduced that not only had his rats learned to associate the sugar water with nausea, they'd also linked it to immune suppression. They'd learned to shut down their immune systems, and as a result, they died.

To Dr. Ader, this explanation made perfect sense. But when he published his findings, immunologists castigated him. Immune responses could not be learned, they insisted, citing the conventional medical wisdom of the day. The immune system functions independently of the mind, the immunologists argued. It simply reacts to germs by attacking them.

Dr. Ader retorted that immunlogists always used military metaphors when discussing the immune system's combat against disease. But soldiers don't function mindlessly. They are under the control of generals who answer to political leaders. Why couldn't the immune system respond directly to the mind? Eventually Dr. Ader teamed up with Rochester immunologist Nicholas Cohen, M.D., and they proved that the psychologist's initial speculation was correct. His rats did indeed learn to shut down their immune systems, which meant that there must be direct connections between it and the mind. Dr. Ader's work helped propel meditation, biofeedback and other mind/body therapies into the medical mainstream. It also established PNI as a legitimate—and exciting—medical specialty.

Today scientists generally understand the mind's mechanism of action on the immune system. The links are both hormonal and neurological. When the body experiences emotional stress, the mind perceives a threat and initiates the fight-or-flight response, a surge of hormone releases that prepares the person for self-defense or escape.

One stress hormone is cortisol, which suppresses the immune system and impairs the lymph system, the special circulatory system where immune cells grow and "hang out" when they're off-duty from battling the body's microscopic enemies. In addition, researchers have discovered direct nerve links to all the places that immune cells grow and cluster: the bone marrow, the thymus gland, the spleen and the lymph nodes.

While attacking germs, the immune system may look like a microscopic guerrilla squad. But like every winning army, the immune system's actions are highly coordinated by a commander-in-chief, the mind.

## Mind/Body Healing at Work

Fundamentally, mind/body healing works by minimizing the distress caused by stress. Over the last 25 years, "stress" has acquired a nasty reputation, but not all stress is bad. Without it, no one would experience the happy shock of a surprise party, the exhilaration of skiing, the nail-biting suspense of a who-done-it thriller or the delicious moment of uncertainty when one lover asks, "Will you marry me?" and the other says, "Yes, I will." All

(continued on page 348)

# The Marvelous Placebo Effect ———

A placebo is a sham treatment that has no inherent medical value. Researchers use placebos to test the effectiveness of new drugs or other treatments. They divide experimental subjects into two groups and give one the real treatment and the other the placebo. To be judged effective, the new treatment must produce significantly greater relief.

Why use placebos? The word's derivation tells the tale. Placebo comes from the Latin for "I will please," and please is what they often do. Study after study shows that in at least 30 percent of cases, placebos *work*. They provide benefits for no medical reason.

In a classic 1955 study, Harvard anesthesiologist Henry K. Beecher, M.D., reviewed 15 studies involving more than 1,000 participants who took either active drugs or placebos for a variety of conditions. He found that on average, 35 percent of placebo-takers reported significant relief. He argued that the placebo effect accounted for the effectiveness of one-third of *all* medical treatments.

Now it turns out that his estimate may have been low. In 1993, Alan Roberts, Ph.D., head of the Division of Medical Psychology at the Scripps Clinic and Research Foundation in La Jolla, California, reviewed pilot studies involving 6,931 people who received one of five experimental treatments for a variety of ailments, including asthma, ulcers and herpes.

Forty percent reported "excellent" results, 30 percent reported "good" results and only 30 percent experienced "poor" results. But in later tests that compared the five drugs with placebos, their effectiveness disappeared, and all five were abandoned—after 70 percent of the initial users reported at least good results. Dr. Roberts says that perhaps as much of two-thirds of drug benefits are due to the placebo effect.

Medical researchers typically treat the placebo effect as an annoyance and take pains to prevent it from polluting their data. But on a deeper level, physicians who hold the classic medical view that the body and mind are separate find the placebo effect downright *embarrassing*. Placebos, they believe, simply demonstrate how gullible people are. Give them *anything*, and at least a third will report benefit—the fools.

The placebo effect is hardly foolish. It's a marvelous example of mind/body medicine at work. Gullibility has nothing to do with it. Placebo effectiveness depends on four factors: user belief, user anxiety, problem severity and physician enthusiasm. Those who are in the greatest discomfort, who feel most anxious and have the greatest faith in the placebo generally report the best effectiveness. In addition, as the doctor communicates more enthusiasm for the placebo, its effectiveness also increases.

This last observation was well-known 100 years ago, before the placebo effect had been identified. Nineteenth-century medical students were told, "Use the new drugs quickly, while they still have the power to heal." Doctors touted new drugs, and thanks to the placebo effect, they often worked wonderfully. But as time passed, concerns about side effects and questions about effectiveness often dampened professional enthusiasm—and the drugs stopped working.

How do placebos actually work? According to a study by researchers at the University of California's San Francisco Medical Center, placebos trigger the release of endorphins, the body's pain-relieving, mood-elevating chemicals.

Parents use the placebo effect all the time. When a child gets a scrape or other boo-boo and bursts into tears, parents often say, "I'll kiss it and make it better." Quite often, it works. The child considers the parent all-powerful, and parental enthusiasm convinces the child that the treatment will provide relief. No wonder it often does. Kissing boo-boos . . . maybe doctors should try it.

these experiences are stressful, but if you can handle them, they cause joy, not distress.

"Nothing in life is inherently distressing," says psychotherapist Alan Elkin, Ph.D., director of the Stress Management Counseling Center in New York City. "Things become distressing only when the stress they engender overwhelms our ability to cope with them. Stress becomes distress when people perceive challenges as threats, when they feel helpless rather than in control, and when their actions feel meaningless rather than a clear expression of personal beliefs or commitments."

*Arthritis.* Joint inflammation is the nation's second most prevalent health problem (after chronic sinus infection), and it is among the most painful.

Beginning in 1978, a Stanford University team led by nurse and health educator Kate Lorig, R.N., Dr.P.H., and James Fries, M.D., professor of medicine, launched the Arthritis Self-Help Course. During six two-hour weekly sessions, participants learned about arthritis and participated in a support group that included mind/body relaxation exercises. After four years and 401 participants, Dr. Lorig compared the program's enrollees with people with arthritis who were nonparticipants. Her alumni reported 20 percent less pain and 40 percent fewer physician visits. The Arthritis Self-Help Course is now offered nationally, and more than 150,000 people with arthritis have participated.

*The common cold.* Many studies have shown that major stressors—divorce, job loss or the death of a loved one—impair immune function and increase susceptibility to disease. But what about life's little joys and heartaches?

Arthur Stone, Ph.D., professor of psychology at the State University of New York Medical School in Stony Brook, asked 100 adults to keep detailed diaries for three months, recording all their daily emotional ups and downs—ups such as compliments from co-workers and hugs from loved ones and downs such as getting stuck in traffic and having to hold while on the phone. The participants also donated daily saliva samples that were analyzed for secretory IgA, a protein produced by the immune system in the mouth and upper respiratory tract that acts as the body's first line of defense against cold viruses. The higher the IgA level, the better the immune function, resulting in extra protection against colds. All "downers," particularly those at work, significantly depressed IgA levels on the day they occurred. Little joys, however, boosted IgA levels for up to two days.

Those IgA changes directly affect cold susceptibility, according to Sheldon Cohen, Ph.D., professor of psychology at Carnegie-Mellon University in Pittsburgh. Dr. Cohen used several standard psychological tests to measure stress levels in 400 people. Then he squirted live cold virus up their noses, hoping to infect them. Compared with the least stressed participants, those who were burn-out cases were twice as likely to catch the cold.

*Diabetes.* In 1978, a woman with diabetes was admitted to Duke University Medical Center in Durham, North Carolina, with a blood sugar (glucose) level so high that she was bleeding into her eyes, threatening her with blindness. Hospitalization brought her glucose level down, but she was under tremendous stress, and her doctor feared her sugar might soar again when she went home. He asked Richard Surwitt, Ph.D., professor of medical psychology at Duke, to teach her stress management skills to help keep her blood glucose under control.

At the time, researchers knew that emotional stress could raise glucose levels in people with diabetes. But no one had ever shown that stress management techniques could keep them under control. Dr. Surwitt had worked almost exclusively with people who had heart disease. He doubted that mind/body medicine had much to offer people with diabetes. But the woman was in a crisis, and there was no harm trying.

For a week, he trained her to relax using biofeedback and progressive muscle relaxation—conscious tensing and relaxing of the major muscle groups. Back home, the woman's blood sugar level remained low. Intrigued, Dr. Surwitt began using mind/body therapies with others who had diabetes, and most gained greater control over their glucose levels. Dr. Surwitt is now the research director of the Duke Neurobehavioral Diabetes Program.

*Headaches.* Headache is one of the leading causes of chronic pain. Kenneth Holyroyd, Ph.D., professor of psychology at Ohio University in Athens, designed a program for managing tension headaches that combines relaxation therapies such as biofeedback and visualization with cognitive therapy. Untrained people showed no improvement, but participants reported an average improvement of 43 percent, with some experiencing complete headache relief. Dr. Holyroyd then reviewed similar studies of migraines and found that while nondrug mind/body approaches were not necessarily curative, they produced significant pain relief in more than half of those who tried them.

*HIV infection and AIDS.* Some people infected with the human immunodeficiency virus (HIV) develop full-blown AIDS quickly. Others take a decade. Now scientists think they know what accounts for the difference.

Two studies suggest that state of mind can affect how quickly HIV infection progresses to AIDS. Jeffrey Burack, M.D., clinical instructor of medicine at San Francisco General Hospital, asked 330 HIV-positive men to complete periodic psychological surveys for six years. Being HIV positive is obviously distressing; anyone with HIV infection can be expected to experience bouts of depression. But Dr. Burack found that compared with the men who reported only brief episodes of mild to moderate depression during their first three years of infection, those who endured prolonged periods of serious depression progressed to AIDS and died twice as quickly.

A study at the University of Michigan in Ann Arbor used a different route to come to the same conclusion. HIV infection slowly destroys certain cells of the immune system known as CD4 cells. Epidemiologist Susan Caumartin, Ph.D., a lecturer in health and behavior at the School of Public Health at the university, discovered that mild to moderate depression does not significantly accelerate the decline in CD4 count associated with HIV, but serious depression does.

*Infertility.* It's very stressful to want a child and not be able to have one. In 1986, nurses working at the infertility clinic at the University of Mississippi Medical Center in Jackson asked Ron Drabman, Ph.D., professor of psychology and director of the clinical psychology residency program, to teach basic stress management skills to their patients. They thought that deep breathing, meditation and guided imagery visualizations might help infertile couples cope with the overwhelming stress, embarrassment and sense of failure many felt.

Dr. Drabman's program did more than relieve several participants' headaches. Four of the 14 couples who tried in vitro fertilization got pregnant on their first try. In vitro fertilization is a high-tech procedure that involves surgical removal of an egg and laboratory insemination, followed by surgical implantation in the uterus. The Mississippi couples' 28 percent success rate may not sound like much, but the first-try success rate for couples unable to participate was just 6 percent. The stress/infertility link centers on the hypothalamus, a gland in the brain that controls the flow and timing of reproductive hormones. The hypothalamus is extremely sensitive to stress.

## The Dark Side of Mind/Body Medicine

Mind/body research demonstrates that depression and emotional stress play significant roles in the development of many illnesses and recovery from them. If that's true, might bad attitudes cause disease? Do people who get sick bring it on themselves? Are the sick at fault?

These are complicated questions that don't have simple answers. When a lifelong smoker dies of lung cancer or a motorcyclist without a helmet crashes and dies of head injuries, it's difficult not to hold them at least partly responsible. But what about people with diseases like multiple sclerosis, rheumatoid arthritis, lupus or most cancers? Nothing as simple as a helmet prevents any of these diseases. Are people who develop them somehow spiritually remiss?

"I've heard people say that 'I create my own reality, and therefore if I get sick, I created the illness.' That really bugs me," comments Joan Borysenko, Ph.D., president of Mind/Body Health Sciences, a Boulder, Colorado, company that produces workshops on mind/body healing. Dr. Borysenko explains that many things can cause illness—microorganisms, accidents, toxic chemicals, diet and so forth. Emotional stress plays a role in causing or aggravating many illnesses, and mind/body therapies often help control or cure them. But to blame illness on a bad attitude ignores the body component of the mind/body continuum. It's the flip side of what, for so long, Western medicine did—ignore the mind. "The mind can certainly influence the body," Dr. Elkin explains, "but it does not absolutely rule it."

"If you have a chronic medical condition," says David Spiegel, M.D., professor of psychiatry at Stanford University and director of the university's Psychosocial Treatment Laboratory, "by all means, learn about it. Work closely with physicians you trust. And do whatever you can to manage your stress and live your life to the fullest." Dr. Spiegel made headlines with a study showing that the emotional lift provided by an ongoing support group doubled the survival time among women with advanced breast cancer. But he admonishes, "Don't get caught up in mind/body if-only's: 'If only I'd had a more positive attitude. If only I'd meditated more or done yoga or attended that support group.' That's nonsense. Like drugs and other treatments, sometimes mind/body approaches don't work. Each of has our own time. We don't die because of a bad attitude. We die because we are mortal."

## CHAPTER 22
# MUSIC THERAPY

In May of 1979, Baltimore psychotherapist and violinist Helen Bonny, Ph.D., felt emotionally burned out. She had too many lectures to prepare for her classes in music therapy at Catholic University in Washington, D.C., too much research to supervise, and too many students to shepherd through final exams, not to mention her commitments to her private therapy clients and her family.

As she toiled away at her desk, Dr. Bonny, then in her mid-fifties, often glanced across the room to her music stand and her beloved violin, the instrument that had been her comfort, her preferred form of meditation and her rejuvenator since she was nine. It was so near, yet so far away. How could her life have become so complicated that she barely had time to play?

But come Memorial Day, that would change. All she had to do was get through the rest of May, and the school year would be over. Then she'd be free to play again. Other people might spend Memorial Day at picnics, but Dr. Bonny vowed that she'd spend the entire day playing Bach, Vivaldi, Haydn, Mendelssohn and Debussy—all her favorites.

But early Memorial Day morning, Dr. Bonny was awakened by crushing chest pain. Gripped by panic, she fumbled for the

telephone and somehow managed to dial her son, who fortunately lived nearby. He rushed her to the hospital, where she was
placed in intensive care. The diagnosis: severe angina, a form of
heart disease caused by narrowed coronary arteries that's often
a warning sign of impending heart attack. For several days, her
condition was critical. She felt helpless, depressed, angry and
disgusted. She wanted her world restored. She wanted her life
back. Most of all, she wanted her music.

While hospitalized, Dr. Bonny asked her son to bring her a
cassette player and tapes of her favorite pieces. When they arrived, she literally hugged them. Some sounded even better than
she remembered, but oddly, several struck her as jarring. As a
musician, she felt surprised: How could she suddenly dislike
pieces she'd loved for decades? As a psychologist, she felt intrigued: Had her illness altered her musical taste? They were fascinating questions, but at the time, she was too sick to ponder
them.

During her convalescence, Dr. Bonny stayed with her sister in
rural Washington. She did not have the strength to play her violin, but her days were filled with taped music. Music had always lifted her spirits. Now, she believed, it was helping her
body heal.

## The Mind/Music Connection

With a master's degree in music education from the University of Kansas and a Ph.D. in music and psychology from the
Union Graduate School, an affiliate of Antioch College in Yellow Springs, Ohio, Dr. Bonny felt that the link between music
and the mind was obvious. But this is not the case for many of
today's physicians. Fortunately, thanks to recent research and renewed appreciation for Nature's cures, music is becoming as
common in some medical settings as it is in concert halls.

Music ranks among Nature's original healers. One of the
world's oldest known medical documents, the *Ebers Papyrus*
(1500 B.C.), prescribes a variety of incantations that ancient
Egyptian physicians chanted to heal the sick. In the Bible, young

David plucked a harp to soothe the troubled soul of King Saul (who, modern psychologists speculate, probably had depression). Apollo, the Greek god of medicine, was also the god of music. And the Greek philosopher Plato wrote that music enhanced health.

Down through the ages, music has been used extensively in many cultures to soothe troubled souls—Russian novelist Leo Tolstoy called it "the shorthand of emotion." But in more recent times music's almost magical hold on the psyche was generally confined to the arts—and largely lost on the emerging science of medicine.

## The Medicine/Music Connection

Fortunately, music never entirely disappeared from medicine. A century ago, with the invention of the phonograph, some hospitals introduced recorded music to help patients sleep and to allay presurgical anxiety.

In 1929, as radio became popular, Duke University Hospital in Durham, North Carolina, made headphones available to all of its patients. The same year, two British researchers studied the effects of radio concerts and gramophone recordings on blood pressure. They found that shortly after the music began, people's blood pressure dropped sharply.

During and shortly after World War II, American veterans' hospitals used music to improve morale among injured, depressed soldiers.

But most physicians on the body side of the mind/body continuum considered music merely a form of entertainment, a diversion to take patients' minds off the tedium of illness and disability. Mental health professionals often felt differently. Starting in the 1940s, music therapy programs were established in several university psychology departments, including Catholic University, where Dr. Bonny taught.

In addition to her teaching, Dr. Bonny conducted research at the Maryland Psychiatric Research Center in Catonsville. For one study, she gave taped musical selections to people with terminal cancer to see if the music could comfort them as they faced death. She used many works of her favorite composers: Bach, Brahms and Beethoven. Some helped the cancer patients, but oddly, most did not.

"It was strange," Dr. Bonny recalls, "I tried all the great symphonies, but only a few worked. I kept wondering why so much great music didn't help these people. I discovered the answer only after I became ill myself."

In her private practice, Dr. Bonny had always used music to help her clients relax. Eventually she began using it to help ease people into a state of deep relaxation similar to the emotional state induced by biofeedback, meditation or hypnosis. "In addition to relaxation," she explains, "music-induced relaxation sharpened my clients' personal insights. I found the same thing with guided imagery. But the combination of music and imagery produced the most profound results. I often watched in amazement as my clients reached deep inside themselves and brought up buried treasure."

It didn't take long before Dr. Bonny gave her approach a name—guided imagery and music (GIM). Today her organization, the Bonny Foundation, offers training in GIM as a tool in psychotherapy. But Dr. Bonny's illness persuaded her that music had value in healing beyond psychotherapy. As she struggled with her angina, Dr. Bonny became an unwitting pioneer in the field of mind/body medicine. Her own experience convinced her that music could help heal the body as well as the mind.

## Healing Tapes: Hospital Tests

Music therapists divide music into two types—"stimulative" and "sedative." Stimulative music has an assertive rhythm that elicits reactions: hand-clapping, toe-tapping, dancing. Everyone is born with rhythm because we all spend months in the womb listening to our mothers' hearts pounding at 70 to 80 beats per minute. Not surprisingly, a great deal of music has a similar rhythm.

In contrast, sedative music is more melodic and soothing. Unlike pharmaceutical sedatives, it does not induce sleep; rather, it promotes feelings of peace and serenity. "Sedative music," Dr. Bonny explains, "has an easy, flowing melody and a tempo similar to that of the resting heart rate. It's pleasing to the ear, not dissonant, and it has no major changes in pitch, dynamics or rhythm. Sedative music supports its listeners. It makes no demands on them."

As she convalesced from her own hospitalization, Dr. Bonny realized that the distinction between stimulative and sedative music solved a few of the riddles in her mind. As great as many stimulative compositions are, they simply didn't meet the needs of the cancer patients in her early studies or her own needs in the hospital. "People who are seriously ill," she says, "need sedative music, pieces like Bach's 'Air on the G String,' Pachelbel's 'Canon in D,' Haydn's Cello Concerto in C and Debussy's 'Clair de Lune.' "

Dr. Bonny assembled tapes of sedative music and tested them on herself during several hospital stays for angina and finally for coronary artery bypass surgery. By 1981, she had a collection of pieces she was convinced had helped her through her illness. But would they help anyone else?

The question intrigued officials at Jefferson General Hospital in Port Townsend, Washington, and St. Agnes Hospital in Baltimore, who agreed to test Dr. Bonny's tapes for six months in their intensive care and coronary care units. Dr. Bonny provided four tapes—three containing sedative, light classical music and one with sedative folk and country ballads, light jazz and swing music calculated to appeal to the patients, all of whom were over 50.

During the study, hospital staff monitored patients' heart rates and blood pressures and surveyed the patients' reactions to the tapes. The results were impressive: The patients showed significantly decreased heart rates and blood pressures, less agitation, sounder sleep, less need for pain medication and, according to a standard psychological test, marked movement from negative to positive emotions.

Surprisingly, the music calmed the hospital doctors and

nurses as well. Many reported decreased job anxiety, increased patience with difficult patients and in general, improved job satisfaction. "The healing power of music is contagious," Dr. Bonny quips.

Dr. Bonny's study is just one of many showing that music has a calming, anxiety-reducing effect. The effect is significant even when the listeners are unconscious. When Jefferson General nurse-anesthetist Noreen McCarron learned of Dr. Bonny's findings, she introduced the tapes into the hospital's surgical suites. It was no surprise when patients reported decreased preoperative and postoperative anxiety. However, their anesthesia requirements dropped by as much as 50 percent when music was played during operations.

## Take One Tape Every Four Hours

Many popular songs say that music "soothes the soul." Truer words were never spoken, er, sung, but few music-lovers understand why.

"At least part of the thrill of music seems to come from the release of endorphins, the powerful opiate-like chemicals produced in the brain that induce euphoria and relieve pain. Administering drugs that block endorphin production significantly blunts the joy of music," explains David Sobel, M.D., regional director of patient education, director of the regional education department at Kaiser Permanente Medical Care Program of Northern California and co-editor (with Robert Ornstein, Ph.D.) of the *Mental Medicine Update* newsletter. Music also reduces levels of stress hormones, such as adrenaline, and has a calming effect on the limbic system of the brain, which plays a role in emotion.

Music is no cure-all, but the latest research shows that this natural therapy has a remarkable number of healing benefits.

*Cancer.* The drugs used to treat cancer are notorious for causing nausea and vomiting. But these side effects have as much to do with anxiety as they do with the toxicity of chemotherapy drugs. Janice Frank, R.N., coordinator of the Brain Tumor Cooperative Group at Montefiore Hospital in Pittsburgh, wondered if a program of taped sedative music and guided imagery similar to Dr. Bonny's GIM might increase the benefits of standard anti-nausea drugs. In a study involving 15 adults who had a variety of cancers, among them breast, lung and ovarian cancer, the music/imagery program significantly reduced feelings of nausea and the number and duration of vomiting episodes.

*Childbirth.* Increasingly, obstetricians and midwives encourage women at term to play music tapes during labor and delivery. "There's good evidence," says Al Bumanis, spokesperson for the National Association for Music Therapy in Silver Spring, Maryland, "that music decreases the need for pain medication in childbirth."

*Chronic pain.* Lani Zimmerman, R.N., Ph.D., associate professor of nursing at the University of Nebraska Medical Center in Lincoln, offered ten different sedative musical tapes to 40 people with severe, chronic pain and encouraged them to choose the one they found most relaxing. Those who expressed no preference were given a tape by Steven Halpern, a composer who specializes in writing music for healing. While listening to the tapes, the people in the study reported significantly less pain.

Other studies show that music reduces hospital patients' need for pain medication by as much as 30 percent. Music also decreases the anxiety and pain of dental work, prompting some dentists to give their patients headphones and taped music in addition to painkilling medication.

*Exercise performance.* Ever wonder why aerobic dance, jazzercise and other music-exercise programs are so popular? "Moving to an even rhythm helps the muscles flex and extend more smoothly," Dr. Sobel explains. "It also increases stamina. If you interview exercisers before and after identical workouts with and without dance or rock music, the ones who exercised to music aren't as tired."

But exercise music should not be too bombastic, according to a University of Tennessee team of researchers, who tested fitness walkers' reactions to three types of sound: silence, light rock and

*(continued on page 362)*

# Turn That Down!
# The Health Hazards of Noise

If your children or neighbors play any music—rock, rap, country, jazz or even classical—at deafening volume, you have an unlikely ally in Pete Townshend, the creative force behind the Who, the high-energy (and high-volume) British rock band. Decades of playing loud music have left Townshend's hearing impaired, spurring him to support Hearing Education and Awareness for Rockers (H.E.A.R.), a San Francisco organization that educates young people about the hazards of amplified music and promotes the use of earplugs at rock concerts.

Loud rock music is just one of many sounds assaulting our hearing. Motorcycles, jackhammers, smoke alarms, burglar alarms, farm and factory noise—in fact, every loud noise—slowly, imperceptibly wear away at hearing.

To make matters worse, the journey to hearing impairment is a one-way ride. "Loud noises destroy the microscopic hairs in the inner ear that transmit sound to the auditory nerve," explains anti-noise activist Arline Bronzaft, Ph.D., professor of psychology at Lehman College of the City University of New York. "They never recover and cannot be repaired."

Today the environmental assault on hearing begins in infancy. Battery-powered high-tech toys expose kids—and everyone around them—to microchip-generated sounds loud enough to injure young ears. Noise exposure grows during the teen years as kids discover personal stereo headphones and heavy metal bands like the aptly named Def Leppard.

Hearing loss is insidious. Today's young rock fans won't notice any ill effects for 20 to 30 years. But what isn't noticed can be measured. Recently audiologists gave hearing tests to 1,000 freshmen at the University of Tennessee. An astonishing 60 percent showed hearing loss typical of those three times their age. How can we protect our hearing? It's simple: Avoid loud noise whenever possible.

Volume is measured in decibels (dB). Normal conversation registers about 60 dB; restaurants, 70 dB; vacuum cleaners, 80 dB; motorcycles, 90 dB; jackhammers, 100 dB; rock concerts, 100 to 130 dB; gunshots, 140 dB. Hearing damage begins with prolonged exposure to sounds louder than about 80 dB, but every loud burst destroys some irreplaceable hairs in the inner ear. "If you know you're going to be exposed to loud noise, wear earplugs," Dr. Bronzaft says. "Inexpensive foam plugs are available at pharmacies. For those occupationally or recreationally exposed to high volume, audiologists can custom-fit super-earplugs for about $100."

## FIGHTING NOISE POLLUTION

The noise problem would be serious enough if it were confined to our immediate personal environment. But it isn't.

During the past 20 years, the background din called "urban hum" has become so loud that experts now consider noise a major pollutant in metropolitan areas. Background noise does more than add to hearing problems caused by loud-volume stereos. It raises blood pressure, ruins sleep and contributes to stress. It also increases the risk of pregnant women for delivering premature, low-weight babies.

Background noise also impairs learning. At one New York City school built next to elevated railroad tracks, trains roared by every five minutes, drowning the adjacent classrooms in noise registering 89 dB. Tests by Dr. Bronzaft showed that, compared with sixth-graders on the quieter side of the building, those in track-side classrooms had reading scores one full grade level lower.

Dr. Bronzaft and the track-side students' parents lobbied the board of education to install sound-absorbing ceilings in the classroom, and they lobbied the New York Transit Authority to fit the tracks with sound-deadening rubber pads. The changes cut track-side noise in half. Two years later, tests showed all students reading at the same grade level.

(continued)

# Turn That Down!
# The Health Hazards of Noise—*Continued*

Noise pollution also drives people bonkers, which is why virtually every community in the country has noise-abatement laws that require reasonable quiet—no construction and no loud music or loud noises of any kind—in residential neighborhoods from about 9:00 P.M. to 8:00 A.M. But some communities are subjected to extraordinary noise levels, particularly those near freeways and the flight paths of the nation's increasingly busy airports.

## THE ROAR OF THE FREEWAY, THE SCREAM OF THE JET

In recent years, complaints about freeway din have spurred the construction of noise-cutting "sound walls" alongside many of the nation's highways. The goal is to keep the noise level within 300 feet of the roadway below 67 dB.

Sound walls work for those who live adjacent to freeways, but they've also created an unforeseen problem for those who live farther away. The high-frequency component of traffic noise bounces off sound walls, exposing those who live up to a half-mile away to freeway din. Engineers insist that this echoed noise adds only an insignificant 1 dB to the background noise level, but some residents, who used to hear just crickets, feel robbed of their peace and quiet.

---

hard rock. The music that boosted endurance and lowered heart rate the most was light rock. Hard rock had about the same effect as silence.

*Heart attack.* Few medical calamities are as frightening as heart attack, the nation's leading cause of death. Working with 80 people newly admitted to coronary care units at three hospitals, Cathie Guzzetta, R.N., Ph.D., professor of nursing at the Catholic University School of Nursing, divided them into three groups. In addition to standard care, one group received nothing extra, another learned a relaxation technique and the

In Marin County, California, a suburb of San Francisco, residents far from the major freeway have protested the construction of sound walls, so far to no avail.

Opposition to aircraft noise has cranked up the volume of the noise pollution debate to the point where it's now reverberating through the federal courts and the halls of Congress. Nowhere is the cacophony louder than in New Jersey, home of Shirley Gaszi, who lives in Cranford, a once-quiet suburb 35 miles from the Newark airport.

One morning in 1987, Gaszi awoke to the unfamiliar sound of low-flying jets roaring overhead every 20 seconds. Without any warning, the Federal Aviation Administration (FAA) had rerouted aircraft inland from the ocean to flight paths over communities like Cranford.

"I haven't been able to use my backyard in years," Gaszi laments. She isn't alone. Residents of 247 New Jersey communities in 18 of its 21 counties complained to the FAA but got nowhere. So Gaszi became executive director of the New Jersey Coalition against Aircraft Noise (NJ-CAAN), one of more than 100 community organizations around the country that monitor—and try to minimize—aircraft and airport noise. They have their work cut out for them. In October 1991, the FAA gave the airlines several additional years to switch to quieter planes.

third received a 20-minute cassette of sedative classical and popular music.

The people who received nothing extra all showed high blood levels of stress hormones and rapid heart rates—reactions that impair the immune system, slow healing and may even aggravate heart damage. The relaxation and music groups, however, both showed significantly lower heart rates and levels of stress hormones. The music group was the least stressed, suggesting that music is even more relaxing than meditation.

*Insomnia.* Canadian researchers introduced a two-hour

program of light, sedative music into a 32-resident geriatric nursing home. After three months, the number of residents who needed sleeping pills fell by more than two-thirds, from 27 to 8.

*Intellectual performance.* Mozart would probably be astonished, but a 1993 experiment done by Frances H. Rauscher, Ph.D., a research fellow at the Center for the Neurobiology of Learning and Memory at the University of California at Irvine, showed that a ten-minute dose of his music temporarily boosts intelligence. Dr. Rauscher had 36 students take a standard intelligence test after listening to either silence, a relaxing guided imagery tape or Mozart's Sonata for Two Pianos in D Major, K. 448. After the period of silence, the students' average score was 110. After the relaxation tape, it was 111. But after they listened to Mozart, it jumped to 119.

Even students who said they didn't like Mozart's music experienced the boost in their test scores. "Listening to complex music like Mozart may stimulate neural pathways that are important in thinking," Dr. Rauscher says. If that's so, other complex musical forms, such as jazz, should have a similar effect, but simple, repetitive forms—folk, country and most rock— might not.

*Migraines.* Loud music can cause headaches, but sedative music at low volume helps treat searingly painful migraines. In one study, after five weeks of using a combination of biofeedback, imagery, meditation and music, people who experienced frequent migraines reported 50 percent fewer attacks.

*Stroke.* Strokes often affect the brain centers that control speech and movement, leaving some people unable to speak and/or walk. Music helps in the rehabilitation of both functions, according to music therapist Christina Lucia, clinical staff member at the Rehabilitation Institute of Chicago and coordinator of the music therapy program at DePaul University.

In the 1960s, stroke specialists noticed that some people who had survived a stroke could sing even though they could not talk, suggesting that talking and singing are controlled by different parts of the brain. They are, but more recent research shows that the brain's talking and singing centers are also connected and that exercising the singing center helps restore the talking center, especially among those with damaged left frontal lobes.

Music also helps stroke survivors to relearn walking. In one study, half of a group of 25 people whose walking was impaired listened to marching music during their rehabilitation sessions. Compared with those denied the marches, the music group made faster progress and showed better retention of what they had learned.

*Surgery.* Other studies have confirmed the finding at Jefferson General that music decreases surgical anesthesia requirements. Japanese researchers have discovered that music before and during surgery reduces levels of stress hormones in the blood that interfere with the effectiveness of anesthesia.

*Work performance.* "Whistle while you work," the song title says, and for good reason. Light, stimulative music gets workers moving and helps boost their productivity. That's one reason that Muzak is played in so many stores. Another is that light stimulative music also boosts something else—consumer spending. "Personally, I can't stand Muzak," Dr. Bonny says, "and I'm offended that it's used to make people spend more. But as manipulative as that is, it's another indication of the power of music on human behavior."

Today, at age 72, Dr. Bonny says, "I'm more enthusiastic about the healing power of music than I've ever been." She plays violin for an hour a day and performs with a string quartet and an orchestra. She continues to promote her GIM program in this country and others, including England, Sweden, Denmark, Switzerland, Lithuania, Australia and New Zealand.

In addition to her work as a psychotherapist, she is particularly interested in bringing music into hospitals. "Our increasingly high-technology health-care system may save more lives than ever," she explains, "but the hospital experience itself has become a major source of anxiety. Patients often feel so alienated that their bodies actually lose some of their innate healing ability. Music preserves and nurtures that ability. Even with the best technology, we still have to heal ourselves, and music helps."

Today, Dr. Bonny's message has found a receptive audience at the highest levels of the nation's medical establishment. "Since 1990," Bumanis explains, "interest in music therapy has exploded." One of the first grants awarded by the National Institutes of Health's new Office of Alternative Medicine went to a study of music's effects on health and healing.

## How to Use Music for Healing

Music-therapy research generally shows that for relaxation, stress management and recovery from illness, soothing sedative pieces work best. And for exercise and productivity, musical selections should be stimulative, but not too bombastic. However, music therapists warn against turning these generalizations into dogma. In studies at M. D. Anderson Cancer Center in Houston, radiotherapy nurse Janet Cook, R.N., discovered that people experienced the greatest anxiety relief when they were allowed to listen to their favorite music, no matter what it was.

"Basically, whatever works, works," Bumanis explains. "When considering selections, the most important element is what the person likes. Classical music is great if you enjoy it, but if I were dealing with an adolescent, I'd probably use rap. For someone from South America, I'd suggest salsa or Cuban music. And for a member of a black church choir, I'd try gospel. Most music-therapy studies have used classical music, not because it's inherently better or more healing than other forms but simply because the participants have generally been older people of European descent who grew up with classical and prefer it."

Musical taste tends to form by about age 25. When creating a healing tape, Bumanis suggests using the music of the person's youth and selecting soft, light pieces, unless the person clearly prefers more percussive styles.

If you're not quite sure what to try, here are a few suggestions. Steven Halpern and Marcey Hamm are two musicians who have devoted their careers to creating healing music, so anything by either would be appropriate. And Janet Cook offers the following list.

*Classical. Bach:* "Air on the G String", "Jesu, Joy of Man's Desiring"; Beethoven: Symphony No. 6 in E Major ("Pastorale"), Sonata in C Sharp Minor ("Moonlight Sonata"), Sonata in C Minor ("Pathetique Sonata"); Brahms: "Lullaby"; Chopin: Nocturne in G; Debussy: "Clair de Lune"; Handel: Water Music; Liszt: "Liebestraum"; Mozart: "Laude Dominum" from the Vespers; Pachelbel: "Canon in D"; Saint-Saëns: "The Swan"; Schubert: "Ave Maria"; and Vivaldi: "The Four Seasons."

*Soundtracks.* Music from *Born Free, Chariots of Fire* and *The Sound of Music.*

*Country-Western.* Willie Nelson: "Stardust" and "Sweet Memories."

*Guitar.* Will Ackerman: "Childhood and Memories" and "Passages"; Alex de Grassi: "Southern Exposure" and "Slow Circle."

*Piano.* George Winston: "Autumn," "December" and "Winter into Spring"; Roger Williams: "Nadia's Theme."

*Symphonic.* Kitaro: "Silk Road Suite."

## CHAPTER 23

# ORNISH THERAPY

*Reversing Heart Disease Naturally*

Dean Ornish, M.D., vividly remembers how his professors reacted when he suggested that heart disease might be reversed. It wasn't that long ago. The time was 1977, and he was a brash young medical student at Baylor College of Medicine in Houston. When he proposed that Nature's cures—yoga, meditation, moderate exercise, group support and an ultra-low-fat diet—might reverse heart disease, his professors laughed. Heart disease *cannot* be reversed, they insisted. Its progression can be slowed with bypass surgery and drugs that reduce cholesterol in the blood. But reverse it? Impossible. With quackery? Ridiculous.

Today those same professors—and cardiologists around the world—no longer dismiss Dean Ornish. He's now an assistant clinical professor and an attending physician at the University of California's San Francisco Medical Center and president of the Preventive Medicine Research Institute in Sausalito. Dr. Ornish has shown beyond scientific doubt that natural therapies can succeed where high-tech medicine has failed.

In three landmark studies, Dr. Ornish's unique combination of natural therapies successfully reversed heart disease—the nation's leading cause of death. The Ornish program does not cure heart disease. It does open clogged coronary arteries, increase blood flow to the heart and reduce chest pain. And it allows those virtually crippled by heart disease to resume normal lives—all for a tiny fraction of the cost of bypass surgery and other high-tech treatments that accomplish much less.

## Gentle Therapy Banishes Pain

"You should have seen me before I started the Ornish program," says 55-year-old Bob Finnell of Redwood City, California, director of a nonprofit educational organization. "I was sick and scared. Two of my coronary arteries were completely blocked and the third was more than 80 percent blocked." (The coronary arteries nourish the heart.)

"I could hardly move without chest pain," remembers Finnell. "Several cardiologists told me that if I didn't have a bypass immediately, I'd be dead in six months. I didn't have that bypass, but today there's a lot more blood flowing into my heart. I have no chest pain. And I'm a much happier person."

Finnell's story is far from unique.

"Even after seven years in the Ornish program, I still can hardly believe the results," says 78-year-old Werner Hebenstreit of San Francisco, a retired businessman. In 1986, his heart disease was so severe that he could barely take a shower without chest pain. "I haven't had chest pain in years," he says. "Recently my wife and I hiked the Grand Tetons and the Canadian Rockies."

## Goaded by Personal Crisis

Dr. Ornish became an advocate of Nature's cures accidentally, because of a personal crisis. As an undergraduate at Rice University in Houston, the pressure of the premedical curriculum sent him into a suicidal depression.

"I think I came as close to killing myself as anyone ever does without actually doing it," he says. He withdrew from school and went home to Dallas. There his sister introduced him to yoga,

(continued on page 372)

# The ABCs of Type-A and Type-B

In the 1950s, San Francisco cardiologist Meyer Friedman, M.D., noticed that the chairs in his waiting room needed re-covering. The upholsterer idly remarked how odd it was that only the fronts were worn: "Your patients sit on the edge of their seats."

Dr. Friedman thought nothing of the observation until years later, when he and fellow cardiologist Ray Rosenman, M.D., began studying stress as a possible risk factor for heart disease. In interviews with dozens of men who'd had heart attacks, they were struck by how many seemed unusually competitive, belligerent and time-pressured.

"They could hardly sit still," recalls Dr. Friedman, director of the Meyer Friedman Research Institute at Mount Zion Medical Center in San Francisco. "They were like runners straining at the starting blocks." That's when he remembered the upholsterer's comment. If life were an endless race and the men were always at the starting blocks, how would they sit? On the edge of their seats.

Dr. Friedman and Dr. Rosenman coined the term *Type-A* to describe those who constantly struggle to accomplish more and more in less and less time. This behavior, Dr. Friedman says, stems from personal insecurity. Type-A's fear they are failures and compensate by driving themselves mercilessly to become successes in their own eyes. But with each new achievement, they raise their goals and push themselves even harder, winding up driven, time-pressured, hostile and impatient, with little time for friends, family and relaxation. Still they remain convinced that their Type-A traits are key to whatever success they have attained. *Type-A* became a household word as a result of two best-sellers that Dr. Friedman co-wrote: *Type-A Behavior and Your Heart* and *Treating Type-A Behavior and Your Heart*.

## TYPE-A DEFINED

Are you Type-A? Here are some typical characteristics of a Type-A person.

- Tries to do two things at once: reads while watching TV, cooks while on the phone, works while eating.
- Interrupts others frequently.
- Yells at the stupidity of other drivers.
- Hates waiting in lines.
- Sits on the edge of seats or leans forward while seated.
- In conversation, often seems preoccupied with something else.
- Overschedules; rarely has free time; has trouble sitting still and doing nothing.
- Pesters waiters ("When will our food be ready?")
- Eats quickly without savoring food; jumps up from the table right after eating.
- Argues with television newscasters.
- Has difficulty accepting criticism.
- When criticized or embarrassed, has fantasies of revenge.
- Plays to win, even in games with children.
- Has often been told by spouse and friends to slow down. Dismisses these exhortations as ridiculous or impossible.

If any of these traits sound familiar, here are some ways you can evolve to Type-B behavior and reduce your risk of heart disease.

**Listen to your spouse and friends.** Stop arguing with recommendations to slow down and relax.

**Don't bite off too much.** Realize that life is a work in progress, always unfinished. Stop trying to do several things at once.

**Cut back your schedule.** Ask yourself which meetings, dates and events on your calendar you will truly care about five years from now. Go to those. Cancel as many of the rest as possible.

**Stop kibitzing.** The next time you see someone doing a task more slowly than you can, do not interfere.

**Practice patience.** Stand in the longest line at the supermarket or drive into the longest line at the bank and use the time to review your progress toward Type-B behavior during the previous week.

(continued)

## The ABCs of Type-A and Type-B—*Continued*

**Learn to value criticism.** When people criticize you, divide their comments into elements with which you agree and disagree. Discuss those you agree with first.

**Lighten up.** When people do you wrong, forgive them.

**Learn to love your leisure.** Read a long novel far removed from your occupation. Visit a museum and banish all thoughts of the objects' monetary value. Appreciate, do not appraise. Write a letter to an old friend. Do not mention your job and use a thesaurus at least once.

**Slow down, you move too fast.** Drive in the right lane and ignore cars that pass you. Instead, reflect on your fondest memories.

**Laugh more.** Laugh at yourself at least once a day.

---

meditation and vegetarianism. He was skeptical at first, but after a few weeks of following her suggestions, his depression began to lift. "I felt better. I had more energy. I could think more clearly," he recalls. Dr. Ornish continued these practices after he returned to school, graduated and went on to Baylor College of Medicine.

When he entered Baylor in 1975, it was a leading center of what was, at the time, the hottest new high-tech treatment for heart disease—coronary artery bypass surgery.

Heart disease develops over several decades as the coronary arteries become narrowed by cholesterol-rich deposits called plaques. This narrowing process is called atherosclerosis. Plaques sometimes rupture, spilling their contents into the bloodstream. If plaque debris gets caught in a coronary artery that's already narrowed by atherosclerosis, blood flow to part of the heart can be completely blocked and part of the heart dies. That's a heart attack.

In bypass surgery, surgeons construct detours around narrowed portions of the coronary arteries, usually using sections of veins taken from the person's legs. With a bypass in place, blood flows into the heart more normally and risk of heart attack diminishes.

## Bypassing the Bypass

Bypass surgery was and is a technological marvel. But it left the young Dean Ornish feeling uneasy. "Bypasses bypass the problem," he explains now. "They don't cure heart disease. They're $30,000 Band-Aids. After a few years, bypasses themselves often develop atherosclerosis, and then people are back where they started—at high risk for a heart attack. Back in medical school, I thought: If heart disease is an overflowing sink, then bypass surgery is a fancy new mop. It seemed that nobody was trying to turn off the faucet."

The young medical student might have kept his doubts to himself, but as he visited and talked with heart disease patients at Baylor, he discovered an emotional bond with them. Many had not only heart disease but also broken hearts—the same feelings of emptiness, isolation, self-doubt and stress that had led Dr. Ornish to contemplate suicide a few years earlier.

Meanwhile, curious new findings were popping up in the medical literature. Studies showed that stress raised cholesterol and blood pressure—both risk factors for heart attack. They also showed that meditation, yoga and exercise lowered blood pressure and that vegetarian cultures in Africa and Japan had remarkably little heart disease. Dr. Ornish was also intrigued by the work of cardiologists Meyer Freidman, M.D., director of the Meyer Friedman Research Institute at Mount Zion Medical Center in San Francisco, and Ray Rosenman, M.D., who showed that the super-stressed Type-A lifestyle was a risk factor for heart attack. (See "The ABCs of Type-A and Type-B" on page 370.)

During his daily meditations, Dr. Ornish envisioned doing a scientific study that would combine moderate exercise with his own personal lifesavers—yoga, meditation and vegetarianism—to see if this combination might arrest or even reverse heart disease. This concept was so important to him that he took a year off between his second and third years of medical school to do his study. He approached cardiologists to find ten people with serious heart disease that he could put to the test.

"What's the name of your study?" one cardiologist asked.

"The Effects of Yoga, Meditation and a Vegetarian Diet on Coronary Heart Disease," Dr. Ornish replied.

"Forget it," the doctor said. "What do I tell my patients—that I'm referring them to a swami? Take my advice: Call it 'The Effects of Stress Management Techniques and Diet Change on Coronary Heart Disease,' and I'd be delighted to refer some patients."

## Pioneers Report Good Results

Dr. Ornish took the advice and recruited ten people with heart disease to participate in the study. For a month, they stopped smoking, took daily walks, learned yoga and meditation, participated in group discussions about heart disease and personal issues and ate a vegetarian diet limited to 10 percent of calories from fat (that's a mere one-quarter of the amount of fat in the average American diet). The diet permitted no red meat, no chicken, no fish, no dairy products, no nuts, no chocolate and no coffee. It allowed all the whole grains, beans and fresh fruits and vegetables participants could eat. There were no calorie restrictions at all.

After only a few days, most of the study participants reported decreased chest pain. At the end of the month, many were pain-free. Sophisticated tests showed increased blood flow to their hearts. In other words, this was the first scientific evidence that these natural therapies might actually help reverse heart disease.

Dr. Ornish's results, published in a medical journal in 1979, were greeted with howls of skepticism. Cardiologists dismissed his ultra-low-fat diet as impossible for the vast majority of Americans. And they rolled their eyes at the yoga, meditation, exercise and group meetings. Besides, they told him, "Everyone knows heart disease can't be reversed."

In 1980, after graduating from medical school, Dr. Ornish repeated his study. This time he recruited 48 people with severe heart disease. Half—the control group—were instructed to follow their doctors' advice. The other half participated in three weeks of yoga, meditation, social support, moderate exercise, an ultra-low-fat diet and no smoking.

By the end of the study, the control group's heart disease had grown worse. But the test group showed a 21 percent drop in cholesterol, a 91 percent reduction in chest pain, a 55 percent improvement in exercise capacity and significantly lower blood pressure, plus reduced anxiety and a greater sense of well-being. What's more, tests showed that their hearts were pumping more normally. The results, published in the *Journal of the American Medical Association* in 1983, caused a minor sensation. Advocates of Nature's cures applauded Dr. Ornish, but critics continued to bash him, saying that most Americans could not eat his ultra-low-fat diet and that despite his results, heart disease can't be reversed.

## The Program Proves Itself

To satisfy his critics once and for all, Dr. Ornish launched a third study, larger, longer and even more scientifically rigorous than the previous two. He recruited 43 men and 5 women. One group—the controls—followed standard recommendations for people with heart disease: no smoking, moderate regular exercise, cholesterol-lowering drugs and a diet containing no more than 30 percent of calories from fat.

The treatment group followed the full Ornish regimen: no cholesterol drugs, no smoking, moderate exercise (walking either for 30 minutes a day or for one hour three days a week), stress management (an hour a day of yoga and meditation) and a strict vegetarian diet with fewer than 10 percent of calories from fat. The treatment group also met twice a week for four hours of group activities: a long walk, yoga, meditation, dinner and a support group.

The people in the treatment group followed the program as well as they could, but no one followed it perfectly. Some had trouble with yoga or meditation. Others thought the support group was silly. One man, a 49-year-old athlete, ate the food, exercised like a maniac and reduced his cholesterol from 294 to 121. But he was extremely competitive, a classic Type-A, and he didn't care for meditation or the support group. A few months into the program, while working out on a rowing machine, he dropped dead of a heart attack.

The man's death was a powerful lesson for everyone in the treatment group. The established risk factors for heart disease—a high-fat diet, smoking, a sedentary lifestyle, high blood pressure and a family history of heart disease—explain only about half of heart attacks. Stress is also a critical factor, though it's often downplayed. The death of the man who was clearly stressed out reinforced Dr. Ornish's message that yoga, meditation and the support group were vital to the participants' health and well-being. After the man's funeral, even the skeptics started meditating and opening up about their feelings.

After a year, those in the control group reported more chest pain and showed increased coronary artery blockage. But in the treatment group, frequency of chest pain dropped 91 percent, and 82 percent of the participants showed significant reversal of arterial blockage. Tests showed that in many participants, blood flow to the heart doubled.

Dr. Ornish published his results in 1990 in the prestigious British medical journal *Lancet*. Since then, reporters and television crews from all over the world have visited Dr. Ornish and talked with people who are actively following his program. They encounter a group of individuals who are highly motivated to reduce stress in their lives and radically change the way they eat. This is a group of Americans who are willing trading in their burgers and fries for things like vegetable sushi, bok choy and broccoli.

## How Hard Is the Diet, Really?

Thanks to Dr. Ornish's studies, cardiologists no longer claim that heart disease cannot be reversed. But many continue to call

Dr. Ornish's ultra-low-fat diet impossible to follow. The American Heart Association (AHA) recommends limiting fat to no more than 30 percent of daily calories, but the Ornish diet contains just 10 percent of calories from fat.

"I don't think most people would be willing to follow it," contends Henry Ginsberg, M.D., associate professor of medicine at Columbia University in New York City and a member of the AHA Nutrition Committee. Adam Drenowski, Ph.D., dean of nutrition at the University of Michigan School of Public Health in Ann Arbor, agrees. "My research has shown that unless people are threatened by death, adherence is impossible."

Not so, say those who follow the program. "We eat well," says Werner Hebenstreit. "I don't feel deprived. It takes longer to chop fruits and vegetables than it does to cook our old way, but whenever that bothers me, I think of all the time I'm saving not having to go to doctors."

Hebenstreit has been on the Ornish program for more than four years. The results he saw after just one year on the program kept him going. After one year, Hebenstreit's crippling chest pain disappeared. Blood flow to his heart was increased by 20 percent. His cholesterol dropped from 320 to 145.

After four years, blockage of his coronary arteries plummeted from 52 percent to just 13 percent. Hebenstreit says he and his wife, who also follows the program, have no difficulty sticking to the diet at home and have few problems eating out. "I just call ahead and talk with the chef. Most are happy to cook our way. When we travel, it's not hard to find low-fat food at Asian restaurants."

"I miss veal," says Victor Karpenko, 71, of Danville, California, "but my wife has a great imagination, and I've been pleasantly surprised by the food we're permitted." When he joined the program, Karpenko weighed 190 and his cholesterol stood at 290. Now he weighs 160 and has a cholesterol level of 130. After one year on the program, his almost totally blocked artery opened up 28 percent. Karpenko says that eating out is sometimes difficult, but he has no problems finding ultra-low-fat items at Asian restaurants. "We had a problem in Spain last

(continued on page 380)

# Cheers!
# A Little Wine Reduces Heart Attack Risk

The French gorge themselves on cheese, butter, cream and pâté, all high in fat. Yet compared with Americans, they have a lower death rate from heart attack. What's going on here?

The reason, some scientists believe, is that they wash down all that fat with red wine. Does that mean you should uncork a bottle of cabernet with your next dinner? Quite possibly.

Wine has been used socially, religiously and medicinally for about 7,000 years. The downside of overindulgence in wine and other alcoholic beverages is, of course, a serious public health problem. Drunk drivers account for thousands of fatalities every year. Alcoholism destroys the liver and the brain, wreaks havoc with many families and is a risk factor for several cancers, including possibly breast cancer. It also elevates blood pressure and is associated with obesity, both risk factors for heart disease.

Currently, most experts agree that alcohol becomes a health threat at three drinks a day or more. (A "drink" is a 5-ounce glass of wine, a 1-ounce shot of liquor or a 12-ounce glass of beer.) Health authorities do not encourage Americans to drink more, and even one drink can impair reaction time when driving.

But among those who raise an occasional glass responsibly, studies show that a little alcohol—up to two drinks a day—is better for the heart than total abstinence. Here are some findings.

Eric Rimm, Sc.D., research associate in nutrition and epidemiology at the Harvard School of Public Health, surveyed the medical records of 51,529 male health professionals going back to 1976. Twelve years later, compared with the nondrinkers, men who imbibed up to two drinks a day had 26 percent fewer heart attacks.

Meir J. Stampfer, M.D., associate professor of medicine at Harvard Medical School, followed the health of 87,526 female nurses starting in 1980. Eight years later, nurses who had about one drink a day had 40 percent fewer heart attacks than the nondrinkers.

How does alcohol reduce heart attack risk? Scientists aren't sure, but moderate alcohol consumption increases the proportion of cholesterol known as HDL, or "good cholesterol," which helps protect against heart attack, and decreases the proportion of LDL—"bad cholesterol"—which increases heart attack risk.

But it's not just the alcohol in beer, wine and liquor that helps prevent heart attack. Researchers have compared Europeans in more than a dozen nations who have similar heart disease risk factors and similar drinking habits. The French have the lowest death rate from heart attack, only one-third that of Scandinavians. The reason, scientists speculate, is that the French love red wine. Studies by French scientists suggest that chemicals unique to red wine help prevent the blood clots that trigger heart attack. In addition, a recent study by Edwin Frankel, Ph.D., adjunct professor of food sciences and technology at the University of California at Davis, suggests that red wine decreases the damage done by LDL.

But don't reach for the burgundy just yet. White wine may confer the same benefits as red. Arthur L. Klasky, M.D., chief of cardiology at the Kaiser Permanente Medical Center in Oakland, California, analyzed the medical records of 81,825 social drinkers for a period of ten years. Wine drinkers had 30 percent fewer heart attacks than beer and liquor drinkers, but wine drinkers who preferred red and those who preferred white had the same heart attack rates. Dr. Klasky also speculates that the "wine advantage" may have nothing to do with what's in the bottle. He notes that compared with beer and liquor drinkers, wine drinkers tend to be better-educated, and as education increases, lifestyles become healthier.

It's still too early to be certain if alcohol, or wine, or red wine reduces heart attack risk, but if you're an occasional drinker, perhaps it's time to cultivate a taste for bordeaux, cabernet and other red wines.

year," he recalls. "Spanish food is fried and oily. So we ate at a lot of Chinese restaurants there."

Dr. Ornish accuses mainstream doctors of a double standard when they object to his diet. "Smoking is one of the hardest addictions to break," he says, "harder than heroin, according to many experts. But doctors routinely advise people to do it, and millions have done it. Doctors tell their patients that much of smoking's damage to their lungs and hearts is reversible—if they quit. They don't say, 'Oh, quitting is too hard, so just cut back from three packs a day to two.'

"In ten out of ten studies—not just ours—people with heart disease who make only the moderate diet and lifestyle changes the AHA recommends get worse. Our program may not be easy, but I have more than 1,000 letters from people around the world who read my book, adopted it and have seen their cholesterol drop and their chest pain disappear."

## Dietary Change Is Not Enough

As difficult as changing one's diet can be, Dr. Ornish has never claimed that dietary change alone will reverse heart disease.

On Dr. Ornish's first day of internship in 1981, a resident took him and another intern on rounds. At the door to one hospital room, the resident said, "Dean, this is a 53-year-old man who had a heart attack three days ago. He's scared and depressed, and he wants to talk to someone, but we don't have time. In the next two hours, we have to see 45 patients. Just go in there, listen to his heart and lungs and get out."

"Medicine is obsessed with numbers," Dr. Ornish says. "weight, blood pressure, cholesterol counts, arterial blockage. But not everything that counts can be counted."

Dr. Ornish has taken a good deal of heat for focusing on what he calls the "spiritual" side of heart disease. But to Dr. Ornish, "spiritual" has nothing to do with seances and ouija boards. "I simply mean feeling connected to other people," he explains, "feeling that you're a part of a larger whole rather than apart from it."

The more the numbers showed that his study participants were improving, the more Dr. Ornish became convinced that the support group element of his program, which couldn't be counted, counted a great deal, possibly the most.

"Heart disease has a deep emotional component," explains Dr. Ornish. "People who develop it often feel isolated and inadequate. They feel they don't have enough and haven't made enough of themselves. That's why we place so much emphasis on group activities: the walks, dinners, yoga and meditation sessions and the support group. A number of studies show that compared with people who feel a sense of connection and community, those who feel lonely and isolated have three to five times the death rate—not only from heart disease but from all causes."

"I always put pressure on myself," Hebenstreit agrees. "I was a classic Type-A: angry, defensive and always in a hurry. I had a big temper and a short fuse. I yelled at the people I was closest to, like my wife. I always interrupted people. I had trouble listening and talking about my feelings. But I've learned to loosen up. Nowadays, very few things bother me. At the first sign of frustration, I smile and start breathing deeply. I'm much more patient, I don't interrupt, and my wife and I get along much better now."

When Bob Finnell first signed up with Dr. Ornish, he concentrated on the program's diet and didn't do much walking or yoga. "I was scared of exercise," he remembers. "I couldn't touch my toes and couldn't do most of the yoga postures." But after six months, he felt much better and was shocked to realize that he actually enjoyed yoga. "I used to get up in the morning feeling like a creaky old barn door," he says. "I'd have to slowly unhinge my elbows and knees, then take a hot shower to loosen up and drink coffee to get going. But doing yoga, I woke up refreshed. My head felt clear and my joints felt fine. For the first time in my life, I enjoyed my body."

As his weight has dropped from the 180s into the 140s and as his cholesterol fell from 235 to 120, Finnell found himself developing a passion for yoga.

"The health-care system has it backward," says Finnell. "The insurers reward sickness, not wellness. When I go to a cardiologist, he bills $165 for 15 minutes, and insurance pays 80 percent of it. When I take a yoga class, none of the cost is reimbursable. I pay 100 percent, $8 to $12 per class. I spend more out of pocket on yoga than on doctors. But yoga has done me a lot more good than any cardiologist. The system ought to pay for prevention."

Finnell jokes that he's gone from being a workaholic to being a yogaholic, but he insists, "It's a mistake to focus too much on the physical changes in Dean's program—the exercise, diet, cholesterol and blood flow. They're important, but I think the emotional changes are more important. If a doctor told me there'd been a big mix-up, that I'd never had heart disease and didn't have to be in the program, I'd still stay in it. The experts can debate whether the Ornish program has prolonged my life, but I know it's enriched it."

## Putting the Therapy to Work

If you have heart disease and would like to try Dr. Ornish's strategy, discuss it with your physician. (Dr. Ornish describes his program in great detail in his book *Dr. Dean Ornish's Program for Reversing Heart Disease*.)

It is possible to prevent heart disease by incorporating many aspects of Ornish therapy into your lifestyle. The key elements of Dr. Ornish's programs fall into the category of Nature's cures. You'll find them—companionship, exercise, low-fat eating, meditation, vegetarianism, walking and yoga—discussed at length in many of the chapters of the book you're holding.

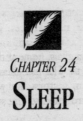

# CHAPTER 24
# SLEEP

## Horizontal Therapy for What Ails You

Yawn! Go ahead. Chances are good that you're sleepier than you think you are. You might even want to stretch luxuriously and go take a nap. Why? Chances are even better that no matter what ails you, sleeping well will help you heal.

"Sleep deprivation is epidemic in our society. Nearly all of us need more sleep than we get. I believe a sudden wave of drowsiness should be taken as seriously as the chest pain that might signal a heart attack," says William Dement, M.D., Ph.D., professor of psychiatry and behavioral science at Stanford University, director of the Stanford Sleep Disorders Clinic and chair of the National Commission on Sleep Disorders Research. "Drowsiness is an urgent warning that should not be ignored, particularly in situations where dozing, inattention or impaired performance could lead to catastrophe. In such situations, stop what you're doing and take a nap. Many cultures honor the afternoon siesta. America should, too."

Like people who are drunk, those who are sleepy often don't realize it and are apt to deny it. In one study, Thomas Roth, Ph.D., director of the Henry Ford Hospital Sleep Disorders Center in Detroit, recruited a large number of volunteers who swore they were not bothered by daytime drowsiness. Yet after they spent an eight-hour night in the hospital's sleep laboratory, tests showed that only 10 percent were optimally alert and 40 percent were living their daily lives in a state of significant sleepiness.

Dr. Roth persuaded those who tested the sleepiest to spend ten hours a night in bed for six consecutive nights. Tests afterward showed major improvements in alertness and intellectual performance. And that brings us to the first health benefit of sleep: Getting enough sleep can save your life.

## Don't Turn into a Statistic

What do the 1989 *Exxon Valdez* disaster, the 1986 space shuttle *Challenger* tragedy, the 1979 near-meltdown of the Three-Mile Island nuclear power plant and thousands of motor vehicle, rail and airline accidents have in common? Answer: Sleepiness.

When the *Exxon Valdez* ran aground in Prince William Sound, Alaska, causing the costliest, most environmentally destructive maritime accident in U.S. history, the news media focused on the captain, who'd been drinking heavily beforehand. But the captain was not on the bridge when the ship struck Bligh Reef. The third mate was actually steering the ship. National Transportation Safety Board (NTSB) investigators concluded: "The cause of the grounding . . . was the failure of the third mate to maneuver the vessel because . . . he was asleep on his feet and failed to respond to the warning light signaling Bligh Reef."

When the space shuttle *Challenger* blew up shortly after liftoff, killing its seven astronauts in front of millions of television viewers, the news media focused on faulty O-rings that failed to control fuel flow. But the Rogers Commission, which investigated the accident, also faulted the sleep schedules of key project managers who made the ill-advised decision to launch the shuttle that day. Two of the three top managers had slept less than three hours apiece on each of the three nights before the launch. "In my opinion," Dr. Dement says, "the project managers were so sleepy, they were unable to assess reports that pointed out possible problems in the O-rings."

The chain of events that culminated in the Three-Mile Island nuclear accident began at 4:00 A.M., when a mechanical failure went unnoticed by drowsy graveyard-shift workers. Nuclear Regulatory Commission investigators blamed the near-meltdown on human error. But the 1993 report of the NCSDR—"Wake Up, America: A National Sleep Alert"—blamed those human errors on sleepiness.

These disasters became major media events, but to understand the real toll of being literally "asleep at the wheel," we must look beyond the headlines to the thousands of little disasters sleep deprivation causes every day. As James Danaher, chief of the Human Performance Division of the safety board, told the research commission, "sleepiness contributes to many car, truck, rail, maritime and airline accidents."

## Good Reasons for a Good Snooze

Prevention of thousands of motor vehicle deaths a year is reason enough for Americans to get more sleep, but a good night's sleep contributes to health and longevity in many other ways as well.

*The common cold.* Ever catch a cold after pulling an all-nighter? "A person with a large sleep debt is much more vulnerable to infections and other illnesses," says Peter Hauri, Ph.D., director of the Insomnia Research and Treatment Program at the Mayo Clinic in Rochester, Minnesota, and co-author of *No More Sleepless Nights.* The reason is that without adequate rest, the body cannot fully recover from day-to-day stresses and the immune system cannot fully defend against disease-causing microorganisms. Surveys show that compared with normal sleepers, people who experience chronic insomnia report more illnesses and slower recovery from them.

*Heart disease.* The connection between sleep and heart disease focuses on something most people dismiss as simply an annoyance—snoring. Quite often that's all it is. But sometimes snoring is a red flag for heart disease—and very few people know it.

# Are You Sleep-Deprived?

Take this simple test developed by William Dement, M.D., Ph.D., professor of psychiatry and behavioral science at Stanford University, director of the Stanford Sleep Disorders Clinic and chair of the National Commission on Sleep Disorders Research. If you answer yes to any question, you need more sleep.

1. Do you have to rely on an alarm clock to get you up in the morning?
2. Do you ever sleep through your alarm?
3. Is getting out of bed a struggle?
4. Do you ever experience powerful waves of drowsiness in school, at work, at the movies or in theaters?
5. Do you ever fall asleep without intending to?
6. Do you ever wonder where your get-up-and-go has gone?
7. Does a single glass of beer or wine hit you unexpectedly hard?

If your bedmate snores loudly, with periods of thrashing and choking silences, and then complains of daytime drowsiness, he or she may have sleep apnea. *Apnea* means a lapse in breathing. People with sleep apnea sometimes stop breathing for up to one minute at a time. Interrupted breathing keeps oxygen from entering the blood and as a result, sleep apnea strains the heart, elevates blood pressure and increases the risk of heart attack and heart failure.

If you've never heard of sleep apnea, you're not alone. "Of the ten million Americans estimated to have the condition," Dr. Dement says, "at least eight million are undiagnosed." Sleep apnea affects more men than women—about 5 percent of the male population and about 20 percent of men over 65.

Sleep apnea typically develops in men during their thirties or forties and in women during their fifties. Risk factors include being overweight and having a small jaw, large tonsils or a deviated nasal septum. "Any adult man who is overweight, snores loudly and falls asleep in meetings, movies or after lunch is almost certain to have sleep apnea," Dr. Dement says. The most effective treatment is weight loss (which also reduces other risk factors for heart disease).

If you suspect that your bedmate might have sleep apnea, encourage him to discuss it with his doctor. It just might save his (or her) life.

*Longevity.* A nine-year study by the California Department of Health showed that adults who slept six hours or less a night had significantly higher death rates from all causes than those who slept seven hours or more. Not surprisingly, motor vehicle accidents accounted for many of the fatalities among those who slept the least, but how people schedule their sleep appears to be as important as how much sleep they get. The study revealed a significant association between untimely death and shift work, the increasingly common practice of working through the night or the even more hazardous practice of switching shifts frequently.

In addition to their higher death rate, those whose jobs call for them to switch shifts—physicians, nurses, police, firefighters, pilots and bus drivers, among others—are five times more likely to experience mental health problems than people who work days. If you do shift work, you might want to reconsider your schedule. If you can't change your sleep schedule, make sure you sleep at least 8 hours out of every 24.

*Recovery.* Why do so many illnesses send us straight to bed? An increased need for sleep is the body's way of orchestrating recovery, says Dr. Hauri. Most growth and most recovery from illness occurs during sleep, specifically during the deepest, or delta, stage. Children spend a good deal of the night in delta sleep because they are growing. As adults grow older, delta sleep diminishes. Many people believe that loss of sound sleep is caused by aging, but it just might be the other way around. A decline in delta sleep may play a key role in the physical decline of aging by limiting the body's ability to repair itself. You may not be able to "sleep like a baby" once you hit 50, but for general well-being and recovery from all illness, few therapies beat a good night's sleep.

*Productivity.* Sleep deprivation hits America right in the wallet by reducing productivity. It impairs the abilities to read, write, react, reason, do math and make decisions—every faculty that contributes to getting jobs done well. People with chronic insomnia are less productive than normal sleepers, and they report 2.5 times as many auto accidents. But you don't have to have insomnia to have sleep deprivation impair your performance. Guess when doctors are most likely to order the wrong medications for hospital patients: at the end of a long, overnight shift. Guess when nurses are most likely to give the wrong medications: ditto. Guess when police are most likely to fire their weapons inappropriately. You get the picture. The list goes on and on.

## The National Snooze Debt

Why don't we notice that we're sleepy? Blame it on Thomas Edison. Before the electric light, most Americans took Benjamin Franklin's advice: Early to bed and early to rise (even if they didn't become wealthy and wise). After electric lighting's arrival, Americans still rose early, but they started staying up considerably later—and as a result, sleeping too little.

There is no "normal" amount of sleep. Sleep needs vary tremendously, and some people *can* get along fine on only four to six hours a night. According to the NCSDR, the vast majority of adults need at least seven hours of sleep a night, and most need eight or more to function optimally. Yet about half the adult population sleeps less than eight hours a night, and 13 percent—some 20 million Americans—get by on seven or less. "Americans spend so much time and energy chasing the American dream," Dr. Dement says, "that they don't have much time left for actual dreaming.

"When you need more sleep than you get," he continues, "you develop a sleep debt, just as you would if you spend more money than you have. Americans simply don't get enough sleep. The problem is so pervasive, it's not even perceived."

Even doctors, who should be telling their patients to get more sleep, are usually laboring under a serious sleep debt. And programs that train medical professionals set them up for it. Medical residents and nurse-trainees often work 24-hour shifts and frequently go 36 hours without sleep. Such schedules inadvertently train them to ignore their own sleep needs.

Is it any wonder that doctors trained to ignore their own sleepiness don't notice it in their patients? A 1991 Gallup survey showed that family physicians failed to diagnose—or even ask about—insomnia in one-third of those with the problem. The average person with more serious sleep disorders had to consult five doctors before being diagnosed.

It's time to wake up to the importance of sleep. A good night's sleep not only feels refreshing, it's also critical to health and longevity.

## How to Get a Good Night's Sleep

"Most people think insomnia means chronic sleeplessness that keeps you up all night," Dr. Hauri says. "Actually, insomnia means any sleep problem. Occasional late-night wake-ups with trouble going back to sleep are not as trying as chronic insomnia, but they're still a threat to well-being."

A 1991 Gallup survey showed that 65 million American adults (36 percent of the population) say they have trouble sleeping. For one-quarter of them, the problem is chronic—and costly. Americans spend about $15 billion a year on sleeping pills and physician care for insomnia, according to the NCSDR. Yet a Gallup survey showed that 85 percent of people with occasional sleep problems never mention them to their doctors. "Insomnia is so common," Dr. Dement says, "it's accepted—mistakenly—as a normal part of older adult life."

When people do mention sleep problems to their doctors, two-thirds of physicians prescribe sleeping pills. Sleep medications can relieve occasional insomnia, but according to the NCSDR, sleeping pills are not the best way to go. Natural approaches work better over the long haul.

The following advice comes from Dr. Dement, Dr. Hauri,

(continued on page 392)

# Sleepy-Time Herbs

Most health-conscious people steer clear of sleeping pills because of concerns about side effects and possible addiction. But, ah, the convenience . . . Wouldn't it be nice if there were a little something you could take to soothe you gently into sleepiness? Actually, there is.

Unlike sleeping pills, herbal sleep aids are nonaddictive, can be used every night and cause no side effects. The amounts recommended here are for healthy adults. Pregnant women and those with medical conditions should consult a physician familiar with medicinal herbs before using these plants. Do not give these herbs to children under age 2. For older children and those over 65, start with low-strength preparations and increase strength if necessary.

**Balm.** Arab physicians began recommending balm, also known as lemon balm, for anxiety during the tenth century. Charlemagne was so impressed with its sedative/tranquilizing effects that he ordered it grown in all the medicinal herb gardens in his vast European realm. Modern researchers have discovered that balm oil has tranquilizing properties. In Germany, where herbal medicine is more mainstream than it is in the United States, balm is widely used as a tranquilizer and sleep aid.

When using commercial preparations, follow package directions. With the bulk herb, use two teaspoons of dried leaves per cup of boiling water. Steep 10 to 20 minutes. Drink one cup before bed. Taste: pleasantly lemony.

**Catnip.** The plant famous for its intoxicating effect on cats has a mild sedative/tranquilizing effect on people. Catnip has been used to treat anxiety and insomnia since ancient times. Scientists have discovered that the chemicals responsible for this plant's amusing effect on cats are quite similar to the natural sedatives in valerian.

When using commercial preparations, follow package directions. With the bulk herb, use two teaspoons of dried leaves per cup of boiling water. Steep 10 to 20 minutes. Drink one cup before bed. Taste: pleasantly minty.

**Chamomile.** This popular beverage tea has been used since ancient times to soothe upset stomachs and jangled nerves. Modern researchers have discovered that chamomile oil has a mild depressant effect on the central nervous system, calming people so they can fall asleep. There are two ways to use this herb as a sleep aid. Either fill a small cloth bag with a few handfuls of the flowers and add it to a hot bath or brew a tea.

When using commercial teas, follow package directions. With the bulk herb, use two to three heaping teaspoons of flowers per cup of boiling water. Steep 10 to 20 minutes. Drink one cup before bed. Taste: pleasant with an aroma of apple.

**Hop.** When German brewers began using this herb to flavor beer around the ninth century, demand soared and farmers began planting large fields with hop. At harvest time, they noticed that hop pickers fatigued easily, and since then the herb has been used as a sleep aid. During the nineteenth century, it was an ingredient in many American sleep aids. But the sedative constituent in hop remained a mystery until scientists isolated 2-methyl-3-butene-2-ol from the plant in 1983.

When using commercial preparations, follow package directions. With the bulk herb, use two teaspoons of dried leaves and flowers per cup of boiling water. Steep five minutes. Drink one cup before bed. Taste: warm and pleasantly bitter.

**Passionflower.** Some misinformed herbalists recommend this gorgeous South American flower as an aphrodisiac. Sorry, but the name has nothing to do with sexual passion; it's a reference to the Passion of the Crucifixion. Passionflower has been used as a tranquilizer/sedative by South Americans for centuries and was adopted by U.S. physicians in the 1830s. Passionflower contains potent tranquilizing chemicals (maltol, ethyl-maltol and flavonoids). In Europe, it's an ingredient in many herbal sedatives.

When using commercial preparations, follow package directions. With the bulk herb, use one teaspoon of dried flowers per cup of boiling water. Steep 10 to 15 minutes. Drink one cup before bed. Taste: pleasant.

*(continued)*

# Sleepy-Time Herbs—*Continued*

**Skullcap.** Chinese physicians have used skullcap as a tranquilizer/sedative for centuries, and it was a popular sleep aid in nineteenth-century America. Some experts continue to debate its merit, but it's an ingredient in many European herbal sedatives.

When using commercial preparations, follow package directions. With the bulk herb, use one to two teaspoons of dried leaves per cup of boiling water. Steep 10 to 15 minutes. Drink one cup before bed. Taste: bitter; add sugar, honey or lemon or mix it with an herbal beverage tea.

**Valerian.** When the elders of thirteenth-century Hamelin, Germany, refused to pay an itinerant flute player for ridding the town of rats, the Pied Piper used his music—and the aroma of valerian—to hypnotize the town's children and lure them away. Valerian has been used as a sedative/tranquilizer ever since. In one experiment, researchers gave 128 people with insomnia either 400 milligrams of valerian root extract or an inactive placebo. Those who took the placebo showed no change in sleep quality, but the herb users showed significant sleep improvement, with no morning grogginess.

When using commercial preparations, follow package directions. With the bulk herb, use two teaspoons of powdered root per cup of boiling water. Steep 10 to 15 minutes. Drink one cup before bed. Taste: earthy and unpleasant; add sugar, honey or lemon or mix it with an herbal beverage tea.

Richard Bootzin, Ph.D., professor of psychology at the University of Arizona, and Donald R. Sweeney, M.D., Ph.D., a lecturer in psychiatry at Yale University School of Medicine and author of *Overcoming Insomnia*. Approximately 80 percent of those who use these kinds of techniques for one month report better, more restful sleep.

**First, see your doctor.** Don't ask your doctor for sleeping pills. Rather, let your doctor rule out the many illnesses that can interfere with sleep. Be sure to mention how much alcohol you consume (alcohol disturbs sleep) and all the medications you take, including over-the-counter medicines (the decongestants in popular cold formulas can cause insomnia). Ask your physician to evaluate you for depression, which often contributes to sleep disturbances.

**Reduce stimulant consumption.** "Caffeine and other stimulants cause more sleep problems than most people realize," Dr. Hauri says. "Many insomniacs are exceptionally sensitive to caffeine and have trouble sleeping after one cup of tea or a chocolate bar in the afternoon." Caffeine is an ingredient in many drugs and soft drinks in addition to coffee, tea and chocolate. Drugs may also contain noncaffeine stimulants. Ask your physician or pharmacist about the possible stimulant effects of every medication you take.

**Limit alcohol.** Many doctors used to advise people who couldn't sleep to drink a cocktail or glass of wine before bedtime, says Dr. Hauri. "But many people find that drinking within a few hours of retiring keeps them from sleeping, and in nearly everyone, drinking late in the evening produces troubled, fragmented sleep."

**Quit smoking.** Where there's smoking, there's often insomnia. Nicotine is a powerful stimulant.

**Watch when you eat.** Bedtime snacks are fine, as long as they're small and light. Don't eat a large, heavy meal within an hour or two of bedtime. Digestive processes can disturb sleep.

**Take your vitamins and minerals.** "Deficiencies in the B vitamins, calcium, copper, iron, magnesium and zinc can all contribute to sleep problems," Dr. Hauri says. Consider taking a multivitamin/mineral supplement that contains some of every essential vitamin and mineral.

**Try tryptophan.** Tryptophan is an amino acid used to make serotonin, a chemical messenger in the brain. Among its many functions, serotonin helps induce sleep. "About 25 studies show that one to two grams of tryptophan help induce sleep in people with mild insomnia," Dr. Hauri says. Tryptophan is now available only with a doctor's prescription and is quite expen-

sive. Milk, however, is rich in tryptophan, a possible explanation
for the popular ritual of a glass of warm milk before bed.

**Ditch the double bed.** When couples sleep in double beds,
each person has no more room than a baby has in a crib. Switch
to a queen-size or king-size bed. Larger beds become especially
important as people age, because older people sleep less soundly
and are more likely to have their sleep disturbed by a restless
bedmate. If you were happy with a queen-size bed ten years ago
but haven't been sleeping well lately, it may be time to move up
tLo king-size.

**Pamper yourself.** You spend one-third of your life in bed.
Invest in that time and you'll probably sleep better. Get comfortable pillows and sheets. Test different types of mattresses.

If you have arthritis or a bad back, try extra pillows or specially shaped therapeutic pillows. If heartburn is a problem, elevate the head of your bed a few inches.

**Be quiet.** For more quiet, try foam earplugs. They're inexpensive and available at most pharmacies. Or consider replacing
your bedroom windows with double-pane, noise-reducing windows. Most people can adjust to steady noise, such as the low
hum of a freeway nearby, but have trouble sleeping through sudden, intermittent noises: a catfight, a motorcycle passing by or
a plane flying overhead. If intermittent noises disturb your sleep,
consider a noise screen—a steady sound that drowns out the periodic ones. Good noise screens include a fan or a radio tuned
between stations.

**Shut out the light.** For a darker bedroom, invest in blackout
drapes, blinds or shades.

**Banish all clocks.** Many people with sleep problems have illuminated digital clocks staring at them all night and making
them anxious, Dr. Hauri says, adding that "for most people, the
bedroom should be a time-free environment."

**Consider sleeping alone.** What if she likes it quiet and dark,
but he can't sleep without an open window that lets in noise and
light? What if he likes a hard foam mattress, but she prefers a
waterbed? Many couples with very different sleep styles feel obligated to share the same bed and bedroom. Perhaps it's not

worth it. Consider twin beds or different bedrooms. You may have to put up with some teasing from friends and family, but who cares? You'll both sleep better, not to mention that you'll probably feel more loving toward one another and have more interest in and energy for sex.

**Never work at going to sleep.** If at first you don't succeed, please do not try, try again. That old adage about repeated tries is sage advice for many things in life, but not for getting a good night's sleep. Sleep is something that finds you, not something you work at doing. If you're having a problem sleeping, get up, find some fairly boring routine activity (a minor household cleaning job should do the trick) and work at it until you feel sleepy. Then go back to bed.

**Get out of bed.** This sounds ridiculous, but many people with insomnia believe that the longer they stay in bed, the more they'll sleep. Not so. If a person who needs seven hours a night stays in bed for nine, the seven hours get spread thinly over the nine and sleep becomes more troubled and less restful.

**Get regular.** Go to bed and wake up at the same time every day, even on weekends. Many people need regular sleep/wake cycles and find their sleep seriously disturbed if they don't stick to them. Sleep/wake regularity is especially helpful for what's known as Sunday night insomnia—a surprisingly common inability to fall asleep as the work week is about to begin. Most people assume they're simply anxious about returning to work on Monday. In fact, Sunday night insomnia typically strikes those who stay up unusually late on Friday and Saturday nights and get up late Saturday and Sunday mornings. By Sunday night, they've set their internal clock to a later hour and in a phenomenon similar to jet lag, they can't fall asleep Sunday night until way past their weekday bedtime. Retiring and rising earlier on weekends usually resolves the problem.

**Adopt bedtime rituals.** Bedtime rituals are a way to wind down and mark the boundary between waking and sleeping. Most people change into pajamas and brush their teeth. If you have trouble sleeping, add a few more rituals to your transition period: Take a hot bath, drink a cup of herb tea or do some light reading. But steer clear of the late TV news. It's usually filled with disturbing images that might keep you awake.

**Try deep relaxation.** In addition to their ritual value, relaxation techniques also help minimize the stress that contributes to sleep problems. Aromatherapy, biofeedback, deep breathing, exercise, listening to music, massage, meditation and yoga can all help in overcoming insomnia. Just don't do any kind of strenuous exercise within a few hours of bedtime. It has a short-term stimulant effect.

**Keep a "to do" pad.** If you toss and turn because you're concerned that you might forget some of the many things you must do the next day, buy a small pad and as a bedtime ritual, jot down all the concerns that might keep you up. Then let go of them until morning.

**Try sex.** At its best, lovemaking is deeply relaxing and has a well-deserved reputation for leading to a good night's sleep. But not all sex works. "It depends on how the sex makes you feel," Dr. Hauri explains. "If you feel loved and well cared for, sex can help you sleep. But if the sex is unsatisfying and takes place in a problematic relationship, it might be the prelude to a very poor night's sleep."

**Stop making excuses.** Think about what you gain from insomnia. Your quick response to this suggestion is probably "I don't gain anything. I hate my sleep problem." Of course you do, but you still might get something from it, such as an excuse for poor productivity or a chance to be the object of sympathy. Ask yourself what might change for the worse if you slept better. Work to resolve those issues, and you just might sleep better.

**Try the Bootzin Technique.** Developed by Dr. Bootzin in the 1970s when he was a professor of psychology at Northwestern University in Chicago, this simple, six-step behavior therapy program helps most of the people who stick with it. Try it for one week, and you'll probably sleep better.

1. Go to sleep only when you feel sleepy. Ignore the clock. Tune in to how you feel.

2. Use your bed only for sleeping and sex. No eating, reading, watching TV, talking on the phone or anything else.

3. If you go to bed but can't fall asleep, get up and leave the bedroom. Stay up—read, watch TV, listen to music, whatever—until you feel sleepy again, then return to bed.

4. Repeat step 3 as often as necessary throughout the night.

5. No matter when you go to sleep, set an alarm for the same time every morning to encourage your body to adopt a regular sleep/wake rhythm.

6. Don't nap during the day.

The first night or two, you may repeat Step 3 several times. But over a few nights, repetitions typically diminish and often disappear. If your sleep problem recurs after a period of sleeping well, simply return to the six steps.

## CHAPTER 25

# TAI CHI AND CHI GONG

## The Flowing, Elegant Healing Therapies

Visitors to China are often amazed when they look out their hotel room windows early in the morning. In parks, squares, plazas and schoolyards, tens of thousands of Chinese of all ages—but particularly the elderly—begin their days with slow, graceful, beautiful choreographed routines called *tai chi chuan* (*tie chee chwan*), generally known in the United States as tai chi.

Practitioners of tai chi say that this centuries-old dancelike exercise, which is derived from the martial arts, clears the mind, relaxes the body, nourishes the spirit, increases energy and contributes to health and longevity.

Over the last 20 years, tai chi has become increasingly popular in the United States—both as a gentle form of meditative exercise and as a way to cope with various illnesses. One such illness is multiple sclerosis (MS), the baffling neurological disease that saps the strength and limits the mobility of an estimated 350,000 Americans, most of them women.

## Moves for Mobility

Angelina Hekking was diagnosed with MS at age 17, but for ten years she functioned fairly normally. Then the San Francisco photographer, now in her late thirties, had a sudden, major exacerbation and wound up in a wheelchair, angry and depressed. Sometimes people with MS spontaneously regain mobility, but typically they do not. Desperate for a way to focus what was left of her mental and physical energy, Hekking learned a tai chi routine, or "form," specially modified for her wheelchair-bound situation. Slowly she regained strength in her legs, and seven months later she was back on her feet. That was nine years ago, and Hekking has not needed a wheelchair since.

Of course, it remains unclear how much tai chi contributed to Hekking's recovery. Occasionally people with MS walk away from wheelchairs without any intervention, but in general, the disease is marked by progressive deterioration. Hekking credits tai chi with her renewed mobility. For several years, she has taught it to other people with MS.

In 1993, Hekking's class came to the attention of Cynthia Husted, R.N., Ph.D., a chemist who does not have MS but who does research on it at the University of California at Santa Barbara. Dr. Husted has practiced yoga and tai chi for many years. In the course of her MS research, many people with the disease have told her that gentle exercise generally helps them.

Dr. Husted decided to investigate tai chi's effects on students in Hekking's class. She recruited about a dozen new participants, and before they learned any tai chi, she assessed their mobility, strength, flexibility, endurance and psychological well-being. After eight weekly hour-long tai chi classes, she reassessed everyone.

"The class was even more beneficial than I'd hoped it would be," Dr. Husted says. "At first most participants had little balance or strength. But as the class progressed, you could see them gaining strength, flexibility and endurance. By the end, they were much surer on their feet. People who walked with canes used them less. One man who began the class in a wheelchair got out of it and performed many of the moves on his feet."

The man who rose from his wheelchair was Charles Levinson, a 45-year-old San Francisco electronics distributor whose 16 years of MS had left him largely unable to use his legs. "At first," he recalls, "the tai chi exercises were largely beyond my physical capabilities. But after a while, I could do them, and as the weeks passed, I began to use my legs more. Since the class ended, I've continued to do tai chi, and I'm able to walk for much longer periods than I could before learning it. I use a walker, but I've walked more in the past two months than I have in the past two years, and recently I began working out on a stationary cycle, which I couldn't do before the tai chi class."

Is there something specific to tai chi that helps people with MS? Or does any regular, gentle exercise help? "All exercise helps," Dr. Husted says, "but the participants in the study agreed that tai chi helps more. I'm not sure why, but I believe the constant movement of tai chi is better for MS than, say, the static postures of yoga."

## Healing with Tai Chi

Tai chi has not been the subject of as much scientific research as yoga, but the few studies that have been published to date point to significant health benefits, particularly for the elderly.

*Balance.* In a 1992 experiment, Diana Bailey, Ed.D., assistant professor of occupational therapy at Tufts University/ Boston School of Occupational Therapy in Medford, Massachusetts, and her colleague Tse Shuk-Kuen recruited nine pairs of similar women ages 65 to 85. One of each pair practiced tai chi; the other did not. Using sophisticated tests, the researchers assessed the women's postural control, their steadiness on their feet and their ability to remain standing when subjected to destabilizing situations, such as a rocking floor. The tai chi practitioners had significantly better postural control, meaning that they were less likely to fall.

This finding has considerable medical importance for those over 65. Falling is a common—and serious—problem in the elderly, especially for women with bone-thinning osteoporosis. Osteoporosis makes the bones brittle, and when elderly women fall, they risk hip fractures, complications from which are the nation's twelfth leading cause of death and a major killer of elderly women.

Weight-bearing exercise, such as walking, helps control osteoporosis, but as women grow older, fear of falling keeps many from getting the weight-bearing exercise they need. All this leads to a vicious cycle: fear of falling, increasingly sedentary lifestyle and increased risk of hip fracture if they do fall. Tai chi can help the elderly stay on their feet, avoid falling and remain physically active, which promotes overall health and well-being.

*Emotional well-being.* Chinese researchers have also found that tai chi elevates mood, reduces anger, relieves fatigue and increases energy as well as other forms of moderate exercise.

*Exercise.* In addition to Dr. Husted's MS experiment, several studies have investigated tai chi's exercise benefits. One, a 1993 Formosan project, showed that a classic, hour-long tai chi routine could raise heart rate and oxygen consumption into the aerobic range, thereby offering the benfits of strenuous exercise, including cardiovascular conditioning.

But most American tai chi students practice one of several shorter forms that take only 10 to 30 minutes. These generally do not provide aerobic exercise, but for many elderly people, that's not bad. Aerobic exercise is often too strenuous for them. A 1991 study reported in the *International Journal of Sports Medicine* showed that tai chi raises heart rate only modestly and as a result "should not be considered dangerous for individuals at risk for heart disease, stroke or other cardiovascular diseases." Chinese researchers echoed this finding in a 1992 study that showed tai chi to be about as strenuous as walking at about four miles per hour, faster than a leisurely stroll but not a running or jogging pace.

These studies suggest that tai chi's modest intensity produces the kind of moderate workout that exercise physiologists often recommend for the elderly and for anyone interested in reducing their risk of heart disease, osteoporosis, arthritis, diabetes, obesity, high blood pressure and other serious medical conditions.

*Immunity.* Like other moderate workouts, tai chi also boosts immune function—causing a 13 percent increase in T-cells, the special white blood cells that attack disease microorganisms.

*Rheumatoid arthritis (RA).* RA is the most severe form of arthritis. Some two million Americans have this painful, potentially crippling inflammatory joint disease. For other forms of arthritis, physicians recommend gentle exercise to help control pain and preserve joint function. But many physicians are reluctant to recommend exercise for people with RA because overexertion can trigger joint inflammation. Tai chi does not. In a 1991 study, 20 people with RA practiced tai chi two hours a week for ten weeks without any aggravation of symptoms. The researchers concluded that tai chi "appears to be safe for RA patients." They also confirmed that tai chi might serve as a safe alternative to other forms of exercise therapy.

*Stress.* The same Chinese researchers who equated tai chi to a moderate-paced walk also measured its ability to reduce stress. They subjected 48 men and women to mentally challenging tests and then showed them a film calculated to upset them. Then the participants were divided into four groups. Each group attempted to destress using one of four activities: tai chi, meditation, a brisk walk or reading. By measuring their heart rates, blood pressure and urinary excretion of stress hormones, the researchers were able to track how quickly the participants recovered from the stress. Tai chi turned out to be as stress-relieving as two better-known stress reducers, meditation and walking. Tai chi would be a good choice for someone who enjoys physically active approaches to stress management but may not be able to take a walk.

## 600 Years Young

*Tai chi chuan* is variously translated as "supreme boxing," "the root of all motion" and "optimal fist-fighting." It is considered a martial art, but unlike the more combative styles—karate and kung fu, with their hard, linear punches and kicks— tai chi is based on fluidity and circular movements. Tai chi masters say that this gentle dance develops the flexibility of a child, the strength of a lumberjack and eventually the wisdom of a sage.

Tai chi was developed by the semimythical Taoist monk Chang San-Feng, who, according to various reports, lived sometime between the eleventh and thirteenth century. One night he dreamed of a snake and a crane in combat. Fascinated by their beautiful movements, he combined the ancient Chinese healing art of *chi gong* (*chee gung*) with the self-defense and fighting moves he observed in his dream, plus the moves of deer, tigers, bears and monkeys. The resulting combinations of movements formed the basis of tai chi.

Over the centuries, several styles of tai chi have evolved. Though they differ from one another, they all are slow, graceful, noncombative, dancelike moving meditations. Most tai chi teachers say it takes about a year to learn one of the 50-move "short forms" popular in the United States. It takes a lifetime to master it.

Tai chi embodies the Chinese idea that life energy, or chi, is divided into two equal, opposite and complementary parts, yin and yang. Tai chi incorporates the yin/yang unity of opposites in many ways: During tai chi forms, the weight shifts repeatedly entirely from one leg to the other, symbolizing emptiness and fullness, two manifestations of yin and yang.

With the addition of various arm movements, these weight-shifting stances become a tai chi form. Each combination of movements has a name, many of them quite colorful, such as play the guitar, the snake creeps down, grasp the bird's tail, the white crane spreads its wings, repulse the monkey and ride the tiger to the mountain.

## How to Learn Tai Chi

Unfortunately, you can't learn tai chi from the printed page. You pretty much have to see the flowing movements for yourself before you can do them correctly. There are several good videos available, including *Tai Chi for Health*, a two-hour instruction film that teaches one tai chi form.

Your best bet, however, is to find a good instructor and take a class. As tai chi is quite popular in America, you may find a class at your local Y or gym. You might also try calling martial arts schools listed in the Yellow Pages and asking the instructors if they know of anyone who teaches tai chi in your area. You might also try asking your doctor.

Tai chi master Martin Lee, author of *Ride the Tiger to the Mountain: Tai Chi for Health* offers these general guidelines for tai chi practice.

*Space.* You need an area that measures seven feet by five feet.

*Clothing.* Wear loose, comfortable clothes.

*Posture.* Stand erect and look straight ahead.

*Relaxation.* Always keep your hands, shoulders and abdomen relaxed and your knees slightly bent.

*Symmetry.* Draw an imaginary line from the top of your head through your navel to the floor. Keep your left foot on the left side of the line and your right foot on the right side.

*Mindfulness.* Be aware of how you are moving and breathing.

*Breathing.* Breathe naturally and regularly. Pay attention to your breathing and let the movements themselves regulate it. Don't hold your breath.

*Pace.* Move slowly. Maintain a constant pace.

*Weight shifting.* Most tai chi moves involve shifting your weight from one leg to the other. When standing on both legs, your weight should be divided equally btween them.

*Practice.* Practice every day, but not shortly after eating.

## Chi Gong: Revving Up Healing Energy

In 1990, after recovering from lymphoma of the hip, Griswold, Connecticut, public relations man Bob Ellal decided to give himself a get-well present, a class in tai chi.

"I'd practiced karate when I was younger, but as the years passed, especially after my cancer, I wanted something gentler and more meditative."

Ellal began studying tai chi in 1992, but he soon developed pain in his other hip. It turned out to be a recurrence of the lymphoma. Ellal told his teacher he'd have to stop practicing tai chi, but instead of bidding him farewell, Ann Chandler of Eagle's

Quest Tai Chi in Hadlyme, Connecticut, urged him to try tai chi's therapeutic ancestor, *chi gong* (sometimes spelled *qi gung* or *chi kung*).

Ellal had never heard of chi gong, but Chandler insisted that it was even gentler than tai chi—and a more powerful healer. Chi gong, in fact, is what tai chi masters practice to keep themselves physically healthy, emotionally centered and spiritually focused. Chandler showed Ellal a few chi gong moves. "They looked like fragments of tai chi forms, stances with modest arm movements but without leg moves. If tai chi is a moving meditation, chi gong is a standing meditation."

In Chinese, *chi gong* means "cultivation of energy," specifically the life energy, chi. Chi is a fundamental concept of traditional Chinese medicine. Chi gong students learn to sense their chi and follow it as it moves around the body. As they become more adept, they learn to strengthen their chi and direct it to areas of their own—or other people's—body that are weak or ailing.

Chi gong is much older than either tai chi or the other martial arts. Chinese medical scholars contend that it was practiced as early as 1700 B.C., almost 3,000 years before the development of tai chi. But only recently has chi gong emerged from the private world of tai chi masters and taken its rightful place in the pantheon of Chinese healing arts. The first World Chi Gong Conference was held in Beijing in 1988.

When Ellal first began practicing chi gong, he didn't know what to think. On the one hand, he felt grateful that it did not involve leg movements because it spared his hip from the tai chi moves that his cancer recurrence had made painful. But compared with the beauty and grace of tai chi, chi gong felt rather mundane. Ellal quickly learned that chi gong's comparatively still waters run quite deep.

Initially, he wasn't sure he'd be able to recognize his chi, let alone be able to direct it to his hip. "But as I repeated the simple forms over and over again and focused on my breathing, my fingertips began to tingle. My teacher said it was my chi. Sometimes I can feel it travel around my body, but it's usually most powerful in my hands. I've been practicing chi gong for two years now, and I still consider myself a novice. But after a half-hour of repeating my forms, my hands become very warm, and they look strangely mottled. If I hold them close together, I can feel the energy radiating from them."

Shortly after Ellal began practicing chi gong, he was hospitalized for four days of chemotherapy. He expected to feel as awful as he had when he'd received chemotherapy for his first bout of lymphoma. But this time he experienced no nausea or other expected side effects, except for hair loss.

Months later he traveled to Boston to receive the ultimate in high-tech cancer treatments, a bone marrow transplant (BMT). This procedure allows cancer patients to receive much higher doses of chemotherapy than their systems could normally tolerate, but at a high price—side effects so severe that they are sometimes fatal.

"The doctors kept telling me to brace myself for terrible fatigue, loss of appetite, fever, nausea and vomiting," Ellal recalls. "I felt a little tired and I ate less, but I pretty much sailed through the experience."

No one knows why Ellal had such an easy time with his BMT, but he credits chi gong. A small but growing number of scientists agree that such results are possible with chi gong.

## Feeling the Body Electric

Chi gong has not been extensively researched, and many mainstream physicians remain very skeptical of Chinese medicine and its concept of life energy. But like the scientists who trace acupuncture's effectiveness to its effects on the nervous system's bioelectricity, the few researchers who have investigated chi gong practitioners say that it concentrates bioelectrical energy.

"The body is made up of matter and energy," explains physicist and biopsychologist Elmer Green, Ph.D., a leading biofeedback researcher who is director emeritus of the Center for Applied Psychophysiology at the Menninger Clinic in Topeka, Kansas. "In the West, we've focused on the matter and have only recently begun to appreciate the importance of the subtle electrical energy field, what the Chinese call chi and the Ayurvedic system calls prana. In Asian medicine, people have two different bodies, a physical body and an energy body. In the West we focus almost all our attention on the physical body and largely ignore the energy side. Our research shows that healers, including those who practice chi gong, can concentrate and manipulate their energy in remarkable ways."

Using sophisticated equipment, Dr. Green measured the electrical fields on the hands of ordinary people and discovered that they varied from 0 to 50 millivolts (1 millivolt is $^1/_{1,000}$ of a volt). Then he measured the fields on the hands of people who worked as traditional healers—chi gong masters, rainforest medicine men and people who practice the laying-on of hands and therapeutic touch. Every self-proclaimed healer Dr. Green tested produced at least 4 volts—80 times more than the average person. One chi gong master produced 200 volts, or 4,000 times more.

Dr. Green also attempted to trace the source of the healers' body electricity. "It seems to come from the central body, the area between the solar plexus and the lower abdomen—the same area the Chinese call *tan dien*, the home of chi, and the Ayurvedic healers call the solar plexus chakra, the seat of prana," he says. Dr. Green's studies have not yet revealed *how* the healers he tested concentrate their electrical energy (or chi or prana or whatever), but he believes that it involves a form of biofeedback. He hopes one day to be able to teach it.

"The ability to concentrate the body's electrical energy is real," Dr. Green says, "and it has many physical effects. It reduces heart rate and blood pressure and it alters brain wave patterns. I don't know if it could help treat cancer, but I certainly wouldn't dismiss the possibility."

Bob Ellal is currently cancer-free, thanks, he says, to excellent mainstream cancer treatment and to chi gong. He practices it every day and appreciates it more and more as the months pass. "Chi gong is repetitive, and people who love the choreography of tai chi might find it boring," he says. "But in its own subtle way, chi gong is beautiful, and I believe it's helping me survive my cancer."

## How to Use Chi Gong

Here are three chi gong exercises as taught by tai chi teacher Larry Johnson, O.M.D. (doctor of oriental medicine).

*Chi gong exercise 1.* Stand with your feet together and your arms at your sides. Slowly rotate your hands so your palms face forward and then form your hands into fists. Inhale as you slowly bend your elbows, raising your fists along the sides of your body to midchest height. Exhale as you slowly extend both fists in front of you. As you extend your fists, rotate them so that by the time your arms are straight, your palms face down. Continue to exhale as you open your fists and raise your fingers so that your palms face forward. Rotate your fingers outward until they point downward. Now inhale as you form fists, then bend your elbows and return them to the sides of your body. Repeat this eight times. When finished, exhale.

*Chi gong exercise 2.* Begin in the position that concludes exercise number 1: feet together, elbows bent, fists at your sides with palms up. Inhale as you slowly raise both arms over your head. As you do so, rotate your fists so that your palms face forward. Exhale as you bend at the waist. Extend your fists downward and touch the ground in front of your toes. (If you can't comfortably touch your toes, reach down as far as you can.) Open your fists, rotate your fingers outward as in exercise number 1, and as you reform your fists, begin to inhale. Return to a standing position, raising and rotating your fists so that they end up over your head, with your palms facing forward. From this position, repeat the exercise eight times. When finished, exhale.

*Chi gong exercise 3.* Begin in the position that concludes exercise number 2: feet together, fists overhead with your palms facing forward. Breathe naturally as you open your fists, rotating your fingers inward so that you end up with your palms flat and your middle fingers touching. Look up at your hands. Hold this position for up to one minute, then sweep your arms down to your sides and look forward.

CHAPTER 26

# VEGETARIANISM

## The Green Way to Better Health

*C*ancer is most frequent among those branches of the human race where carnivorous habits prevail." These words appeared in *Scientific American* more than 100 years ago, in January 1892. It has taken a century for their wisdom to sink in, but today they are echoed by Walter Willett, M.D., Dr.P.H., chair of the Department of Nutrition at Harvard University and one of the nation's foremost researchers on the health effects of diet: "If you look carefully at the data, the optimum amount of meat you should eat is zero."

Strong words, but the evidence is hard to deny. Dr. Willett's 1990 analysis of data from the Nurses' Health Study, an ongoing investigation of the diet and lifestyle of more than 87,000 nurses, showed that consumption of beef, pork and lamb significantly increased women's risk of colon cancer. Two years later, Dr. Willett was a co-author of another study showing a connection between meat and colon cancer in men. And in 1993, as a co-author of a study based on long-term follow-up of 51,529 male health professionals, he helped show that a diet high in meat is associated with an increased risk of prostate cancer.

Meat-eating has also been persuasively linked to an increased risk of death from heart disease. In a landmark study comparing

25,000 Seventh-Day Adventists, whose religion requires vegetarianism, to meat-eating Americans (omnivores), researchers at Loma Linda University in California discovered that eating meat once a day tripled the risk of fatal heart disease by age 64. Seventh-Day Adventists also have unusually low rates of most cancers. Why? The answer again seems to be their meatless diet, as a growing body of evidence suggests that meat's high fat content is the main problem. The worst fat, healthwise, is the saturated variety, and meat is loaded with it, accounting for about 35 percent of the saturated fat Americans consume.

## Where's the Beef?

If you've read this far, chances are that you eat less meat than you did years ago. If so, you're not alone. U.S. beef consumption has fallen about 25 percent since the mid-1970s. But during the same period, consumption of chicken and turkey has almost doubled. Skinless poultry breast meat is low in fat, but the skin and dark meat and the many food items made from them—chicken franks, turkey meatballs and so forth—are high in fat (including saturated fat). In addition, if you prepare a skinless chicken breast with butter, cream, sour cream or other high-fat ingredients, even this "healthy" meat can pack the fat wallop of a cheeseburger.

The upshot is that while red meat consumption has plummeted, American fat consumption has hardly budged. Average Americans today get 34 percent of their calories from fat and 12 percent from saturated fat, a decline of just 2 percent since 1978. (For more on the health hazards of eating too much fat, see Low-Fat Eating on page 291.)

The many health hazards of meat-eating (and a high-fat diet in general) have given Dr. Willett a major beef, as it were, with the new Food Pyramid released in 1993 by the U.S. Department of Agriculture (USDA) to replace the venerable but outdated Four Food Groups—the cornerstone of the nation's nutrition education efforts since the 1950s. The USDA Pyramid places the foods that are best for health along the wide base, with those you should eat less often positioned toward the narrower top.

Meat falls in the upper middle portion of the Food Pyramid, along with fish, poultry, beans, eggs, nuts and dairy products. Recommended consumption of these items is two to three servings a day. Meanwhile, Dr. Willett and an increasing number of nutrition experts contend that even one daily serving of meat substantially increases the risk of heart disease and cancer. So what's with the USDA?

Unfortunately for the public health, the USDA does more than provide nutrition information. Part of its mission involves protecting and promoting the nation's livestock industry. An early draft of the Food Pyramid, based solely on nutrition and health considerations, placed meats farther up the pyramid, in a category of foods that should be eaten only now and then. But the meat and dairy lobbies persuaded the USDA to place these items closer to the base of the pyramid and recommend daily consumption.

This move infuriated Dr. Willett, his colleagues at the Harvard School of Public Health and officials of the World Health Organization. They devised a competing pyramid based on the traditional diet of southern Italy and Greece, regions whose residents have long life expectancies and historically low rates of heart disease, cancer and stroke (which together account for two-thirds of U.S. deaths).

While it does not exactly ban meats, the Mediterranean Pyramid recommends a semivegetarian diet and places red meat at the very top, to be eaten at most only a few times a month. In the Mediterranean Pyramid, poultry and fish have also been moved up, with fish recommended no more than a few times a week and poultry once a week or so.

## Up with Veggies

A continent away from Dr. Willett, Gladys Block, Ph.D., professor of epidemiology and nutrition at the University of California at Berkeley School of Public Health, came to a similar conclusion following a very different route. Instead of investigating how bad meat is for health, she has focused on how good

# Taming Tofu

Tofu is the food many Americans love to hate. They condemn the cheeselike soy product as bland and tasteless and invoke its supposed shortcomings as an indictment of vegetarianism in general.

There's a germ of truth in tofu-phobia. Right out of the container, it is bland and tasteless. But so is pasta, and pasta dishes rank among many people's favorites. Tofu has a very mild flavor and acquires the taste of anything cooked with it. Like pasta, it can be used in hundreds of ways: Hide it in spaghetti sauce or refried beans. Crumble it with eggs or egg substitute in a morning scramble. Use it in muffins, soups or salads. Or cover it with barbecue sauce and slap it on the grill. The possibilities are endless.

Still leery of tofu? Then try the meat substitutes made with its close relative, soy protein. Yves' Soy Burger Burgers look and taste so much like beef hamburgers that on a bun with ketchup and relish, you might not be able to tell the difference. Yet they contain no meat and have only three grams of fat per burger, a small fraction of what most beef patties contain. Yves' and other soy products are available at health food stores and some supermarkets.

In addition to the convenience of soy foods as meat substitutes, several studies show that diets high in tofu and soy products may also help prevent cancer. Soybeans are high in chemicals called isoflavonoids. A 1993 Finnish study linked high blood levels of isoflavonoids to a lower risk of prostate cancer.

Soy foods also contain phytoestrogens, plant versions of the female sex hormone estrogen. According to Claude L. Hughes, M.D., assistant professor of obstetrics and gynecology at Duke University in Durham, North Carolina, high blood levels of phytoestrogens help protect women against osteoporosis and breast and ovarian cancer.

fruits and vegetables are. In 1992, Dr. Block, formerly an epidemiologist at the National Cancer Institute (NCI), collected all the studies published through 1991 that correlated diet with rates of the major cancers (lung, breast, colon, cervical, ovarian, bladder, throat, oral, pancreatic, prostate and stomach)—nearly 200 reports in all.

Every single study showed that as fruit and vegetable consumption increased, cancer risk decreased, not just for the cancers most often linked to dietary fat—colon, breast and prostate—but for all the major cancers. Compared with those who consumed the most fruits and vegetables, those who ate the least had twice the cancer risk.

On the other side of the world, studies by T. Colin Campbell, Ph.D., also showed that the healthiest diet is vegetarian (or close to it). Dr. Campbell, a nutritional biochemist at Cornell University in Ithaca, New York, along with researchers from Oxford University in England and two universities in China, investigated the diets of 65,000 rural Chinese for the China Health Project.

Contrary to the American dinner-table myth that children should clean their plates because "there are people starving in China," rural Chinese who are poor by U.S. standards and have nowhere near our access to technological medicine eat more nutritiously and are healthier than most Americans. They're not starving, but they eat very little animal protein and as a result have much lower rates of heart disease, cancer, diabetes and osteoporosis. "Humans are basically a vegetarian species," Dr. Campbell notes, "animal foods are not really healthful, and we need to get away from eating them."

The studies by Dr. Willett, Dr. Block, Dr. Campbell and others have become the pillars supporting the NCI's recently launched "strive for five" program—an effort to reduce Americans' cancer risk by persuading them to eat at least five servings of fresh fruits and vegetables a day.

Five servings is the healthy minimum, but Dr. Block encourages people to strive for eight or nine. To get nine servings of fresh fruits and vegetables a day, you'd have to add some fruit to your cereal each morning, have a salad and two vegetables at both lunch and dinner and have two fruit or vegetable snacks a day. There's really only one way to do that—become some kind of vegetarian.

# The Many Kinds of Vegetarian

What's a vegetarian? The simple answer is that it's someone who does not eat meat. But life in the 1990s is more complicated. There are many different kinds of vegetarianism. Some "vegetarians" even eat meat occasionally.

In 1992, *Vegetarian Times*, a leading magazine in the field, commissioned a research firm to find out how many Americans consider themselves vegetarians, what they eat and why. About 13 million Americans—5 percent of the population—identify themselves as vegetarians, but they come in almost as many varieties as apples.

Vegans (*VEE-guns*) are the strictest vegetarians. They eat only plant foods: fruits, vegetables, grains, beans and nuts. They shun all animal foods: red meat, poultry, fish, seafood, milk, cheese and eggs. Vegans represent about 4 percent of vegetarians, or some 520,000 Americans.

Ovo-lacto-vegetarians add eggs (ovo), milk (lacto) and other dairy products to a vegan diet. They represent about one-third of vegetarians.

Semivegetarians start off as ovo-lactos and then include some flesh foods in their diet. About two-thirds of those who proclaimed themselves "basically vegetarians" in the survey said they continue to eat poultry and fish. About one-third eat them weekly. Two-thirds of self-proclaimed vegetarians eat no red meat, but about 20 percent indulge in meat about once a month.

Vegetarians eating meat? Isn't that a contradiction? Not really; now that vegetarianism has shed its cult status and gone mainstream, the single biggest factor in people becoming vegetarians is increased health consciousness.

Just as low-fat eaters indulge in the occasional piece of cheesecake, semivegetarians consume the occasional chicken breast or cheese soufflé. Semivegetarianism may not be *best* choice for health, but its increasing popularity shows that a plant-based diet has become trendy. Not too long ago, according to Chicago vegetarian Judy Krizmanic, when you said you were a vegetarian, people looked at you funny. Now they ask for recipes.

# From "Unsafe" to Optimum

As recently as the mid-1970s, most nutrition experts actively discouraged vegetarianism as a one-way ticket to malnutrition and serious health problems. Vegetarians, the experts insisted, can't get enough protein, iron and calcium. They risk brain damage from vitamin B12 deficiency. And if they're foolish enough to subject their innocent children to their food fanaticism, the kids are destined for stunted growth.

What a difference 20 years makes. Today we know that it's easier to eat a healthful diet as a vegetarian than as a burger-fries-and-shake meat-eater, largely because most vegetarians consume less fat than the typical omnivore. Nonetheless, friends and family of newly converted vegetarians often raise the old arguments against abandoning meat, so let's review the evidence.

*"Vegetarians can't get enough protein."* Twenty years ago, thanks to a series of best-selling books by nutritionist Adele Davis, protein was king of the nutrients. Davis promoted protein relentlessly, and millions of Americans came to believe that it was impossible to get enough without eating meat. But in recent years, the pendulum has swung the other way. Now nutritionists insist that Americans eat too much protein, considerably more than the body requires. If that protein comes from meat, it's also burdened with unhealthy baggage—fat. Meanwhile, plant foods contain plenty of protein. Even vegans can get all they need from vegetables, nuts and beans. The Recommended Dietary Allowance (RDA) for protein ranges from 28 grams for young children to 63 grams for adult men. This protein requirement can be met easily by eating plant foods. Two tablespoons of peanut butter contain 8 grams of protein (the same as a glass of milk). A cup of pasta has 7 grams, and a cup of lentils has 18.

""Protein has become a nonissue," says Suzanne Havala, R.D., a dietitian in Charlotte, North Carolina, and author of the 1993 American Dietetic Association position paper endorsing vegetarian diets as healthful. "If you eat a reasonable variety of foods, you would find it difficult to avoid eating enough protein. In fact, as long as you consume enough calories to meet your en-

# The Joy of Juicing

Some people who are attracted to vegetarianism hesitate to embrace it because they fear they'll find their food selections limited and get bored. That's a possibility, but vegetarianism can actually expand the range of foods you eat—or drink. Consider juicing. It's a quick, convenient way to broaden your vegetarian horizons while enjoying tasty, satisfying, nutritious drinks.

For best results, juicing requires a juicer, a kitchen appliance similar to—but distinct from—a blender. Blenders liquefy by chopping at high speeds, producing a combination of some juice mixed with a great deal of pulp. For drinks made with low-fiber fruits, such as grapes and watermelons, blenders create palatable beverages. But for most other fruits and all vegetables, juicing in a blender produces a slushy liquid that's too fibrous and pulpy to enjoy.

Juicers, on the other hand, are specifically designed to extract the liquid from fruits and vegetables. The juice contains most of the food's vitamins, minerals and other nutrients. The leftover pulp is the fiber. Discard it (or use it in compost).

Of course, the body needs fiber. It aids digestion and helps prevent some cancers. In addition, many Americans don't get enough. But most vegetarians don't have to worry about a fiber deficiency

ergy needs, you'd have to work hard to devise a protein-deficient diet."

*"Vegetarians can't get enough iron."* Meat is high in iron, but you don't have to eat steaks to consume adequate amounts. In the China Health Project, Dr. Campbell discovered that even Chinese who consume little or no meat have healthy iron levels. Other studies of vegans agree. Plant foods provide plenty of iron. Meanwhile, meat-eaters may get too much iron. A 1993 Finnish study linked excessive iron intake to an increased risk of heart attack.

*"Vegetarians can't get enough calcium."* We've heard it all our lives: Drink milk for strong bones and teeth. Dietitians rec-

because a good vegetarian diet provides plenty. Juicing sacrifices a certain amount of fiber in the interest of variety, taste and nutrition.

Juices pack incredible nutritional punch. One pint of mixed vegetable juice contains the vitamin and mineral equivalent of two meal-size salads. One pint of fresh carrot juice contains 20,000 international units of beta-carotene, a precursor of vitamin A. This is four times the Recommended Dietary Allowance set by the Food and Drug Administration but in line with the generous amount now promoted by many nutritionists as a daily optimum.

Most juicers cost $20 to $300; they are available at stores that sell small appliances, at health food stores and by mail order through companies that advertise in vegetarian publications.

If you'd like to become more of a juicer but don't want to make your own, Stephen Blauer, author of *The Juicing Book,* recommends several commercial brands that are available in health food stores and some supermarkets: After the Fall, Apple and Eve, Heinke's, Lakewood, R. W. Knudsen, Walnut Acres and Winter Hill.

No matter whether you make your own juices or buy them, juicing is a delicious, nutritious complement to any diet. Raise a glass and toast your health.

ommend that Americans consume 1,200 to 1,500 milligrams of calcium a day. Milk, cheese, yogurt and other dairy foods are high in calcium: One cup of milk contains 300 milligrams, one ounce of mozzarella cheese has 145 milligrams and a cup of nonfat yogurt contains a whopping 450 milligrams.

But many plant foods are also high in calcium. One cup of cooked mustard greens has 104 milligrams; a cup of cooked bok choy supplies 158 milligrams; one cup of tofu has 517 milligrams; five dried figs provide 135 milligrams; and one cup of cooked kale offers 170 milligrams. No wonder several studies have shown that even a vegan diet provides enough calcium and other minerals.

Calcium is particularly important for women because after menopause, they often develop osteoporosis, a loss of calcium from bone tissue that may lead to "dowager's hump" and life-threatening hip fractures. And vegetarianism helps prevent osteoporosis by reducing total protein intake.

"Diets high in protein, especially animal protein, increase calcium excretion in the urine," says Neal Barnard, M.D., author of *Food for Life*, an analysis of the health benefits of vegetarianism, and president of the Physicians Committee for Responsible Medicine, a professional organization in Washington, D.C., that promotes preventive medicine through nutrition. "The amino acids that form proteins increase the blood's acidity. To neutralize this effect, the body releases calcium from the bones, which winds up in the urine. The dairy industry has used osteoporosis as a marketing tool, but countries that consume large amounts of milk and dairy products actually have the highest rates of hip fracture."

*"Vegetarians risk neurological damage from vitamin B12 deficiency."* Vitamin B12 is found primarily in meats and animal foods. Not surprisingly, levels in vegetarians, particularly in vegans, are low. On the other hand, the RDA for B12 is tiny, just two micrograms (two-millionths of a gram), and because humans evolved largely as vegetarians who ate meat only now and then, the body evolved the ability to store vitamin B12, typically socking away a two-year supply. So yes, B12 can be a problem for vegetarians, but it's no crisis, and actual risk of neurological damage is small—much smaller than the risk of heart disease, cancer, obesity and other health problems from a diet high in animal foods. To be on the safe side with vitamin B12, take a supplement. Most multiple vitamin formulas contain the RDA.

*"Vegetarianism stunts children's growth."* Several studies have shown that this simply is not true. Kay Stanek, R.D., Ph.D., associate professor of nutritional sciences at the University of Nebraska in Lincoln, compared the body measurements and nutrient intakes of omnivorous children ages 10 to 12 with those of a similar group of children who had been ovo-lacto-vegetarians from birth. Neither group showed any nutrient deficiency prob-

lems, and both the vegetarians and omnivores had similar height ranges, demonstrating that vegetarianism does not stunt growth. The only health hazard observed in the children was obesity. It was more of a problem among the omnivores.

From the early 1970s through the late 1980s, evidence piled up debunking the old arguments against vegetarianism and supporting its value in preventing and treating a number of serious diseases. That's why in 1988, the American Dietetic Association (ADA) stopped calling vegetarian diets unbalanced. In 1993, the organization endorsed vegetarianism as "healthful and nutritionally balanced when properly planned," even for pregnant and nursing women. "It's actually easier to eat a balanced diet as a vegetarian than as an omnivore," Havala says. "As a meat-eater, you have to worry about dietary fat and all the health problems associated with it. As a vegetarian, all you have to do is take a vitamin B12 supplement."

In addition to its protection against heart disease and cancer, some studies suggest that a vegetarian diet may help treat food sensitivities, rheumatoid arthritis, multiple sclerosis and systemic lupus erythematosus. (For details about dietary treatment for these conditions, see Elimination Diets on page 150.)

"Vegetarianism," Dr. Barnard says, "is the best way to eat." It also saves money. Dr. Barnard estimates that going vegetarian saves the average family of four about $40 a week, or $2,100 a year.

## The Pure Foods Factor

Every vegetarian recognizes the downside of red meat. It's bad for health. It wastes natural resources. And it can be downright dangerous. In 1993, *Escherichia coli* bacteria contaminated hamburgers at a Jack in the Box restaurant in the Pacific Northwest. Five hundred people got sick and three died. In 1994, seven Californians became severely ill with *E. coli* infections that were traced to hamburger they bought at a local supermarket. Then there's brucellosis, a flulike bacterial illness transmitted from pigs to humans in pork-processing plants. An

## Going for the Green

Everyone has a family member or friend who's taken the plunge. Why do Americans (in ever-increasing numbers) become vegetarians? In 1992, a national survey asked the nation's 13 million vegetarians why they'd given up meat. Here's what they said.

Health reasons: 46 percent
Animal welfare, objections to killing: 20 percent
Not sure: 18 percent
Influence of family and friends: 12 percent
Environmental concerns: 4 percent

outbreak of 18 cases in North Carolina in 1992 focused renewed attention on the shortcomings of USDA controls on the movements of brucellosis-infected animals.

But what about dairy products, chicken and fish? They're not as hazardous as beef, pork, lamb and veal, but they're not exactly health-promoters either.

The best-known problem with dairy products is the fat they contain. Whole milk derives 50 percent of its calories from fat, more than twice the proportion now considered optimal for prevention of heart disease and cancer. Fortunately, dairy foods' fat content is easy to fix. Just buy nonfat or 1 percent milk (17 percent of calories from fat) and nonfat yogurt, sour cream and cheeses.

Unfortunately, many ovo-lacto-vegetarians don't watch their fat consumption. At Hammersmith Hospital in London, British researchers used high-tech magnetic resonance imaging to determine levels of saturated and unsaturated fat in human fat tissue. Ovo-lacto-vegetarians had the same saturated fat levels as the meat-eaters. Only the vegans showed low levels of saturated fat.

Beyond their fat levels, ovo-lacto-vegetarians face other problems. According to the Centers for Disease Control and Prevention in Atlanta, dairy products (mostly eggs) account for 14 percent of food poisonings in the nation. A 1989 *Wall Street Journal* investigation also showed that 40 percent of milk samples from ten major cities were contaminated with antibiotics and other drugs used to promote cattle growth. Dairy foods have also been linked to an increased risk of infant colic, allergies, asthma, sinus problems and rheumatoid arthritis. Finally, compared with plant foods, dairy products (and poultry and fish) contain significantly higher levels of pesticide residues.

What about poultry? Ounce for ounce, poultry skin and dark meat contain almost as much fat as beef. But even if you eat only skinless poultry breast meat, which is very low in fat, you may be getting something else you don't want—*Salmonella* bacteria, a major cause of food poisoning. Nine percent of the nation's 400,000 yearly cases of food poisoning, some 30,000 severe—and sometimes fatal—illnesses, are caused by poultry. When investigators inspected chicken packages at supermarkets, they found one-third contaminated with *Salmonella*. Anyone who eats poultry should wash it thoroughly and wash everything that comes in contact with it.

Contamination is also a problem with fish and seafood. Aquatic creatures live in what Dr. Barnard calls "civilization's sewer." Among the contaminants in fish and seafood are the toxic pollutants known as polychlorinated biphenyls (PCBs). A 1992 investigation by Consumer Reports discovered PCB contamination in 43 percent of salmon samples, 50 percent of whitefish and 25 percent of swordfish.

## Organically Grown Produce: The Advantages

Of course, animal foods don't have a monopoly on chemical contamination. Plant foods may also carry pesticide residues. In 1993, the Environmental Working Group, a Washington, D.C.–based consumer organization, analyzed 24,000 samples of fruits and vegetables and discovered that half contained pesticide residues. A 1991 study by the USDA showed similar results: 58 percent of 2,900 samples showed pesticide residues.

Pesticide applications to U.S. food crops soared from near zero in 1940 to more than one billion pounds in 1987. Fear of exposure to even trace amounts of these chemicals is the major reason that a growing number of Americans now spend more than $1.5 billion a year (up from about $175 million in 1980) on organically grown produce.

Scientists generally agree that occupational exposure to large doses of pesticides poses a health hazard. In a 1991 study, NCI researchers showed that farmers have unusually high rates of Parkinson's disease and several cancers. But what about consumers' nonoccupational exposure to trace amounts of these chemicals? Is chemically grown produce hazardous to those who eat it?

This issue is passionately controversial. The USDA, the Food and Drug Administration, the chemical and agricultural industries and many scientists insist there is no evidence of a human health hazard from ingesting trace amounts of pesticide residues. Plants defend themselves against insects and disease by producing toxic, carcinogenic chemicals similar to commercial pesticides. According to Bruce Ames, Ph.D., chair of the biochemistry department at the University of California at Berkeley, there are more natural carcinogens in fruits and vegetables than on them.

Environmentalists counter that something must be causing rising cancer rates and that short of banning all pesticides, buying organic is a prudent approach to limiting exposure to toxic chemicals. As for the carcinogens in plants, pesticide critics contend that over the millions of years of human evolution, we adapted to plants' natural toxic chemicals, but we have few if any defenses against the many synthetic pesticides and industrial pollutants introduced since World War II.

The jury is still out, but several studies suggest a health hazard from nonoccupational pesticide exposure. In 1992, Frank Falck, M.D., Ph.D., assistant clinical professor of surgery at the University of Connecticut School of Medicine in Farmington, analyzed the tissue of 50 women who had suspicious breast lumps removed for biopsy. The lumps that turned out to be cancerous contained significantly more DDE, a chemical breakdown product of the pesticide DDT (now banned but environmentally persistent and still with us). Subsequently, Mary Wolf, M.D., professor in the Division of Environmental and Occupational Medicine at Mount Sinai School of Medicine in New York City, analyzed archived blood samples of 14,000 women. Compared with those who did not develop breast cancer years later, those who did showed significantly higher blood levels of DDE.

Finally, a 1994 pilot study by Danish researchers showed that compared with Scandinavian men who ate chemically grown food, those who ate organic food had substantially higher sperm counts. Sperm are the most delicate cells in a man's body. As a result, they are the most sensitive to toxic chemicals. This study was small (30 men) and it has not been confirmed by other research, so its findings must be viewed cautiously. But many studies have shown that since the 1930s, the average sperm count worldwide has declined by about 40 percent. Pesticides came into wide use after 1945. Perhaps there's a connection.

## How to Go Organic

In light of these studies, it's surprising that few studies have compared the health consequences of eating organic and conventionally grown produce, but here's what scientists know now.

Any fruits and vegetables are better than none. In Dr. Block's study, those who ate the fewest plant foods had the highest cancer rates, and those who ate the most produce had the least cancer. "The studies I reviewed used off-the-shelf, nonorganic fruits and vegetables," she explains. "Don't let fear of pesticide residues stop you from eating fruits and vegetables. Eat organic if you like, but even if your fruits and vegetables are conventionally grown, eat them. In fact, eat more of them."

The main source of pesticides in the American diet is not produce but meat. The Environmental Defense Fund measured pesticide contamination of breast milk in 1,400 nursing women in 46 states. Compared with levels found in the vegan women, the meat- and dairy-eaters' levels were twice as high.

"Most pesticides are fat-soluble," Dr. Falck explains. "If you eat plants that have been treated with them, you ingest a tiny amount of residue that accumulates in your fatty tissues, such as female breast tissue. But the real problem develops when you eat animal fat. Food animals accumulate pesticides in their fat tissues throughout their lives. By the time people eat them, they have much higher levels than any of the feed plants they ate. When people eat the meat, they consume most of the pesticides the animals ate. The higher up the food chain you eat, the more toxic chemicals you ingest."

The cleanest produce is organic. Even organically grown fruits, vegetables, grains and beans may pick up some pesticide contamination because of chemicals in groundwater, in the air from neighboring nonorganic farms or from fumigation of trucks and warehouses. But compared with conventionally grown produce, organic fruits and vegetables are significantly cleaner.

In one study, researchers compared breast milk samples of omnivorous women with those of women from The Farm, a religious community of vegans in Tennessee where residents grow most of their own food organically. The breast milk of the women from The Farm showed contamination levels averaging only 2 percent of the levels found in the milk of the omnivorous women.

If you opt for organic fruits and vegetables, the good news is that they're more available than ever. Health food stores, farmers' markets and even some supermarkets now carry items called organic. But are they really? Or do unscrupulous merchants simply slap the organic label on chemically grown food to be able to charge more for it? The Center for Science in the Public Interest, a Washington, D.C.–based nutrition advocacy organization, offers some suggestions.

**Do some local research.** Contact your state agriculture department or local extension service for referrals to organic growers in your area. Contact the farmers and ask how they grow their produce and where they sell it.

**Meet your greengrocer.** Talk with your health food store or supermarket produce manager. Ask for organic produce.

**Exercise a little skepticism.** Unless you trust the vendor, don't place much faith in handwritten signs. Look for a certification label. Labels include "Farm-Verified Organics," "Organic Crop Improvement Association," "Organic Growers and Buyers Association" and "California Certified Organic Farmers." As this book goes to press, only California has a government-regulated organic certification program. The other certification labels are granted to members of voluntary associations who pledge to uphold certain voluntary standards. But any label is more trustworthy than a handwritten sign.

**Buy your produce by mail.** It's easier than you think. *Green Groceries: A Mail Order Guide to Organic Foods* by Jeanne Heifetz lists dozens of organic growers who ship nationally. Pick those closest to you for the freshest items and lowest shipping costs. Root vegetables—carrots, turnips and rutabagas—are excellent mail-order choices. They ship well, and when conventionally grown, root vegetables tend to accumulate higher levels of pesticides than other vegetables.

**Grow your own.** No matter where you live, you can grow at least some of your own fruits and vegetables organically. To learn how, subscribe to *Organic Gardening* magazine.

If you don't buy organic, you can still minimize your exposure to pesticides by heeding the following suggestions.

**Scrub up.** Wash all fruits and vegetables with a dilute solution of dishwashing liquid and water. Use a vegetable brush. Chop spinach, broccoli, cauliflower and celery before washing.

**Peel waxed produce.** Apples, cucumbers and eggplants are often waxed, and pesticides can be sealed in with the wax.

**Toss a few.** Discard the outer leaves of cabbage and lettuce.

**Support your local farmers.** Buy foods in season and encourage your supermarket to stock locally grown items, which are less likely to be waxed and treated with postharvest pesticides during transport and storage.

**Look for produce from the West.** It's less likely to contain fungicides than produce grown in the more humid East.

## The Etiquette of Going Vegetarian

Going vegetarian poses few problems when you cook for yourself. But what do you say when family and friends offer you turkey for Thanksgiving? Or baked ham at Christmas? Or a burger or T-bone at a Fourth of July barbecue? Paul Amato, Ph.D., professor of sociology at the University of Nebraska at Lincoln, noticed that when he became a vegetarian, the choice, which he viewed as purely personal, had surprising ramifications for those he knew and loved. He mentioned his social discomfort to another vegetarian, graduate student Sonia Partridge, who'd had similar experiences. Intrigued, they surveyed 320 vegetarians and discovered that when people declare themselves vegetarians, sparks often fly.

"Among family members," Dr. Amato says, "the news usually gets an initial negative reaction." Nearly two-thirds of the vegetarians he and Partridge surveyed said their parents initially expressed disapproval. Only 10 percent of parents were supportive. Parents disapproved of their children becoming vegetarians independent of the child's age and whether or not the new vegetarian lived at home.

Why do parents disapprove? Dr. Amato cites several reasons: They might believe the old (and incorrect) nutritional arguments against vegetarianism. They might experience the choice as a rejection of their values, their nutritional beliefs or their cooking. They might worry that their child has joined some bizarre religious cult. They might feel inconvenienced by the need to accommodate a vegetarian during holidays or family get-togethers. Or they might be willing to be accommodating but feel uncomfortable cooking vegetarian dishes.

The survey showed that compared with parents' disdain, friends, siblings and children tend to accept new vegetarians more readily. One-third expressed complete approval, another third gave mixed messages—saying they approved but teasing new vegetarians about the decision—and one-third expressed strong disapproval.

In a follow-up study, Dr. Amato located ex-vegetarians and

asked why they'd gone back to eating meat. More than half said they'd succumbed to social pressure, particularly from friends. Fear of social awkwardness is also a big reason that many people who consider themselves vegetarians have the occasional poultry, fish or meat dish at parties and holiday gatherings.

"There's no question," Dr. Amato says, "that at first, becoming a vegetarian can strain one's social relationships. But over time, vegetarians and the people they care about accommodate each other, and most of the problems subside."

Compared with life's major traumas—death, disability, divorce, moving, job loss or financial crises—going vegetarian is not that big a deal. If loved ones believe you're risking your health, give them a copy of this book. If they're unfamiliar with tasty vegetarian cuisine, give them a vegetarian cookbook, such as *Eat More, Weigh Less* by Dean Ornish, M.D., which contains dozens of vegan recipes developed by some of the country's top chefs.

If they seem puzzled by your decision, just give them time. Family and friends who have a deep personal commitment to meat—cattle ranchers or owners of burger franchises—may never forgive you, but in Dr. Amato's survey, most vegetarians said their loved ones adjusted within a year and that their relationships sustained no permanent damage.

Sometimes going vegetarian improves relationships. As parents, siblings and friends age, their physicians are increasingly likely to tell them to cut down on fat and red meat. The "family vegetarian" often becomes a key resource for those who must change their diets for health reasons.

## CHAPTER 27

# VISION THERAPY

### Gentle Help for Eye Problems

Laura Taxel's twin toddlers, Nathan and Simon, were wonderful, beautiful, energetic boys—and a little clumsy. They kept spilling their juice, not by knocking over their cups but by dropping them as they reached out to place them on the table. It was as though they couldn't judge where the table was. Taxel, a freelance writer in Cleveland Heights, Ohio, also noticed that occasionally the boys' left eyes seemed to drift off on their own, but she recalls, "I didn't think it was a big deal."

A few years passed, and the boys' clumsiness persisted. Worse, they had difficulty identifying letters and doing other close-focus tasks that prepare kids to read and write. Fortunately, the Taxels' HMO offered childhood eye screening, so Taxel took her sons to see the HMO optometrist. "She placed a card over their left eyes, and they could see fine with their right eyes," she recalls. "Then she placed the card over their right eyes, and neither of them could see much with their left eyes. They were almost blind in one eye. It was terrible. I cried."

The optometrist diagnosed Nathan and Simon with "lazy" left eyes that prevented them from focusing both eyes simultaneously on the same target object. As a result, their brains were presented with two different images, one from each eye. When this happens, the brain ignores input from one eye—in the twins' case, the left—and "sees" only with the other.

One-eye (monocular) vision impairs depth perception and the ability to do close-focus tasks. Worse, over time, the eye that the brain ignores atrophies and may become permanently blind. Laura and her husband, Barney, a photographer, quickly became frantic. What could they do to keep the boys from losing sight in their left eyes?

## Eyes Need Each Other

The optometrist said that within the HMO, the Taxels had only one option—conventional medical treatment, which meant eye surgery. But if they were willing to go outside the HMO and pay out of pocket, they could try a more natural approach, vision therapy. Vision therapy, also called vision training, eye training or orthoptics, involves noninvasive eye exercises and other techniques that retrain the eyes to work together and in the process correct any glitches in the brain's processing of visual information to restore normal two-eye (binocular) vision. Vision therapy is the little-known specialty of a small but growing number of eye-care professionals known as behavioral optometrists.

Before deciding on any treatment, the Taxels consulted two ophthalmologists to see if the optometrist's diagnosis was correct. It was, but both doctors dismissed the suggestion of vision therapy as "nonsense" and "voodoo." They insisted that surgery was the only way to go. The operation involved cutting some of the muscles that controlled movement in both eyes to "balance" them. They warned that any delay in having the surgery might aggravate the boys' condition and risk left-eye blindness.

Frightened and confused, the Taxels gathered information from ophthalmologic and behavioral optometric organizations and consulted more ophthalmologists, several vision therapists and veterans of both forms of treatment. What they learned was, in Laura Taxel's words, "a real eye-opener."

Ophthalmology is a surgical specialty, and surgeons are trained that "to cut is to cure." Most ophthalmologists dismiss vision therapy because they are unfamiliar with it. That's unfortunate, because many experts feel that vision therapy works better than surgery for the problem the Taxel boys had and for many other problems as well.

That was what a team of researchers led by Bradley Coffey, O.D., professor of optometry at the Pacific University College of Optometry in Portland, Oregon, discovered when they reviewed 59 studies of lazy eye treatment that tracked a total of 3,856 people. Of those who had surgery, 46 percent were cured. The success rate for vision therapy was 59 percent.

Other investigators have reported even better results for vision therapy. In 1992, Indian researchers used vision therapy on 30 people with lazy eye for periods ranging from eight weeks to one year. They reported significant improvement in 75 percent.

"We talked with several parents whose children had had the surgery," Taxel recalls. "It corrected the cosmetic aspect of the problem. The affected eye stopped drifting noticeably. But it sometimes took up to three operations for the kids to be able to read and do close-focus work competently. We figured that if vision therapy didn't work, we could always try surgery. But why opt for something so invasive and traumatic when the natural approach made more sense to us and had a better success rate?"

## Basic Training for Vision

The Taxels took Nathan and Simon to David Munson, O.D., a behavioral optometrist in nearby Chagrin Falls. One hour a week for a year, Dr. Munson had the boys play a series of deceptively simple hands-on children's games, like marbles, and engage in additional behavioral optometric activities, such as focusing on beads placed at various distances along a string, to coax their eyes into better coordination and persuade their brains to pay attention to information from their left eyes. There was also homework in the form of vision exercises that involved the whole family.

"It was work," Taxel says, "but at the end of the year, both boys showed tremendous improvement. Now, four years later, they read above grade level, and they're playing musical instruments. That's really significant to me because when we were considering surgery, one of the ophthalmologists said that even if the operations were successful, they might never be able to read music, because it's harder than reading words. Today they both read music quite well."

## Vision Quest

The conventional wisdom on vision is that for most people, seeing carries a price—eventual blurring of far or near vision or both. When the eyes lose their ability to see distant objects clearly, that's nearsightedness, or myopia, a condition that an estimated 60 million Americans develop as children or teens. Later, typically after age 40, close objects become the problem in a condition called presbyopia.

But not to worry: Glasses or contacts can correct the problem, and if those who are nearsighted also develop presbyopia as they age, bifocals are the answer. Or are they?

Maybe not, according to a small, largely unpublicized group of eye-care professionals who, since about 1910, have championed a different—and until recently heretical—view of vision.

Chief among these renegades was William H. Bates, M.D., an ophthalmologist who developed his Bates Method in the 1920s. Dr. Bates believed there was more to vision than the physical act of seeing. About half of vision, he said, was "mental," a mind/body process of interpreting visual information. Unfortunately for Dr. Bates, he declared vision a mind/body experience 70 years before mind/body medicine became medically fashionable, at a time when the vast majority of physicians viewed the mind and body as completely separate. Dr. Bates's fellow ophthalmologists dismissed his view as "spiritualistic."

But Dr. Bates didn't stop there. In his 1940 book, *The Bates Method for Better Eyesight without Glasses*, he claimed to have discovered the answer to a great ophthalmological mystery—the cause of refractive errors, the technical term for the process that

# Cure for a President's Daughter

How would you like to take a bad report card home to the President?

President Lyndon Johnson's daughter Luci was very bright and worked diligently in school, but she had trouble reading and writing and earned only D's.

She had all sorts of tests—including an eye exam that rated her vision 20/20. No one could figure out why she was such an underachiever. By age 16, Luci felt so frustrated that she seriously considered dropping out of high school.

Finally, in desperation, the White House physician referred her to a Washington behavioral optometrist, who diagnosed a binocular disorder. Luci's eye movements were uncoordinated, which made it difficult for her to focus on reading and writing.

"There I was," she recalls, "the daughter of a president, and I had a major visual problem that went undiagnosed for years."

For several months, the optometrist led Luci through a series of vision therapy exercises, many of which were so deceptively simple that they seemed silly to her. But slowly her eyes began working as a team. Her reading and writing abilities improved—and so did her grades. "In a year and a half, I went from D's to B's, and later, in college, I made the honor roll. It was thrilling." Her physical coordination also improved significantly.

Luci was so impressed with vision therapy that she went to work for the optometrist who cured her. "I saw a little boy who was hav-

causes nearsightedness and farsightedness. From Dr. Bates's day to our own, the vast majority of ophthalmologists and optometrists have believed that for unknown reasons, in nearsightedness, the eyeball somehow becomes too long. Light from distant objects focuses not on the retina, the nerve-rich area in the back of the eye that connects to the optic nerve, but in front of it, causing distant objects to look blurry. In farsightedness, light focuses behind the retina, blurring close objects.

ing difficulty in kindergarten transformed from an angry failure into a happy, successful student," she recalls. "I saw teens go from failing grades to the honor roll as I'd done. I saw young men eager to be military pilots improve their vision to the point where they achieved their wish. And I saw one little girl who'd had two unsuccessful operations to correct crossed eyes achieve a marked degree of control."

Today Luci Johnson Nugent is the national honorary chairwoman of Volunteers in Vision, an organization that helps visually disadvantaged children. She urges parents to look for the following signs of possible vision problems.

- Do your child's eyes frequently "run," as if crying?
- Do your child's eyes seem to move independently of one another, even occasionally?
- Does your child experience headaches, nausea or blurred vision after reading for only a short time?
- Does your child ever complain of seeing double?
- Does your child ever squint or omit words or letters when writing?
- Does your child seem uncoordinated? One indication is a need to touch things to understand or interpret information about them.

If you answered yes to any of these questions, consult a behavioral optometrist for a complete vision examination.

Dr. Bates had a different idea. He believed that nearsightedness and farsightedness were caused by chronic stress on two sets of muscles in the eye—the ciliary muscles that control the shape of the lens and the six muscles surrounding the eyeball that move it up and down and left and right.

In his book, Dr. Bates wrote, "All abnormal action of the muscles of the eyeball is accompanied by straining effort to see. With relief of this strain, the action of the muscles becomes normal, and all errors of refraction disappear." Dr. Bates claimed that simple stress-relieving eye exercises, his Bates Method, allowed the formerly nearsighted and farsighted to take off their glasses for good and see clearly without them.

Dr. Bates might have remained an obscure figure had it not been for Aldous Huxley, the British philosopher who wrote the novel *Brave New World*. Huxley had terrible vision, and during the 1930s he embraced the Bates Method. Huxley was never able to throw away his glasses, but he claimed that using the technique improved his vision considerably.

Huxley became so enamored of the Bates Method that he touted it in a 1942 book, *The Art of Seeing:* "Ever since ophthalmology became a science," he wrote, "its practitioners have been obsessively preoccupied with only one aspect of the total complex process of seeing—the physiological. They have paid exclusive attention to the eyes, and none to the mind, which uses the eyes to see." American ophthalmologists scoffed at Huxley, especially after he visited the United States and at public appearances revealed how poor his improved vision still was. Critics of the Bates Method wrote it off as a fraud.

The irony of the Bates controversy was that it involved ophthalmologists, who rarely deal with refractive errors. The diagnosis and treatment of nearsightedness and farsightedness are usually the province of optometrists.

Around the time that Dr. Bates developed his method, a St. Louis optometrist named A. M. Skeffington became convinced that Dr. Bates was on the right track. He began experimenting with Bates-style eye exercises and discovered that they could treat many vision problems, possibly even freeing some people from glasses. Dr. Skeffington was a founder of behavioral optometry and helped popularize the forerunners of the eye exercises used in vision therapy today. He also helped establish the Optometric Extension Program (OEP), an organization that promotes vision therapy. About 3,700 of the nation's 26,000 optometrists (14 percent) are members.

Unfortunately, few people have ever heard of vision therapy. "It's the best-kept secret in eye care," says vision therapy specialist Donald Getz, O.D., a behavioral optometrist in Van

Nuys, California. "The few people who know anything about it think it's the Bates Method. But Bates is outdated. He focused only on the eye muscles. Today we know that in addition, vision therapy works by retraining the way the brain processes visual imagery. It's more like visual biofeedback than vision calisthenics. Using today's methods, we get better, more permanent results than Bates did."

## Seeing Is Believing

Today's vision therapy helps treat many vision-impairing eye conditions.

*Crossed eyes (strabismus), lazy eye (amblyopia) and binocular disorder (mild amblyopia).* In addition to causing cosmetic problems—the eyes look funny—these disorders interfere with reading and close-focus work and may lead to blindness of the weaker eye. They are also surprisingly common. According to a report in the *Journal of the American Optometric Association*, about 5 percent of schoolchildren have strabismic eyes, and up to 8 percent have some degree of amblyopia. Each year in the United States, the National Society to Prevent Blindness estimates 127,000 new diagnoses of amblyopia. Six months of vision therapy produces substantial, long-lasting improvement of these conditions in about 75 percent of cases, according to a review of more than 200 studies done by Allen Cohen, O.D., professor of optometry at the State University of New York College of Optometry in New York City.

*Focusing problems (vergence and accommodative disorders).* Normal eyes hold objects in focus and automatically refocus when they shift from one object to another that's closer or farther away. People with focusing problems can't do this, and their constant struggle to keep their eyes focused leads to chronic eye stress that often causes headaches, fatigue, double or blurry vision and a burning sensation in the eyes.

Researchers at the Ohio State University College of Optometry used vision therapy to treat 96 people with focusing problems. Fifty-three percent were cured. Symptoms were significantly reduced, though not eliminated, in 43 percent. Only 4 percent showed no benefit.

*Jerking eye (ocular-motor problems).* This condition interferes with smooth eye movement, causing the eyes to jerk from point to point. It impairs reading ability and anything else that requires fluid eye movements. Stephen Miller, O.D., director of clinical care for the American Optometric Association in St. Louis, says vision therapy "usually cures ocular-motor problems."

*Learning disabilities.* "Many children diagnosed with learning disabilities or dyslexia don't really have them," Dr. Getz says. "They often have learning-related vision problems, and vision therapy can help them—if they're diagnosed and treated by a behavioral optometrist. Unfortunately, many are not."

In a 1994 study, Gary Sigler, Ed.D., associate professor of applied psychology at Eastern Washington University in Cheney, and Spokane behavioral optometrist D. Todd Wylie, O.D., worked with three children, two age eight and one ten, who had severe problems with reading. One had been diagnosed as dyslexic. After two months of vision therapy, the children's reading abilities improved dramatically.

The OEP publishes materials that alert educators to the visual components of many learning problems and helps them select young people who might benefit from optometric evaluation and vision therapy. Some children's classroom behavior problems also have a visual component that may respond to vision therapy.

*Balance.* Good vision is critical for good balance because vision, our dominant sense, provides the brain with a great deal of information about the body's position. At Acadia University in Wolfville, Nova Scotia, Bill McLeod, Ph.D., director of the School of Recreation and Physical Education, and Edward Hansen, Ph.D., professor of psychology, tested the balance of 20 male and female students and then trained them in Eyerobics, a visual-skills training program that uses vision therapy exercises to improve depth perception, peripheral vision, reaction time and spatial judgment. After Eyerobics training, the researchers retested the participants' balance and found significant improvement.

*Athletic performance.* "Keep your eye on the ball" is standard advice in baseball, basketball, tennis, volleyball and many other sports. The problem is that sometimes even world-class athletes can't do it well enough to remain competitive.

With the help of vision therapy, they can. "I've worked with the U.S. Olympic volleyball team," Dr. Getz says, "and I've gotten especially good results for professional tennis players. I flash lights at them and time how long it takes them to respond. At first it may take them one-tenth of a second. But after a while, they start responding in one one-hundredth of a second, ten times faster. The difference between a tenth and a hundredth of a second may not sound like much, but when you're playing professional tennis, it's the difference between seeing the ball leave your opponent's racquet and not seeing it until it's already on your side of the court."

*Traumatic brain injury.* Some people who sustain head injuries in auto or other accidents largely recover, except that they experience blurred or double vision. "They're often told they have to live with it," Dr. Getz says, "but vision therapy can often help them see better."

## Bye-Bye Myopia?

What about Dr. Bates's assertion that his eye exercises could eliminate the need for lenses to correct myopia?

Almost a century after the good doctor first made this claim, it remains highly controversial. Ophthalmologists and many optometrists scoff at it, but Dr. Bates's book is still available, and a small band of vision specialists continues to tout the Bates Method. A few weekend and home-study courses—notably the Cambridge Institute for Better Vision and Vision WorkOut—offer Bates-inspired programs that even carry money-back guarantees. The Cambridge Institute "guarantees that your vision will improve when you use the Program for Better Vision. See for yourself. Use the Program for 60 days. If you are not com-

# No More Computer-Screen Eyestrain

Twenty years ago, before the arrival of personal computers, people who did close-focus work, such as jewelers, embroiderers and avid readers, often complained of eyestrain, a stinging sensation often accompanied by blurred vision, headache and a dry, gritty feeling in the eyes.

In recent years, as millions of office workers traded in their typewriters and adding machines for video display terminals (VDTs) attached to desktop or laptop computers, eyestrain has become a national epidemic.

Actually, *eyestrain* is a misnomer. It's not the eyes that become strained but rather the ciliary muscles, which control the focusing mechanism of the eyes' lenses, and the external muscles that move the eyes up and down and from side to side. The eye muscles evolved in a world of varied eye uses: some close-focus work (cooking, eating and crafts), some middle-distance tasks (farming and building) and some far-distance work (hunting).

We still use our eyes for middle- and far-distance tasks, but for much of the workday, record numbers of Americans are staring at VDTs, engaged in only close-focus work. Deprived of the variety that allows them to function at their best, the eye muscles tense up and tire, hence eyestrain. Here's how to prevent it.

**Let there be light.** Make sure your workspace is comfortably lighted—neither too dim nor too bright.

**Get set.** Arrange your workspace so that you can look beyond the screen to the other side of the room. Confining your visual horizons to just your cubicle is a one-way ticket to eyestrain. Arrange your workspace so that when you look up, you can look into the distance.

---

pletely satisfied for any reason, return it for a full refund." Vision WorkOut makes a similar promise.

Strong words, but notice that the Cambridge Institute doesn't guarantee anyone a future without glasses.

"Many of our 30,000 clients have been freed from glasses,"

**Reduce glare.** Make sure your VDT screen is free of glare. No light should reflect directly off the screen into your eyes. If your office lighting makes glare inevitable, tilt the screen, cover offending lights or windows or invest in an inexpensive cloth mesh anti-glare shield that attaches to the VDT and diffuses the light it reflects.

**Look down.** Sit so that your eyes are 24 to 36 inches from your VDT screen and looking slightly down at it.

**Look away.** After a few minutes of staring at the screen, treat your eyes to some middle- and far-distance time by looking across the room or across the street. To remind yourself to look away from your screen, adopt a ritual: look away every time the phone rings or whenever you type certain letters: q, x, z or k.

**Think blink.** In a 1993 study, Japanese researchers studied 104 office workers who worked on computers for about three hours a day. When they were engaged in relaxed conversation, they blinked an average of 22 times per minute. While reading printed material, they blinked 10 times a minute. But at their VDTs, they blinked only 7 times a minute. In addition, computer users kept their eyes unusually wide open. Computer users' wide-eyed lack of blinking contributes significantly to the gritty, dry-eyed feeling of eyestrain. The more wide open the eyes, the more moisture evaporates from their surface. Blinking replaces that moisture, but as the blink rate declines, dry eyes stay dry.

**Exercise your eyes.** About once every half-hour, take a break from your screen and do the exercises described elsewhere in this chapter.

says Cambridge Institute executive director Martin Sussman. "Many have passed driver's license eye tests without them. Of course, if a person sees very poorly to begin with, we can't promise they'll shed their lenses. What we promise is that using all the optometric measures of vision—acuity, focusing ability and eye coordination—they'll see better without their glasses and suffer less from eyestrain."

Surprisingly, few studies have investigated vision therapy for myopia correction, but those that have, mostly case reports, have produced intriguing results.

At the Chinese University of Hong Kong, psychologist Jin-Pang Leung recruited a moderately nearsighted male college student into a program of intensive vision therapy. After several months, his visual acuity improved significantly, though not enough to change his eyeglass prescription. Meanwhile, a 1991 review of several case reports documents considerable success for vision therapy treatment of myopia; in some cases there was enough improvement to eliminate the need for corrective lenses.

Additional indirect evidence comes from population studies. When public education first came to northern Alaska, researchers examined the eyes of 197 Inuits (Eskimos) in Barrow. Among the parents, who had never attended school, only two had myopia, but among their school-going children, 60 percent had it. This study and others with similar though less dramatic results have fueled optometric speculation that the way the eye focuses on close tasks plays a significant role in the development of myopia and that vision therapy may be able to retrain the eye/brain focusing system to prevent or reverse nearsightedness.

Ophthalmologists and optometrists in general don't recommend vision therapy for myopia. There are exceptions, however.

Dale Freeberg, O.D., a Hawthorne, California, optometrist who specializes in myopia, attended a Cambridge Institute weekend seminar in the early 1980s and was so impressed that he volunteered to help Sussman create his home-study course. "I've never received a dime from the Cambridge Institute," he says. "I just think it's a good program. It can significantly correct myopia, though many people will still have to wear glasses. Personally, I recommend whatever works. I've had the best success with a combination of vision therapy and rigid gas-permeable contact lenses. But exercises like the ones the Cambridge Institute recommends are good for everyone. They relax the eyes and sharpen visual acuity. I believe that in many cases, they can also minimize or even eliminate myopia."

The American Optometric Association's Dr. Miller isn't so sure: "In my opinion, the home vision-improvement programs make extravagant claims. If you wear corrective lenses, do not assume that vision therapy will eliminate them. However, some people who think they're nearsighted actually have a condition called pseudomyopia, a type of focusing problem that may respond to vision therapy, so some people might benefit."

Dr. Getz believes vision therapy can help nearsightedness—if the person is trained when myopia first develops. "Vision therapy works best for young people who are just beginning to become myopic," he says. "Then we can often halt the progression of nearsightedness and free them from glasses. But wearing glasses tends to cement myopia. Vision therapy exercises are good for everyone's eyes because they're relaxing, and they may reduce nearsightedness somewhat, but it's unrealistic to suggest that they will always eliminate the need for lenses."

The bottom line: Vision therapy is no sure cure for nearsightedness, but it can't hurt, and it just might help.

## Vision Therapy Exercises

Vision therapists recommend more than 200 different eye exercises and often administer them with simple aids: glasses with different-colored lenses, eye patches, bull's-eye targets and beaded strings. What follows are simple vision therapy exercises that anyone can do at home.

*Palming.* This helps relax tired eyes. Briskly rub your hands together for 15 seconds or so until they feel warm. Close your eyes and cup your warm palms over them. Make sure your palms are cupped enough so they don't touch your eyelids. Your fingers should overlap and rest on your forehead. Holding this position, breathe deeply and regularly for a few minutes.

*Look away.* If you do close-focus work—reading, sewing, wiring or computer work—tack the front page of a newspaper to a wall about eight feet away. Every ten minutes or so, take a short break from your work and look at it, scanning the large headline type, the smaller subheads and the fine print. This helps maintain your focusing ability and minimizes the blurred vision many close-focus workers experience at the end of the day.

*Follow your thumb.* Several times each day, hold your thumb out at arm's length and move it in slow circles, crosses, Xs and in-and-out motions. Without moving your head, follow it with your eyes. Keep it—and the rest of the room—in focus as much as possible.

*Bead and string.* Thread three colored beads along a piece of string or yarn about six feet long. Fasten one end to a wall at eye height and hold the other to the tip of your nose. Slide one bead close to the wall, the second about four feet from your nose and the third about a foot away from you. Look at the farthest bead. You should see two strings forming a V with the bead at its point. Next focus on the middle bead. You should see two strings forming an X with the bead at its cross point. Then look at the nearest bead. You should also see an X. If your eyes work as a team, as they should, you will always see two strings crossing when you focus on a bead. If not, you may see only one string, suggesting that your brain is suppressing information from your weaker eye. If you see only one string, consult a behavioral optometrist.

*Call the ball.* Write letters or numbers of various sizes on a softball, kickball or soccer ball. Hang it from the ceiling on a string and give it a push in any direction. As it swings, call out the letters or numbers you see.

The Optometric Extension Program Foundation markets dozens of visual exercise items, from low-tech flashcards aimed at day care children to sophisticated computer systems for behavioral optometrists who specialize in athletic eye/hand coordination. If you'd like to delve deeper into vision improvement, contact the OEP at 1921 East Carnegie Ave, Suite 3L, Santa Ana, CA 92705, for a catalog or a referral to a behavioral optometrist near you.

## CHAPTER 28

# VISUALIZATION, GUIDED IMAGERY AND SELF-HYPNOSIS

*Tapping into the Healing Power of Your Mind*

In 1987, Karen Olness, M.D., professor of pediatrics at the Case Western Reserve Medical Center in Cleveland, injured her thumb in a skiing accident. The injury required surgery, which was fine with Dr. Olness, but she had a major problem with her surgeon's plan. He wanted to anesthetize her.

Of *course* he wanted to anesthetize her—anesthesia is standard American surgical procedure. But Dr. Olness had a different idea, a mind/body approach to pain control known variously as visualization, guided imagery and self-hypnosis.

"My surgeon was understandably dubious," she recalls. He might have refused a nonphysician, but he knew of Dr. Olness's medical specialty. For more than 20 years, she'd practiced and taught hypnotherapy, and she was one of the field's leading researchers. He reluctantly agreed to allow her to use self-hypnosis—provided that an anesthesiologist was on hand with standard anesthetics just in case.

Sitting in the operating room with her hand extended on the operating table, Dr. Olness closed her eyes, breathed deeply and quickly entered a state of deep relaxation similar to the one achieved in meditation. But unlike the passive, accepting, spectator frame of mind that's adopted during meditation, she imagined the farm where she grew up: "In my mind, I felt what it was like to lie in the grass, gaze up at the heavens and see a bit of the barn out of a corner of my eye."

As the surgeon cut into Dr. Olness's thumb, she felt no pain. She was awake and fully aware that she was in surgery, but at the same time she felt far removed from the experience. When the surgeon had finished, he signaled Dr. Olness, who quickly returned to a normal state of consciousness, opened her eyes, walked out of the operating room unassisted and had lunch with a friend. "I felt great," she recalls. "I had no anesthesia hangover."

Dr. Olness has no special gift for visualization—anyone can learn to use it. If you doubt it, try this simple experiment: Imagine a basket of fresh lemons. In your mind, take one, slice it open and inhale its lemony aroma. Now squeeze some of the tangy, sour juice onto your tongue. Chances are that your salivary glands are now oozing. Congratulations—you can use visualization to improve your health.

You may never opt for "mental anesthesia" when you need surgery, but Martin Rossman, M.D., clinical associate professor of medicine at the University of California's San Francisco Medical Center and author of *Healing Yourself: A Step-By-Step Program for Better Health through Imagery*, estimates that visualization techniques can help treat "90 percent of the problems people bring to primary care doctors."

## From Mesmerism to Visualization

Visualization has an undeservedly speckled reputation, based on its strange history. Since prehistoric times, shamans and traditional healers around the world have used the power of suggested mental images in healing, but the technique was largely unknown in the West until 1778, when Viennese physician Franz Anton Mesmer opened a practice in Paris.

Dr. Mesmer was one of many physicians of that era who believed in "magnetic healing"—the idea that placing magnets on injured parts of the body helped cure them. But unlike other magnetic healers, who treated people individually, Dr. Mesmer worked with groups whose members sat holding hands while his assistants gave them massages and verbal suggestions punctuated by musical tones.

Many participants experienced strong reactions: crying, laughing, shrieking and agitation. Finally Dr. Mesmer himself would appear, a charismatic figure wearing a long silk robe and waving a magnetic wand. He too gave his patients massages and verbal suggestions. But Dr. Mesmer's words had a calming effect, and many participants claimed that the treatment helped resolve all manner of physical and emotional complaints.

Dr. Mesmer and his treatment, "mesmerism," became quite popular—and controversial. In 1784, the French Academy of Sciences investigated him. (Among the investigators was American scientist/statesman Benjamin Franklin, who was living in Paris at the time.) The committee lambasted mesmerism, saying that it involved nothing more than the power of suggestion. Dr. Mesmer was ruined, but his influence lives on.

He is considered the father of hypnosis. He gave the English language the term mesmerize, meaning "to entrance." And indirectly he played a role in the genesis of one of America's homegrown religions, Christian Science. In 1862, Phineas P. Quimby, a Portland, Maine, physician who used mesmerism in his practice, cured Mary Baker Eddy, founder of Christian Science, of severe back pain by using suggestion. The experience shaped the young woman's view that illness is all in the mind.

Eventually mesmerism became known as hypnotism. Unfortunately, hypnotism became notorious for its use in nightclub acts, where outlandishly dressed hypnotists would swing pocket watches in front of people, say the words, "You're getting sleepy" and then order the hapless individuals—often the hypnotists' confederates—to embarrass themselves by doing things they supposedly couldn't remember when they woke up.

In fact, hypnosis has nothing to do with getting sleepy. It doesn't

# Can Visualization Cure Cancer?

In 1978, radiation oncologist O. Carl Simonton, M.D., and Stephanie Matthews-Simonton published Getting Well Again. In their book they claimed that visualization exercises could, in some cases, shrink tumors and allow people with advanced cancers to survive considerably longer than their physicians thought possible, presumably by stimulating their immune systems to fight the cancer more effectively. The book stirred tremendous controversy. People with cancer snapped it up, but their doctors raised serious questions about the Simontons' research methods, and many scoffed at their results.

Seven years later, in 1985, psychologist Jeanne Achterberg, Ph.D., a former colleague of the Simontons, published Imagery in Healing, which made even more remarkable claims. Dr. Achterberg claimed to have developed a scale for evaluating the effectiveness of tumor-fighting imagery.

In her view, optimal anti-cancer visualizations involved vivid images of small, weak, confused cancer cells overwhelmed by big, aggressive, powerful white blood cells. Dr. Achterberg claimed that by evaluating a cancer patient's imagery, she could predict with as-

produce a "trance." It's actually a form of heightened concentration. "You're perfectly aware of what's going on around you," Dr. Olness explains. "You simply choose not to focus on it."

If you work with a hypnotherapist, you're never under that person's control. "No one can make you do anything you don't want to do," Dr. Olness says, "which is why hypnosis has a poor track record for helping people quit smoking."

Contrary to the nightclub hypnotist's classic line, "When I snap my fingers, you'll wake up and have no memory of this experience," most people remember everything that happens while they're in the deeply relaxed hypnotic state. And no one has to snap any fingers to rouse you from hypnotic relaxation.

tounding 100 percent accuracy who would survive and who would die within two months.

Again, many people with cancer embraced the book, while most cancer researchers called Dr. Achterberg's claims outrageous. But were they so outrageous? Since her book appeared, other researchers have produced similarly intriguing results.

Over an eight-year period, Bernauer Newton, Ph.D., director of the Newton Center for Clinical Hypnosis in Los Angeles, taught self-hypnosis to 280 people with cancer. He was mostly interested in helping them cope with the rigors of surgery, radiation and chemotherapy, and he found that the combination of meditative relaxation and imagery contributed to their quality of life.

Dr. Newton also rated the group based on his own impressions of their commitment to hypnosis. Of the 105 people "most committed" to self-hypnosis at the time of his analysis, 54 percent were still alive. Of the 57 "least committed" to it, only 18 percent were still alive. Clearly, factors other than hypnosis may have affected their survival. But visualizations seem to enhance the quality of life for people with cancer—and just might add to their longevity as well.

"You can return to normal awareness whenever you choose," Dr. Olness says.

Fortunately, while entertainers were distorting hypnosis, a few physicians and psychologists quietly continued to explore its uses in healing. In 1949 American hypnosis researchers formed the Society for Clinical and Experimental Hypnosis, and in 1957 hypnotherapists founded the American Society of Clinical Hypnosis. But during the 1970s, as mind/body approaches to healing became more popular, many professionals abandoned the nightclub-tainted term hypnosis in favor of *visualization, imagery* or *guided imagery.* Feel free to call this natural cure whatever you like.

# The Healing Power of Images

Can something as simple as deep relaxation and imagination affect illness? Some physicians continue to express doubt, but among those familiar with the field, the answer is unequivocally yes. Here are several areas where it's been shown to help.

*Anesthesia.* Dr. Olness is not the only person who has used visualization in place of anesthesia. Philip Ament, D.D.S., Ph.D., a Buffalo, New York, dentist and psychologist, has used a similar technique with dental patients who are unable to tolerate full chemical anesthesia. After they have become deeply relaxed, he suggests that they visualize themselves becoming numb. Quite a few have had dental surgery using subtherapeutic amounts of chemical anesthesia plus visualization for pain control.

*Habit control.* "Young people have greater medical success with hypnosis than adults," Dr. Olness says, "because they are more in touch with their imaginations." Using relaxation and imagery, she has helped kids overcome bed-wetting, thumb-sucking, hair-pulling and habitual coughs.

*Chronic illnesses.* "I've seen hypnosis stabilize blood sugar levels in diabetics, reduce the frequency and severity of asthma attacks and even decrease bleeding in hemophiliacs," Dr. Olness says. (A person with hemophilia lacks a blood component that promotes clotting.) Dr. Rossman reports similar benefits: reductions in allergy symptoms, blood pressure, irregular heartbeats (arrhythmias), autoimmune diseases and stress-related urinary, reproductive and gastrointestinal complaints.

*Immune enhancement.* Dr. Olness measured a component of the immune system, immunoglobulin A (IgA), in the saliva of 57 children ages 6 to 12, then divided the children into three groups. One group simply played. Another learned deep relaxation. The third viewed a video on the immune system, then learned deep relaxation and was asked to visualize their bodies producing more IgA. The groups that played and learned deep relaxation showed no change in IgA. But the visualization group experienced a significant increase in IgA.

*Migraine headaches.* Dr. Olness randomly assigned 30 children with migraines to receive one of three treatments: a placebo (an ineffective, dummy pill), propranolol (a common migraine medication) or hypnosis. Only the hypnosis group reported a significant decrease in their migraines. Visualization can also help adults who have migraines, but Dr. Olness cautions that it often takes up to two months of daily practice to begin to experience noticeable benefits.

*Stage fright.* Performance anxiety affects many actors, athletes, public speakers, job seekers preparing for interviews and students studying for exams. Visualization can help by preventing the anxiety-induced reactions that develop in anticipation of performing: nausea, hyperventilation, sweaty palms and so forth.

*Surgical recovery.* In a review of 18 studies, Robert Blankfield, M.D., professor of family medicine at Case Western Reserve Medical Center, found that for people having surgery—hysterectomy, hemorrhoid removal, abdominal surgery and coronary artery bypasses—hypnotherapy decreased their postsurgical nausea and pain, accelerated healing and allowed them to leave the hospital sooner.

Many people try hypnosis or visualization to help them quit smoking. The technique works for some, but not for many. David Spiegel, M.D., professor of psychiatry at Stanford University and director of the university's Psychosocial Treatment Laboratory, taught self-hypnosis to 266 people who said they wanted to quit smoking. Half the smokers quit for a week after learning the technique, but after a year, only 25 percent remained smoke-free.

"It's a misconception that hypnosis and other imagery techniques work wonders for people trying to kick poor health habits," Dr. Olness says. "These techniques work by harnessing your imagination. If you can't imagine giving up smoking or overeating or alcohol—whatever—then imagery techniques probably won't help you."

## The Body Listens

How does visualization work? Scientists still aren't certain, but some studies show that imagery used for pain relief stim-

(continued on page 452)

# Are Prayers Answered?

"Dear God, please (fill in the blank)."

Prayer is probably the world's most widely practiced visualization technique. Those who pray often begin with a relaxation ritual—attending a house of worship or kneeling by the bed. Then they conjure a personal image of a God or some Higher Power and ask that the requests in their prayers be granted.

Many people feel profoundly calm after praying, and no wonder. Prayer is deeply relaxing, and those who do it regularly are, in effect, meditating. But science cannot explain some intriguing studies showing that to a degree that goes way beyond coincidence, prayer sometimes works.

In one study, Randolph Byrd, M.D., a cardiologist at San Francisco General Hospital, randomly divided 393 patients in the hospital's coronary care unit into two groups. Fundamentalist Christian home prayer groups prayed daily for the recovery of one group. Neither the patients nor their doctors or nurses knew which patients received prayers and which did not. After ten months, Dr. Byrd reported some surprising findings. The prayed-for patients were:

- Significantly less likely to require antibiotics (3 patients versus 16)
- Significantly less likely to develop pulmonary edema—a condition in which the lungs fill with fluid because the heart cannot pump properly (6 versus 18).
- Significantly less likely to require insertion of a tube into the throat to assist breathing (0 versus 12).
- Less likely to die (but this difference was not statistically significant).

When Dr. Byrd's results were published in the Southern Medical Journal, they caused a sensation. Many called his study scientific proof that prayers are answered. But skeptics remained unimpressed, saying that none of the patients recovered and that Dr. Byrd, a fundamentalist, may have somehow biased his findings.

If this were the only study showing statistically significant benefit for prayer, it might be ignored. But it isn't. In his 1994 book, *Healing Words,* Larry Dossey, M.D., former chief of staff at Humana
Medical City in Dallas and now co-chair of the Panel on Mind-Body
Interventions of the Office of Alternative Medicine at the National Institutes of Health in Washington, D.C., reviews over 100 experiments,
most published in parapsychological literature, on the effects of
prayer/visualization. More than half showed an effect on everything
from seed germination to wound healing.

- In several experiments, volunteers visualized stimulating or re-
  tarding the growth of bacteria and fungi and achieved significantly positive results from as far as 15 miles away.
- At the Mind Science Foundation in San Antonio, Texas, researchers took blood samples from 32 volunteers, isolated their
  red blood cells (RBCs) and placed the samples in a room on the
  other side of the building. Then the researchers placed the RBCs
  in a solution designed to swell and burst them, a process that can
  be measured extremely accurately. Next the researchers asked
  the volunteers to pray for the preservation of some of the RBCs.
  To help them visualize, the researchers projected color slides of
  healthy RBCs. The praying significantly slowed the swelling and
  bursting of the RBCs.
- In another study at the Mind Science Foundation, volunteers in a
  room on one side of the building were asked to visualize volunteers in a room on the other side of the building becoming calmer
  or more agitated. Meanwhile, the "receivers" were hooked up
  to biofeedback-type equipment to gauge their reactions. The results showed that the "influencers" exerted a statistically significant effect on the receivers' moods.

It's difficult to determine what, if anything, these studies mean.
Anyone who has ever prayed knows that prayers often remain unan-

*(continued)*

# Are Prayers Answered?—*Continued*

swered. But Dr. Dossey, who rejected his childhood religious training as an adult, believes that something is going on. Medical ethics demand that physicians do everything in their power to help those in their care. After reviewing the scientific literature on prayer, Dr. Dossey came to believe that he is ethically obligated to pray for them.

These days, Dr. Dossey arrives at his office about a half-hour before it opens, enters a meditative state and asks "the Absolute" that his patients achieve "the best possible outcome."

---

ulates the release of endorphins—the body's pain-relieving chemicals.

In addition, a recently developed imaging technology—positron emission tomography—shows that it doesn't matter whether people actually perform an activity or just vividly imagine it. The same parts of the brain become activated either way. This should come as no surprise to anyone who enjoys movies. The process of settling into theater seats relaxes moviegoers and puts them in a receptive frame of mind. Then the big screen overwhelms them with intense sight and sound images. It's no wonder that chase scenes make viewers feel anxious or that love scenes provoke sensual arousal.

Many physicians still pooh-pooh visualization, but they use it every day—whenever they say, "Take this. It will help." Those words inspire belief in the treatment—a vision of relief and healing and quite often what's known as a placebo response.

*Placebo* is Latin for "I will please." In medicine, a placebo is a dummy treatment known to have no healing effect. Nonetheless, when given placebos for any condition from minor colds to life-threatening illnesses, about one-third of people report benefit.

The placebo effect first came to light more than a century ago. When new drugs were introduced, physicians touted them, and they seemed to work magnificently. But as time passed and side effects appeared, professional doubts arose. Physicians toned down their enthusiasm, and the treatments produced less dramatic results.

This phenomenon of diminishing benefits was well recognized at the time. In nineteenth-century medical schools, aspiring doctors all learned the adage, "Use the new medicines quickly, while they still have the power to heal."

Every medication, whether useful or not, triggers some placebo benefits. When researchers realized that placebo responses could cloud their studies, they developed the "placebo-controlled" trial. Half the people in a study get the new treatment and half get a placebo. To be judged effective, the group taking the new treatment must report a significantly better response than the placebo-takers.

Today physicians who view medicine as a science rather than an art often view the placebo response as an embarrassment, proof of people's gullibility: You tell them that a worthless pill works wonders, and one-third report relief. But physicians who understand mind/body medicine appreciate the placebo response as a manifestation of visualization.

People with medical problems are typically anxious. A physician says, "Take this. It will help." Independent of the treatment's actual benefits, people are apt to relax a bit, newly secure in the knowledge that an expert believes their condition can be treated successfully. They are also likely to visualize feeling better and the return of good health. The mind/body aspect of the placebo response may also explain why some people respond to faith-healing.

Physician-inspired visualizations of the negative sort can also cause harm. A doctor who describes a heart problem as "a time bomb waiting to explode" or who tells a person, "You have only a few months to live" triggers vivid images that may create a self-fulfilling prophecy.

In a 1993 study, David P. Phillips, Ph.D., professor of sociology at the University of California at San Diego, showed how detrimental such negative health visualizations can be in an analysis of the birth years and death dates for 28,000 Chinese-Americans.

In Chinese culture, each birth year is linked to "bad luck" for certain organs and diseases. Dr. Phillips discovered that a Chinese-American with leukemia who was born in a year considered bad luck for cancer died on average four years sooner than a similar Chinese-American with leukemia who was born in a year not associated with cancer. Because the year had no effect on white people, it was clear that Chinese-Americans' expectations were playing a role in the outcome of their illnesses.

Visualizations clearly have powerful effects on health. The question for physicians is not whether they're using imagery in medicine but *how wisely* they are using it.

## Opening a Window to Better Health

What is a visualization image? Dr. Rossman says it's a "flow of thoughts you can see, hear, feel, smell or taste. Imagery is a window into your inner world, the currency of daydreams, memories, plans and possibilities. It's the language of the arts, the emotions and, most important, the deeper self."

A small number of people interested in this powerful natural therapy consult health professionals to learn how to do it. But the beauty of visualization is that it's easy to do yourself. Some people follow written directions. Others use self-recorded or prerecorded cassette tapes. All three approaches—professional therapy, written instructions and tapes—produce similar results.

## Beginning Deep Relaxation

Any visualization begins with deep relaxation, similar to the state induced by meditation. The following exercise, based on autogenic training and progressive muscle relaxation (both pioneering relaxation techniques developed during the 1930s), has been adapted from the work of William Fezler, Ph.D., a psychotherapist in Beverly Hills and author of *Total Visualization: Using All Five Senses.*

Begin by practicing this technique for ten minutes one to three times a day.

# Affirmations: Quick Visualizations for Self-Confidence

You're about to face a tax audit or ask the boss for a raise or meet your future in-laws for the first time. You want to feel relaxed, but more important, you need to feel confident. Never fear: affirmations to the rescue.

Affirmations are quick mini-visualizations. They're similar to a form of positive self-talk known as cognitive therapy in that they help correct distorted, self-deprecating thinking. But cognitive therapy is reactive—you catch yourself in negative self-talk and immediately replace it with positive thoughts. Affirmations are more anticipatory.

An affirmation is simply a thought that helps you see yourself in a more positive light—and then act on that vision. Affirmations begin with the word "I," as in "I filled out my tax forms properly." They should be positive: "I make an enormous contribution to this company." They should also be definite—not "I hope I like my daughter's beau" but "My daughter has very good taste in men." Finally, they should focus on the present—not "I'm working to control my temper" but "I can handle any situation without losing my temper."

Here's a list of useful affirmations. If these don't suit your needs, develop your own.

- I am lovable.
- I am patient.
- I am generous.
- I am forgiving.
- I am intelligent.
- I am successful.
- I am self-confident.
- I am strong.
- I am playful.
- I express myself well.
- I enjoy my life.
- I handle money well.
- I feel comfortable on airplanes.
- I use my time wisely.

1. Sit in a comfortable chair with your hands in your lap and your feet on the floor.
2. Fix your eyes on a spot across the room where the wall meets the ceiling.

3. Begin counting slowly from 1 to 100.

4. As you count from 1 to 10, breathe slowly and deeply, and focus on your eyelids. Tell yourself, "My eyelids feel very heavy. They are getting *heavier* and *heavier* every moment, and the more weighty they become, the more deeply relaxed I feel. My eyes feel so heavy that by the time I reach 10, I'll be forced to close them."

5. Continue the exercise with your eyes closed.

6. From 11 to 20, focus on how tightly your eyes are shut: "My eyes are locked. My eyelids are so *heavy* that I couldn't lift them even if I wanted to."

7. From 21 to 30, concentrate on your toes. Feel them grow heavy and relaxed: "My toes feel so heavy that I couldn't move them if I tried."

8. Take a moment to return your attention to your eyelids and experience how heavy, tightly shut and relaxed they feel.

9. Then return to your toes and notice how relaxed they feel.

10. From 31 to 40, follow the relaxed heaviness in your toes as it rises to engulf your legs.

11. Take a moment to check in with your eyelids and toes, and at every subsequent step feel how every body part you have previously relaxed becomes even more so. Then return to the part you're working on, in this case, your legs, and feel them become numb, heavy and completely relaxed.

12. From 41 to 50, focus on your fingers and hands.

13. From 51 to 60, concentrate on your arms.

14. From 61 to 70, direct your attention to your pelvis and abdomen.

15. From 71 to 80, focus on your chest.

16. From 81 to 90, concentrate on your shoulders and neck.

17. From 91 to 100, relax your face.

18. Then feel yourself moving into a state of deeper and deeper relaxation.

19. Finally, count to 3, telling yourself: "When I reach 3, I will open my eyes and feel completely relaxed and totally refreshed as though I've just awakened from a great night's sleep."

Practice this deep relaxation training for a week or two until you can ease into it comfortably whenever you want to. This exercise also contains a beginning visualization component, the idea that your body is getting heavy. Once you feel comfortable with this mini-visualization, you're ready for a more elaborate visualization exercise.

## Beginning Visualization: The Beach

Dr. Fezler developed this visualization to help relieve anxiety.

Enter the state of deep relaxation that you've been practicing. Now, in your mind's eye, see yourself walking along a beach at five o'clock on a July afternoon. It's hot but not as oppressive as it was a few hours ago, before the thunderstorm. The rain washed everything clean and now the air smells crisp and fresh. The sun is sinking toward the horizon but has not yet begun to set. It's a blazing yellow, framed against a brilliant blue sky. You can feel its warmth on your face and arms.

You are barefoot. With every step, your toes dig into hot, dry sand. You stroll to the water's edge. The hot, dry, yielding sand becomes cool, wet and firm.

About 40 yards out, huge blue-green waves break into a carpet of white foam that slides shoreward and laps at your toes, tickling them. The steady crash of the waves is punctuated by the shrieks of seagulls wheeling overhead and the murmur of a pleasant breeze.

You walk toward the sinking sun, reveling in its warmth as it turns from yellow to orange. You climb a sand dune. Your feet dig in for each step and get covered up to your ankles. The top of the dune is covered with soft, low-growing pink, white and yellow flowers. You gaze out to sea. The water is calm—God's mirror—and the sun's reflection shines pure silver.

The sun begins to set. The sky turns orange, then red, crimson, scarlet, gold, amber and finally purple. You're engulfed in the warm purple haze of twilight. You look up and see thousands of stars. They call to you. You inhale deeply and taste the warm, salty air. The starlight grows brighter. You float upward toward it and merge into the oneness of the Universe.

## Visualizations for Specific Health Concerns

Because visualizations like The Beach are deeply relaxing, they can help minimize stress-related medical conditions. Dr. Fezler has used The Beach successfully to help clients with chronic pain, phobias, stuttering, sex problems and drug abuse.

But what if you have a specific illness? Then visualizations typically focus on the organ, system or body part that's affected.

A 24-year-old man with serious asthma consulted Dr. Rossman, hoping to use imagery to reduce his need for medication. Dr. Rossman taught him basic relaxation and imagery skills and then suggested a specific image—envisioning his bronchial tubes and lungs as relaxed and wide open, with air moving through them freely.

The man practiced this visualization for 20 minutes twice a day. "Soon," Dr. Rossman says, "he decreased his drug dosage, and as he became adept at visualization, he was able to go for months without an asthma attack."

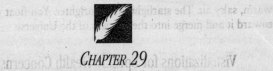

## CHAPTER 29

# VITAMINS AND MINERALS

## The New Science of Sensible Supplementation

**M**ention "vitamins" and "science" in the same breath, and the name that immediately springs to mind is Linus Pauling, Ph.D. The iconoclastic Palo Alto, California, chemist spent more than 20 years before his death in 1994 touting the benefits of enormous doses of vitamin C for everything from the common cold to cancer.

Dr. Pauling may be gone, but his legacy lives on. He was the only person ever to win two unshared Nobel Prizes—for chemistry in 1954 and the Peace Prize in 1962 for work promoting disarmament. The journal *New Scientist* once included him along with Albert Einstein, Charles Darwin and Isaac Newton as one of the 20 greatest scientists who ever lived. But in 1970, when Dr. Pauling's book, *Vitamin C and the Common Cold*, appeared, his scientific admirers became flabbergasted. At the time, the entire medical profession agreed that given a reasonable diet, vitamins were completely unnecessary and therefore marketers of supplements were hucksters. How could the great Dr. Pauling have become a vitamin nut?

Dr. Pauling not only flouted the scientific consensus on vitamins, he also violated protocol by taking his case directly to the public instead of confining his opinions to the research journals. Most of his colleagues ridiculed him as a crackpot.

# Sweet Vindication

Linus Pauling lived long enough to enjoy a hearty last laugh. When he died at age 93, he'd outlived scores of his critics, and studies done since the 1970s have largely vindicated his views on vitamin C—though not his advocacy of taking up to 18,000 milligrams a day. Thousands of physicians who once scoffed at supplements now take large doses of vitamins A, C and E themselves to prevent cancer and heart disease, and increasingly, they advise their patients to do the same.

When Dr. Pauling was diagnosed with prostate cancer in 1991, some of his critics seized on his illness as proof that his vitamin regimen does not prevent cancer. But Dr. Pauling never said that supplements conferred immortality. He simply said that they significantly postpone cancer, heart disease and other serious conditions while extending the healthy life span. They certainly seem to have done so in his case (not to mention that physicians consider prostate cancer virtually inevitable in men over 90).

Though Dr. Pauling lived to see his views on supplements become mainstream, several years before his death the spotlight of supplement notoriety turned from him to another researcher across San Francisco Bay. Gladys Block, Ph.D., a mother of two grown children, worked at the National Cancer Institute (NCI) for nine years before moving to the University of California at Berkeley School of Public Health in 1992 to become a professor of epidemiology and nutrition.

Dr. Block is soft-spoken, not at all as flamboyant as Dr. Pauling was. "Pauling was provocative," she reflects. "He urged people to take 18,000 milligrams of vitamin C. I take 2,000 to 3,000. He's written books for the public. I've stayed within the scientific literature. And I've been very careful to appear rational to the scientific community, to move people along at a pace they can handle."

In early 1992, Dr. Block moved quite a few researchers along with a major review of nearly 200 previous studies correlating diet with rates of most major cancers (lung, breast, colon, cervical, ovarian, bladder, oral, throat, pancreatic, prostate and stomach). Every single study showed that those who consumed large amounts of fresh fruits and vegetables were less likely to develop cancer than those who did not. Compared with those who consumed the most fruits and vegetables, those who ate the least had twice the cancer risk. Why?

"Antioxidants," Dr. Block explains. "Fruits and vegetables are high in antioxidant nutrients, notably vitamins A, C and E. These nutrients play a key role in preventing the oxidative damage we now know contributes to both cancer and heart disease. I think antioxidant nutrients are profoundly important in reducing risk of these diseases." (We'll get to how supplements fit into this picture in just a moment.)

"Antioxidants" and "oxidative damage" may sound like a mouthful, but the science behind Dr. Block's assertions is not difficult to understand. It all begins with oxygen, which is absolutely essential to life. As oxygen circulates throughout the body, fueling our cells, some oxygen molecules lose an electron and become highly reactive—and chemically unstable. These altered oxygen molecules are known as ions or free radicals. To regain stability, they snatch electrons from other molecules, damaging them. This is oxidative damage.

Over time, this damage can alter DNA, the body's repository of genetic information, and lead to cancer. Oxidative damage also plays a major role in the buildup of atherosclerotic plaques, the deposits that narrow arteries, restrict blood flow and trigger heart attack. Normal biological processes produce a certain number of free radicals, but more are produced by exposure to things like cigarette smoke and toxic chemicals. Vitamins A, C and E come to the rescue by graciously donating electrons to these free radicals so they don't have to steal them from the body's cells. That's how these vitamins protect the body from oxidative damage.

## Antioxidants to the Rescue

Scientific understanding of antioxidants has evolved slowly over the last 15 years. The fine points remain controversial, but researchers now generally agree on the big picture. That picture came into sharper focus in 1993 when three large studies persuaded most remaining scientific skeptics that antioxidant nutrients are indeed critical to the prevention of cancer and heart disease.

One was a population study sponsored by the NCI involving 30,000 residents of a province in north-central China. The province was selected because it has one of the world's highest rates of esophageal and stomach cancer. Participants in the study took either a daily placebo (blank pill) or one of several possible supplement combinations. Five years later, the placebo group and all but one of the supplement groups had experienced no change in deaths from these two cancers. But in one supplement group, the death rate declined 13 percent. That group had taken a combination of vitamin E, beta-carotene (a form of vitamin A) and the trace mineral selenium—all antioxidants.

The other two studies, both by Harvard researchers, tested vitamin E for prevention of heart disease. One study tracked 39,000 male health professionals for four years. Those whose diets included the most vitamin E developed the least heart disease—36 percent less than those who consumed the least vitamin E. In addition, those who took a supplement containing 100 international units of vitamin E for at least two years were 37 percent less likely to develop heart disease than those who took no supplement.

The other study tracked 87,000 female nurses for eight years. Compared with those whose diets provided the least vitamin E, those who consumed the most were 34 percent less likely to develop heart disease. And compared with the nurses who took no vitamin E supplement, those who took 100 international units daily for two years were 41 percent less likely to develop heart disease.

The 100 international units of vitamin E used in the two Harvard studies is seven times the Food and Drug Administration's (FDA) Recommended Dietary Allowance (RDA) for vitamin E (15 international units). For years, most physicians have talked themselves hoarse telling the public that it's unwise—and possibly dangerous—to consume more than the RDA of any nutrient. Yet soon after the Harvard studies were published, thousands of doctors who once scoffed at "megadoses" were themselves taking 100 to 400 international units of vitamin E—up to 25 times the RDA—and recommending it to their patients with heart disease as well.

Over the last few years, a growing number of physicians and nutritionists have come to accept—in fact, endorse—supplements. This represents a profound shift in mainstream medicine's view of this popular natural approach to optimal health. Gone are the days when physicians and most nutritionists argued that a balanced diet provided all the necessary nutrients and that supplements were at best a waste of money and at worst a cynical fraud.

"The problem with that belief," Dr. Block explains, "is that most Americans don't eat a balanced diet. Large segments of the population, rich and poor, don't get 100 percent of the RDAs. Besides, as far as many scientists, myself included, are concerned, the RDAs for many nutrients are set way too low."

Even before Dr. Block's study showing that fresh fruits and vegetables protect against cancer, the NCI was urging Americans to "strive for five"—five servings of fresh fruits and vegetables every day. Unfortunately, surveys show that only about 9 percent of Americans get their five, and a recent one-day analysis of the diets of 12,000 Americans showed that 41 percent ate no fruit at all and only 25 percent ate a fruit or vegetable rich in the antioxidant vitamins A or C.

Dr. Block counts herself and her children among those who don't always eat five servings of fresh fruits and vegetables a day. "I get three or four," she says, "five if I focus on it, but sometimes I don't. And I know my sons don't get five a day. It's not terribly difficult to get your five—fruit in your cereal at breakfast, a salad for lunch, one fruit snack a day and a salad and vegetable with dinner. But unfortunately, Americans don't eat that way."

Instead, millions of Americans wake up to scrambled eggs, grab a burger for lunch, snack on potato chips and have pizza for dinner. In addition, about one-quarter of the population smokes, about one-third are dieting at any given moment, and everything from alcohol to birth control pills robs the body of essential nutrients. Dr. Block urges everyone to strive for five, but she's also a pragmatist who understands that it simply isn't happening.

How can Americans fill the nutritional gap that might save them from premature death from cancer and heart disease? "Supplements," Dr. Block says. "They're a safe, convenient, inexpensive way to get the nutrients most Americans aren't getting from food."

Dr. Block is by no means alone in this opinion. "Oxidative damage is a major mechanism of destruction in many diseases," says Sheldon Saul Hendler, M.D., Ph.D., assistant clinical professor of medicine at the University of California, San Diego, and author of *The Doctor's Vitamin and Mineral Encyclopedia*. "Antioxidants aren't just 'supplements' anymore. They're rapidly becoming the cutting edge of medicine."

"The scientific journals are filled with studies showing the benefits of antioxidants," says Shari Lieberman, Ph.D., a clinical nutritionist in New York City and co-author (with Nancy Bruning) of *The Real Vitamin and Mineral Book*. "I don't know anyone familiar with the scientific literature on antioxidants who doesn't take them."

## RDAs, Megadoses and Supplement Safety

Supplement critics have spent a great deal of energy wringing their hands over the alleged toxicity of vitamins and minerals. Let's debunk that myth right away. The American Association of Poison Control Centers reported that in one five-year period, the total number of accidental fatalities from legal, FDA-approved prescription and over-the-counter drugs was 1,132. The total number from supplements during the same five-year period was 0—that's right, zero, nada, zilch. Since that time there have been a couple of fatalities—5 deaths among children who took large doses of iron supplements that were left out by parents unaware of their potential toxicity.

"Extremely large doses of some supplements, such as iron and vitamin D, can cause problems," Dr. Block says, "but by and large, supplements are safe, even at doses substantially above the RDA."

The myth is that the RDAs are the gold standard of nutrition—get 100 percent of the RDAs for all the vitamins and minerals that have them and you're covered. In fact, current RDAs are extremely controversial. Growing numbers of scientists say they're too low and should be increased, in some cases substantially.

The first RDAs were established in 1943 by the Food and Nutrition Board of the National Academy of Sciences (NAS). At the time the RDAs were defined as "the intake of essential nutrients . . . adequate to meet the known needs of practically every healthy person." But the nutritional needs of, say, a pregnant woman are different from those of a 75-year-old man, so the RDAs were further divided into categories that reflect age, gender, pregnancy and nursing a baby. In the early 1970s, when the FDA introduced its first attempt at nutritional food labeling, the agency selected the highest level for each nutrient in the 1968 edition of the RDAs to create its own standard, the U.S. Recommended Daily Allowances (USRDAs).

In 1994, the FDA revised its nutrition labeling program and replaced the USRDAs with Daily Values (DVs) for vitamins, minerals and other nutrients. Food labels now state the percentage of the DV for selected vitamins and minerals, such as vitamins A and C, iron and calcium.

The RDAs have been updated periodically, most recently in 1989, but recent updating attempts have been fraught with controversy. Traditional NAS scientists say the RDAs should remain more or less where they have been, at levels that prevent nutrient-deficiency diseases such as scurvy, beriberi and rickets. But a growing number of scientists say they should be raised to a level Dr. Lieberman calls the optimal daily requirement—the levels the latest studies show help prevent cancer, heart disease and other health problems.

As recently as 1987, the American Dietetic Association

## What the Experts Take

Ever wonder which vitamins and minerals all those scientific researchers and experts actually take? Here are the answers.

Gladys Block, Ph.D., professor of epidemiology and public health nutrition at the University of California at Berkeley School of Public Health. "I take a daily multivitamin and mineral supplement plus 2,000 to 3,000 milligrams of vitamin C, 400 international units of vitamin E and 1,000 milligrams of calcium."

Sheldon Saul Hendler, M.D., Ph.D., assistant clinical professor of medicine at the University of California, San Diego, and author of *The Doctor's Vitamin and Mineral Encyclopedia*. "Every day I take an inexpensive multivitamin/mineral insurance formula containing all of the 11 vitamins and 7 minerals for which there are RDAs. My supplement contains 100 percent of the RDA or a little more. In addition, I also take 400 international units of vitamin E for prevention of heart attack."

Shari Lieberman, Ph.D., a clinical nutritionist in New York City and co-author (with Nancy Bruning) of *The Real Vitamin and Mineral Handbook*. "I take a daily multivitamin/mineral supplement containing 5,000 international units of vitamin A, 50,000 international units of beta-carotene, 50 milligrams of the B vitamins (except for 1,000 milligrams of niacin), 3,000 milligrams of vitamin C, 400 international units of vitamins D and E, 1,000 milligrams of calcium, 150 micrograms of iodine, 25 milligrams of iron, 500 milligrams of magnesium, 25 milligrams of manganese, 200 micrograms of selenium and 50 milligrams of zinc."

(ADA) maintained the traditional view. An ADA publication at that time insisted: "The RDAs represent the best current assessment of safe and adequate intakes. There are no demonstrated benefits of supplementation beyond these allowances." But in July 1993, at a hearing convened by the NAS Food and Nutrition Board to solicit expert opinions on the next round of RDA revisions, ADA president Susan Calvert Finn, R.D., spoke in

David Sobel, M.D., regional director of patient education and health promotion for the Kaiser Permanente health maintenance organization in Oakland, California. "I take a multivitamin and mineral supplement, plus 20,000 international units of beta-carotene, 1,500 milligrams of vitamin C and 400 international units of vitamin E."

Bonnie Liebman, director of nutrition at the Center for Science in the Public Interest in Washington, D.C. "I'm nursing a baby these days, so I'm taking a multivitamin and mineral supplement in consultation with my physician. After I wean my baby, I plan to take an adult insurance formula and probably additional antioxidants."

Trish Ratto, R.D., coordinator of Health Matters, the University of California at Berkeley wellness program for faculty and staff. "I hate pills and can't get them down, so no, I don't take vitamins. I did when I was pregnant, but it was a struggle. Of course, I understand the value of antioxidants, so I'm very good about eating fresh fruits and vegetables. I eat more than five servings a day, including lots of cantaloupe just about every day. It's packed with vitamin A."

The late Linus Pauling, Ph.D., who was president of the Linus Pauling Institute for Medicine, Palo Alto, California. In the years before his death, Dr. Pauling was taking the regimen recommended in his 1986 book *How to Live Longer and Feel Better:* a daily insurance formula plus 15 milligrams of beta-carotene, 18,000 milligrams of vitamin C and 800 international units of vitamin E.

favor of raising many RDAs considerably—to the levels shown to prevent cancer in the Chinese study and heart attack in the two Harvard studies.

"Supplement conservatives continue to warn the public against taking more than 100 percent of the DVs, as if those figures represent the upper boundary of safe consumption," Dr. Block says. "But they don't. With some nutrients—the antioxidants, for example—it's clearly better for the public health for people to take much more."

But how much more? No one knows for sure, which is why supplementation continues to be controversial. But as a guide to optimal nutrition, the DVs look more like *minimum* daily requirements. "Take vitamin C," Dr. Block explains. "The DV is 60 milligrams a day. But studies of early human diets show that our ancestors probably consumed close to 300 milligrams a day, and people who follow the NCI's 'strive for five' recommendations can easily consume up to 500 milligrams. So we have one government agency, the NCI, in effect recommending an intake of vitamin C eight times higher than what traditionalists at the NAS and FDA consider the maximum safe amount. It's time the traditionalists looked beyond scurvy and considered nutrients' role in preventing the diseases we're dying of today. The research is there, and it's compelling."

To its credit, the FDA now allows supplement labels to state that consumption well above the RDA helps prevent osteoporosis and that large doses of folic acid help prevent neural tube birth defects, serious malformations of the spine and brain. In addition, as this book is written, the FDA seems to be warming up to approving large doses of beta-carotene and vitamins C and E for prevention of cancer and heart disease. Currently the RDAs and DVs remain unchanged, however, which leaves many consumers confused about the safe limits of sensible supplementation.

For an overview of how supplements can help treat individual conditions and diseases, see "Prevention and Treatment with Supplements" on page 474.

## Taking Supplements without Getting Taken

Walk down the supplement aisle at most health food stores, pharmacies and, increasingly, supermarkets, and it's almost impossible not to feel overwhelmed by the dozens—sometimes hundreds—of brands and combinations. Should you select a multivitamin/mineral combination (known in the trade as a multi) or a dozen bottles of single-nutrient supplements or a multi plus a few additional singles? Should you buy natural supplements or synthetic? Regular or timed-release? A store brand or a national brand? Tablets or capsules? Regular minerals or chelated? Less than 100 percent of the RDA, 100 percent, or more, and if so, how much more? Energy formula? Stress formula? Women's formula or men's?

David Sobel, M.D., regional director of patient education and director of the regional education department at Kaiser Permanente Medical Care Program of Northern California, takes supplements daily, but he hates buying them. "It's such a hassle," he sighs, "so many brands, so many combinations."

Dr. Sobel's sentiments probably ring true to most of the 70 percent of Americans—some 175 million people—who take supplements at least occasionally.

"The selection is huge," says Bonnie Liebman, director of nutrition at the Center for Science in the Public Interest (CSPI) in Washington, D.C., a consumer advocacy organization that specializes in food and nutrition issues. "The choices are confusing. And few consumers know much about what they're buying. As a result, they often spend much more than necessary for supplements that may not meet their needs."

Fortunately, you can take supplements without getting taken. Here's what the experts advise.

**Think food first.** Supplements absolutely, positively do not replace food, and they cannot undo the damage caused by a chronically poor diet. "Before you buy supplements," Dr. Block advises, "fill your shopping cart with fresh fruits and vegetables—and eat them. Buy organic produce if you like. But the data clearly show that any fresh fruits and vegetables help prevent cancer. Get your five servings a day, and then take your supplements as extra added wellness insurance."

**Forget brand names.** All vitamins are essentially the same. "Only about a half-dozen drug companies, such as Hoffmann La Roche, actually make vitamins," Dr. Hendler explains. "They supply all the hundreds of companies that sell them. What you're paying for is basically packaging and advertising. Personally, I buy the cheapest vitamins I can find. They're just as good as the expensive brands."

**With three exceptions, ignore the word "natural."** Chemically, there's no difference between the vitamin C (ascorbic acid) in an orange or a red pepper and vitamin C synthesized in a laboratory. Some "natural" vitamins are extracted from plants, such as vitamin C from rose hips. But frequently packagers mix a tiny amount of a natural vitamin with a large amount of the synthetic and market the combination as "natural."

The three exceptions to this rule involve vitamin E, folic acid and calcium. Natural vitamin E (d-alpha-tocopherol) is absorbed better than the synthetic vitamin (dl-alpha-tocopherol). If the label says "with d-alpha," you may wind up with a tiny amount of the natural vitamin mixed with lots of the synthetic. Select a supplement that contains only d-alpha.

As for folic acid and calcium, *avoid* natural forms and go with the synthetic. Synthetic folic acid is more easily absorbed. And natural calcium may actually be hazardous. Natural calcium sources include bone meal and dolomite, both of which may be contaminated with lead, a highly toxic heavy metal that impairs thinking and can cause mental retardation in children. Calcium carbonate, a laboratory creation, is the way to go.

**Don't get taken in by hype.** Want more energy? Stress management? Sexual ecstasy? Longevity? Immune enhancement? Freedom from illness? Some supplement labels promise their products can do everything except raise the dead—and maybe that too, if you take enough.

Biochemically, vitamins and minerals play important roles in virtually every body system and process. So yes, they are involved in energy production, stress reactions, sexual enjoyment and everything else. But by themselves, supplements don't eliminate fatigue, alleviate stress or make you a great lover. Some supplements can help prevent and treat specific medical conditions, but brands that claim to keep you young, beautiful, energetic, mellow and sexy offer more hype than hope.

**Ignore the bells and whistles.** Don't fall for claims of "newly discovered" vitamins. There aren't any. (New discover-

ies won't be announced on labels from obscure vitamin manufacturers.) Don't pay more for supplements that claim to be
sugar-free or starch-free. Unless you're on a severely restricted
diet, the little bit of sugar and starch in some supplements
doesn't matter.

Don't pay extra for "chelated" (*KEY-lated*) minerals. Chelation combines minerals with other substances, often amino
acids. Proponents claim that chelation increases the amount of
the minerals that actually gets absorbed into the bloodstream.
They call this increased absorption rate bioavailability. Technically, the claim may be true, but ordinary minerals are absorbed just fine and don't need any help to get into your
bloodstream.

Unless a health professional advises otherwise, steer clear of
timed-release supplements. Timed-release products may not provide the steady flow of nutrients users expect. In some cases,
they can even cause problems. Timed-release niacin can be far
more toxic to the liver, for example, than the standard niacin
supplement. Besides, it's usually cheaper to take a few pills a day
than one timed-release supplement.

**Make sure the pills dissolve.** Look for a dissolution statement on the label. To do any good, supplements must dissolve
completely in the digestive tract. Some don't.

Many vitamin companies claim that their supplements offer
"guaranteed bioavailability" and "complete absorption." Possibly they do, but then again, maybe not. How can you tell for
sure?

Recently the U.S. Pharmacopoeia (USP), the organization
that sets the nation's drug-composition standards, adopted a
voluntary supplement-dissolution standard saying that vitamins
should disintegrate in the digestive tract within 45 minutes.
Look for a label statement like the one Leiner Health Products
uses on the store brands it formulates for Safeway, Kmart and
Wal-Mart, among others: "This product is specially formulated
to pass a rigid 45-minute laboratory dissolution test." *Dissolution* means "dissolve." *Disintegration* means "break into tiny
pieces." Forty-five-minute dissolution is what you want.

**Look for an expiration date.** "An expiration date is no guarantee of freshness, but it suggests that the packager understands that vitamins have a finite shelf life," says dietitian Trish Ratto, R.D., coordinator of Health Matters, the faculty and staff wellness program at the University of California at Berkeley. Steer clear of supplements within six to nine months of their expiration dates. They've probably been in the bottle for several years and may be past their prime.

**Start with an "insurance formula."** Multivitamin/mineral supplements—sometimes called insurance formulas—contain some of every vitamin and mineral. They're convenient and economical. They take up less shelf space than a dozen bottles of single-nutrient supplements. And it's easier to swallow one pill than a dozen. In addition, compared with taking a few single-supplement nutrients, insurance formulas are better for you.

"Few people understand that vitamins and minerals work together synergistically," Dr. Lieberman explains. "The whole is greater than the sum of the parts. Nature packages nutrients together in foods, and it's best to take them that way in supplements. Unfortunately, medicine has a long history of looking for 'magic bullets,' and this has carried over to supplementation, with people looking for the one magic nutrient that supposedly helps solve their problems. The big ones now are vitamin E to prevent heart disease and calcium to prevent osteoporosis. But by themselves, vitamin E and calcium are not enough. Vitamin E works better if you take it along with vitamin C. Take calcium alone and bone loss slows. But take calcium with vitamin D, manganese, zinc and copper, and you get increased bone mass. I always advise people to start with an insurance formula and then take additional supplements if they need them to treat or prevent specific conditions."

In addition, some minerals compete with each other. Iron interferes with the body's ability to absorb zinc. Zinc interferes with copper absorption. Your best bet is an insurance formula that contains all the essential minerals.

**Supplement your insurance formula.** Insurance formulas have breadth but possibly not enough depth for your personal needs. If you have a family history of cancer or heart disease, you may want to take larger doses of antioxidants. In addition, some minerals are simply too bulky to fit into a single pill. The optimal daily requirement for calcium is 1,000 to 1,500 milligrams a day, but it's impossible to get that much from an insurance formula. Magnesium is also too bulky to fit into a single pill. Women of childbearing age should take 400 micrograms of folic acid to reduce the risk of neural tube birth defects, but insurance formulas may not provide that much.

**Look for beta-carotene instead of vitamin A.** The body converts beta-carotene into vitamin A, so for all practical purposes, they're the same thing. However, long-term use of vitamin A at doses above 50,000 international units a day may cause problems. Beta-carotene is nontoxic even at high doses, so stick to that. Beware of labels that say vitamin A "with" beta-carotene. If the label doesn't specify, you can't be sure how much of each you're getting.

**Look for at least 25 micrograms of biotin.** Biotin is the most expensive vitamin, and many packagers skimp on it. Biotin content is a quick, easy way to compare insurance formula pricing. Buy the cheapest one that contains adequate biotin.

**Go easy on the iron.** Unless your physician advises otherwise, don't take more than 100 percent of the RDA for iron. People with iron-deficiency anemia and women with unusually heavy menstrual flow may need more than 100 percent, but most people don't. At high doses, iron can cause problems. In addition, a recent study suggests that high blood levels of iron may increase risk of heart disease. Yet some supplements contain several times the RDA.

**Take care with calcium.** Different calcium compounds have different levels of bioavailability. Calcium carbonate is 40 percent calcium, but other forms of calcium contain considerably less. Look for the words *calcium* or *elemental calcium* on the label.

**Check for selenium.** For years some researchers have touted this trace mineral as a cancer preventive. That view gained considerable credence when the NCI's study in China showed that it helped prevent deaths from esophageal and stomach cancer.

**Vegan vegetarians may need extra B12.** If you consume no animal products, you may become deficient in vitamin B12. This deficiency can damage the nervous system, so make sure your supplement contains at least the DV for B12.

**Keep supplements away from children.** This is especially true for iron, often taken to treat iron-deficiency anemia or iron loss from heavy menstrual flow. Although iron—and supplements in general—are safe for most adults at the optimal daily requirement, it takes only a few tablets of a high-potency iron supplement to kill a child. An estimated 5,000 children swallow toxic doses of iron supplements every year; a few die. In the typical case, an adult carelessly leaves iron supplements on a bathroom or kitchen counter. Don't do this.

**Watch your wallet.** Ten dollars a month should do it. "If you pay more than $10 a month for your supplements," CSPI's Liebman says, "you're paying too much."

## Prevention and Treatment with Supplements

As the physician trade journal *Medical World News* editorialized not too long ago: "Vitamins aren't just supplements anymore. They're emerging as disease-fighters."

Supplement therapy by itself is rarely sufficient to treat illness, but it may be used in addition to standard medical care. If you have any of the conditions listed below, consult your physician about the advisability of taking supplements therapeutically. Here's a summary of the latest findings.

*AIDS.* In one study done at the University of California at Berkeley School of Public Health, researchers looked at the progression to AIDS in men who tested positive for HIV, the virus that causes AIDS. Some of these men ate poorly, while others ate a diet high in fresh fruits and vegetables. Over six years, those in the good-diet group were significantly less likely to progress to AIDS. Iron, the B vitamins and vitamins C and E were particularly protective.

These results were confirmed by another study. A researcher at Johns Hopkins University in Baltimore analyzed diet and supplement diaries kept by 281 men who had tested positive for HIV. The diaries had been kept for up to almost seven years. Compared with men who had a low intake of vitamins A and C, thiamin (B1) and niacin, those with a moderate to large intake had 40 percent less risk of progressing to full-blown AIDS.

*Allergies.* When the body produces histamine, the result is the nasal symptoms of hay fever or the welts of hives. That's why antihistamines are prescribed to treat allergies. In one study, a researcher at the Food and Nutrition Laboratory of Arizona State University in Tempe gave people with hay fever daily vitamin C supplementation (2,000 milligrams). Their histamine production dropped 38 percent.

*Alzheimer's disease.* In one study, 30 people with early Alzheimer's took either a placebo or a combination of zinc (90 milligrams), selenium (2 milligrams) and evening primrose oil (6 grams). After 20 weeks, the supplement group scored significantly better on a battery of mental-function tests.

*Arthritis.* In one study, a group of 189 people with arthritis were given a standard anti-inflammatory medication. Some were also given a daily supplement containing thiamin (100 milligrams), vitamin B6 (100 milligrams) and vitamin B12 (0.5 milligram). After just seven days, those in the supplement group reported significantly less pain.

*Autism.* For 30 weeks, researchers at the University of Alabama in Birmingham gave a daily vitamin C supplement (1,000 milligrams per 20 pounds of body weight) to 18 children with autism. Compared with untreated children, the vitamin-takers exhibited significantly less autistic pacing, rocking and spinning.

*Bladder cancer.* In one study, 65 people with bladder cancer were given standard therapy. Half also received two daily doses of vitamin A (40,000 international units), vitamin B6 (100 milligrams), vitamin C (2,000 milligrams) and vitamin E (400 international units). Almost two years later, tumors recurred in 80 percent of those given standard therapy but in only 40 percent of those who took the supplements. Average survival time was 19 months in the standard-therapy group and 33 months in the vitamin group.

*Breast cancer.* Eating foods rich in vitamin A—among them carrots, cantaloupe and spinach—reduces risk of breast cancer, according to Harvard researchers. They surveyed the diets of 87,000 nurses and analyzed their breast cancer incidence eight years later. The women who consumed less than 6,600 international units of vitamin A a day showed 20 percent increased risk.

*Cervical cancer.* Folic acid appears to offer some protection against cervical cancer because it reduces risk of infection by the human papillomavirus, according to C. E. Sutterworth, Jr., M.D., professor in the Department of Nutrition Sciences at the University of Alabama in Birmingham. This virus is strongly associated with cervical cancer.

*Colon cancer.* Researchers have been following the diets of 26,000 health professionals for many years. They've discovered a link between colon cancer risk and folic acid consumption. Compared with those who consumed the least folic acid, those who consumed the most developed colon cancer one-third less frequently.

*The common cold.* Several studies by Elliot Dick, Ph.D., chief of the Respiratory Viruses Laboratory at the University of Wisconsin in Madison show that taking 500 milligrams of vitamin C four times a day (a total dose of 2,000 milligrams) significantly reduces the duration and severity of cold symptoms. Another study showed that sucking on zinc gluconate lozenges (one 24-milligram lozenge every two hours, up to eight a day) also significantly reduced the duration and severity of cold symptoms.

*Depression.* In a four-week study of depressed elderly people at the University of Arizona in Tucson, researchers gave everyone participating in the study a standard antidepressant medication. Half of the group also took daily supplements of thiamin (ten milligrams), riboflavin (ten milligrams) and B6 (ten milligrams). Compared with people who took only the antidepressant, the vitamin group showed less depression and experienced improved functioning.

*Fibromyalgia.* Fibromyalgia is a form of arthritis that causes tenderness at various points around the body, plus other symptoms. Researcher Abraham Guy, M.D., of Torrance, California, gave 15 people with fibromyalgia either a daily placebo or a supplement containing magnesium (300 to 600 milligrams) and malic acid (1,200 to 2,400 milligrams). After eight weeks, the placebo group reported a slight increase in symptoms. The supplement group reported a significant decrease.

*Heart attack survival.* In one study, 460 people hospitalized due to heart attacks received intravenous magnesium for periods ranging from 20 minutes to 72 hours. Compared with 470 who did not receive the mineral, there were 54 percent fewer deaths in the magnesium group.

*Heart disease.* A four-year Harvard study of 39,000 male health professionals showed that compared with those who took no vitamin E supplements, those who took 100 international units a day for two years reduced their heart attack risk by 37 percent. An eight-year Harvard study of 87,000 female nurses showed 49 percent fewer heart attacks.

*High blood pressure.* In a study done at the Medical College of Georgia in Atlanta, 21 people with elevated blood pressure took 1,000 milligrams of supplemental vitamin C every day for four weeks. Their average blood pressure declined significantly.

*High cholesterol.* In a study done at the Division of Cardiovascular Diseases at the Mayo Clinic in Rochester, Minnesota, 47 men and 7 women who were enrolled in the clinic's cardiac rehabilitation program received standard diet and exercise recommendations. Fifty-five men and 8 women received the same information and in addition took a daily 2,000-milligram niacin supplement. After seven months the standard-care group showed no change in total cholesterol, but the vitamin group showed a 9 percent decrease. If you want to take niacin to combat high cholesterol, you should do so only under the supervision of your doctor. Niacin can cause unpleasant side effects, and taking timed-release niacin can damage the liver.

*Immune enhancement and infection resistance.* In a yearlong study at Memorial University of Newfoundland, healthy people over 65 received either a daily placebo supplement or a multivitamin/mineral containing 100 percent of most RDAs and about 400 percent of the RDAs for vitamin E and beta-carotene.

Compared with those taking the placebo, the supplement group showed significantly enhanced immune function, half as many illness days (23 versus 48) and significantly fewer days on antibiotics (18 versus 32).

*Low birthweight and preterm delivery.* Both preterm delivery and low birthweight increase the risk of infant mortality and other medical problems. Researchers at the University of Medicine and Dentistry in Camden, New Jersey, evaluated zinc consumption in 818 pregnant women. Those with the lowest zinc intake (less than six milligrams a day), had twice the risk of delivering babies with low birthweight and three times the risk of preterm delivery.

*Lung cancer.* In addition to standard chemotherapy, Finnish researchers gave people with lung cancer a daily supplement containing vitamin A, beta-carotene, vitamin E, thiamine, riboflavin, vitamin B6, vitamin B12, niacinamide, vitamin D, vitamin C, calcium, manganese, magnesium, zinc, copper, selenium, chromium and potassium. Nutritional therapy significantly reduced the side effects of chemotherapy and radiation, and compared with those who took no supplements, those who did survived significantly longer. If you're undergoing treatment for cancer and would like to take vitamin and mineral supplements, please discuss it with your doctor.

*Infertility.* Zinc deficiency has been associated with fertility impairment. In a study at the University of Rochester Medical Center in New York, 64 infertile men took a daily zinc supplement (400 milligrams) for anywhere from two months to two years. The zinc significantly improved their semen quality.

"Zinc worked for me," Dr. Hendler says. "My wife and I couldn't have children for years because I had poor semen quality. Then I started taking zinc supplements. Within a few months, my wife was pregnant."

*Memory loss.* Under the direction of Dutch researchers, 38 healthy men in their seventies took daily vitamin B6 supplements (20 milligrams) for three months. Compared with untreated men, those who took the vitamin showed improved long-term memory.

*Menstrual discomfort.* Ten women with normal menstrual cycles had their menstrual symptoms evaluated by research psychologists at the U.S. Department of Agriculture's Human Nutrition Research Center in Grand Forks, North Dakota. Then for about six months they took a daily supplement containing calcium (either 587 or 1,336 milligrams) and manganese (either 1 or 6 milligrams). At the higher dose of both minerals, the women experienced significantly less pain, moodiness and water retention.

*Migraine.* Since the mid-1980s, several researchers have suggested that low blood magnesium levels might contribute to migraine risk. Alexander Mauskop, M.D., director of the New York Headache Center in New York City, compared magnesium levels in people who had frequent migraines or tension headaches with those who do not often have headaches. Those who had migraines were twice as likely to have low magnesium levels. Dr. Mauskop suggests that people who get migraines have their magnesium levels tested. If they're low, he advises, they should take a daily supplement.

*Neural tube and other birth defects.* The FDA recently approved folic acid supplementation for pregnant women to prevent spinal malformations and the birth of babies without brains. The Centers for Disease Control and Prevention in Atlanta recommend that all women of childbearing age take 400 micrograms of folic acid a day.

In a study of 4,000 pregnancies, Hungarian researchers showed that combining a folic acid supplement with supplemental vitamin C, copper, manganese and zinc reduced not only the risk of neural tube defects but that of other birth defects as well.

*Oral cancers.* Researchers with the American Health Foundation in New York City compared the diets and supplement use of 400 people with cancers of the mouth and esophagus to a similar number of people who did not have these diseases. They concluded that vitamin E consumption had a significant protective effect against oral cancer, and vitamins C and E had a protective effect against esophageal cancer.

*Osteoporosis.* The FDA already allows the manufacturers of calcium supplements to claim benefits in preventing osteoporosis.

Magnesium also helps, according to Israeli researchers who gave women past the age of menopause 250 to 750 milligrams of the mineral daily for two years. Compared with untreated women, whose bone density declined 1 to 3 percent, bone density in the magnesium group increased 1 to 8 percent.

Vitamin D also apparently has some benefit. A study of 138 elderly women done at Cambridge University in England showed that those with the highest blood levels of vitamin D had the lowest risk of osteoporosis. Vitamin D helps bone tissue absorb calcium.

*Pregnancy-induced hypertension (PIH).* About 10 percent of expectant mothers develop PIH—high blood pressure of pregnancy, a potentially life-threatening condition. In one study of 1,167 pregnant women, those who took 2,000 milligrams of calcium a day had a 30 percent lower risk of PIH than those who did not.

*Retinitis pigmentosa.* This hereditary degenerative eye disease begins with vision impairment at night and progresses to tunnel vision or blindness. In a study done at the Massachusetts Eye and Ear Infirmary in Boston, 600 people with retinitis pigmentosa were divided into two groups. One took a large daily dose of vitamin A (15,000 international units), while the other took only a trace amount. Six years later, the high-A group showed significantly less vision loss.

*Smoking.* Some of the lung damage caused by smoking is oxidative. Danish researchers found that ten days of supplementation with the antioxidant vitamins C and E reduced oxidative lung damage to smokers' lungs by about 50 percent.

*Tinnitus.* Tinnitus, chronic ringing in the ears, is a frustrating condition that doctors have difficulty treating. At the Institute for Noise Hazards Research in Ramat-Gan, Israel, researchers compared people with tinnitus and other forms of hearing impairment. Those with tinnitus were significantly more likely to show low blood levels of vitamin B12. B12 supplementation provided some tinnitus relief for several people in the study.

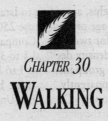

# CHAPTER 30
# WALKING

## Terrific Exercise, One Step at a Time

Our ancestors did not set aside time to exercise. They simply led physically active lives. They walked almost everywhere they went. They also chopped wood, pumped water, gardened and tended farm animals—all activities that involve a great deal of walking.

Walking upright on two legs is a key attribute that separates humanity from other animals. It's no exaggeration to say that walking was humanity's original exercise. But because it was so fundamental, walking was taken for granted. When the ancient Greeks convened the first Olympics, foot races meant running, not walking. The same mindset was still firmly in place more than 2,000 years later during the mid-1970s, when the personal fitness movement was in its infancy. One of the big early fitness books was Jim Fixx's *Complete Book of Running*—not walking.

In just the past few years, walking has finally gained respect—thanks to an avalanche of recent research on the many health benefits to be gained from surprisingly little nonstrenuous exercise. (All this wonderful research is detailed in Exercise, on page 169.)

"Strenuous aerobic workouts are still best to get into optimal cardiovascular condition," explains John Duncan, Ph.D., associate director of the Cooper Institute for Aerobics Research in Dallas. "But to reduce weight, cholesterol and blood pressure and to make you feel better, strenuous workouts are not necessary. Modest exercise programs confer similar benefits—if you make them a regular part of your life." Guess which "modest exercise program" was used in most of these studies. That's right—walking. Humanity's original exercise is still one of the best.

A regular walking program confers an enormous number of physical and psychological benefits, according to health educator Robert K. Cooper, Ph.D., president of the Center for Health and Fitness Excellence in Bemidji, Minnesota, and author of *Health and Fitness Excellence: The Scientific Action Plan.* Walking elevates mood, improves posture, helps treat mild to moderate depression, bolsters self-confidence, helps control stress and anxiety and improves coping abilities. Walking also reduces risk of heart disease, stroke, high blood pressure, obesity and diabetes. It improves recall, reaction time, sleep quality and enjoyment of sex—even resistance to the common cold. Two of the main benefits of walking deserve special mention—weight control and bone building.

## Walk It Off

"The name of the game in weight loss is burning more calories, using up stored fat," says former chemical engineer Rob Sweetgall, author of *Walking Off Weight* and president of Creative Walking, a Clayton, Missouri, organization that helps corporations, schools and hospitals develop fitness walking programs. "Some people think walking isn't a calorie-burner, but they're wrong. With a daily brisk walking program and a low-fat diet, you can burn enough calories to lose weight." In fact, walking often burns as many calories as other activities that seem more strenuous.

For a person of average weight (150 pounds), a game of basketball burns anywhere from 360 to 660 calories an hour. Bicycling at 5 miles per hour burns 240 calories an hour. A game of tennis (doubles) burns 360 calories an hour. On the other hand, a brisk walk (3.5 miles per hour) burns 360, and a fast walk (4 to 5 miles per hour) burns 420 to 480.

"If walking is the way you exercise," Sweetgall says, "the key to weight-loss success is walking for *distance,* not speed. Walking longer distances at a moderate pace is more effective than walking shorter distances more quickly. At a moderate pace, chances are you'll do more walking more often, with fewer injuries. For weight loss, I recommend 45-minute walks seven days a week. Walking three or four days a week, most people can maintain their weight. But to lose weight, it's usually necessary to walk every day."

For weight loss, Sweetgall suggests a "cruising pace." At this pace you move along at 3 to 3.5 miles per hour and you won't feel winded and sore after 45 minutes. If you can't yet walk for 45 minutes all at once, no problem. Three 15-minute walks burn the same number of calories—approximately 270—as a single 45-minute walk. If you walk this much every day, you'll burn about 1,890 calories a week. Each pound of stored fat contains about 3,500 calories, so with this program and a low-fat diet, you should lose about 2 pounds a month, or 24 pounds in a year.

## Shoring Up Brittle Bones

Once past menopause, one out of every four women has osteoporosis—a condition that leads to brittle bones and increased risk of fractures, including hip fractures that may be life-threatening. Osteoporosis strikes both sexes, but it's much more common and severe in women.

Bone is living tissue, and as with other tissue, the body constantly creates new bone to replace bone that has worn out. In those under 35, a well-nourished body replaces all the bone it loses. But after 35, people begin to lose more bone than they naturally replace. The process of bone loss begins slowly and imperceptibly, but it accelerates over time.

Because bone loss begins many years before the first signs of osteoporosis appear, preventive efforts should begin well before age 30. Key elements of osteoporosis prevention include calcium supplementation and regular, weight-bearing exercise, such as walking.

Regardless of calcium intake, weight-bearing exercise—walking, gardening, dancing or anything that puts weight on the hips, knees and ankles—has been shown to increase bone mass and density. In one study, Miriam Nelson, Ph.D., a research scientist at Tufts University in Boston, recruited 36 women in their fifties and sixties and divided them into two groups. Half took brisk 45-minute walks four times a week, the other half did not. She also gave half of each group 800 milligrams of calcium a day. After one year, regardless of their calcium intake, all the walkers increased their spinal bone density by an average of 0.5 percent, compared with a 7 percent loss in spinal bone density for the nonwalkers.

"Even without supplemental calcium," Dr. Nelson says, "walking helps preserve bone. It's an effective way to slow osteoporosis."

## Walking Away from Illness

As if all this weren't enough to make you want to walk every day for the rest of your life, the list goes on. Many people lace up their walking shoes to help them recover from injuries or manage chronic illnesses. Here are a few more of the conditions that walking can help.

*Arthritis.* As part of a study, John Allegrante, Ph.D., associate director of education, epidemiology and health sciences research at the Cornell Multipurpose Arthritis Center at the Hospital for Special Surgery in New York City, recruited 102 people with arthritis of the knees. He assessed how far they could walk before experiencing significant pain. He then placed half the group on a regular walking program.

Eight weeks later, the nonwalkers showed no change in arthritis pain or medication use, and their ability to walk pain-free had deteriorated by an average of 20 yards. The walkers, on the other hand, reported a 27 percent decrease in pain and less medication use. They also experienced a 75-yard *increase* in their pain-free walking ability.

"Regular, moderate exercise is a key element in managing most types of chronic arthritis," explains San Francisco family practitioner Anne Simons, M.D., assistant clinical professor of family and community medicine at the University of California's San Francisco Medical Center and author of *Before You Call the Doctor.* "It gently works the major joints through their range of motion. It helps keep them lubricated. It strengthens bone. And it strengthens the muscles around arthritic joints for better joint support."

If you have arthritis, consult a physician before starting a walking program. For tips on using walking to manage arthritis, contact the Arthritis Foundation, 1314 Spring Street, N.W., Atlanta, GA 30309.

**Back problems.** After Arnold Levick, D.D.S., of Albuquerque, New Mexico, had back surgery, his physician said he could strengthen his back muscles by walking. Dr. Levick, a longtime nonexerciser, was surprised to hear the prescription for exercise. "I thought walking would hurt my back," he explains. Instead, it helped. Dr. Levick started slowly and soon fell in love with walking. After a while, a friend who was a racewalker suggested he try competing. Eventually he earned a place on New Mexico's Senior Olympics racewalking team for his age division (55 to 59). "As for my back," Dr. Levick says, "it's much better."

**Diabetes.** An estimated 12 million Americans have diabetes. It develops if the body either stops producing the hormone insulin or becomes unable to use the insulin it does produce. Without insulin, the body can't process blood sugar (glucose), the cells' main energy source.

There are two types of diabetes: Type I (insulin-dependent), which requires insulin injections, and Type II (non-insulin-dependent), which usually does not. Type II accounts for about 85 percent of diabetes. It can usually be controlled through diet and weight loss.

A ten-year study involving 1,400 people with the disease—the Diabetes Control and Complications Trial, reported in

1993—showed that regular moderate exercise helps control blood glucose levels in both Type I and Type II diabetes. What kind of exercise? The American Diabetes Association (ADA) recommends walking. For more information on walking's benefits, contact the ADA at 1600 Duke Street, Alexandria, VA 22314.

*General healing.* If you have any chronic medical condition, a walking program might help. Discuss the possible benefits with your physician. As long as walking doesn't aggravate your condition, it's almost guaranteed to help because it has antidepressant effects and boosts self-esteem.

*Heart disease.* Walking is a key element in Ornish therapy, the scientifically proven approach to not only managing heart disease but reversing it. "In addition to being good for the heart and circulatory system," explains Dean Ornish, M.D., president of the Preventive Medicine Research Institute in Sausalito, California, "walking can be done in groups. It allows social contact. Social support is another important element of our program." (To learn about Dr. Ornish's full program for reversing heart disease, see Ornish Therapy on page 368.)

*High blood pressure.* Not too long ago, high blood pressure—a risk factor for both heart disease and stroke—was for the most part treated solely with medication. If exercise was recommended, it was only as an aid to weight loss, which helps reduce blood pressure. In severe hypertension, drugs are still necessary, but recent studies have shown that for mild to moderate cases, exercise is beneficial even if people don't lose weight.

"I'd certainly recommend a regular, moderate walking program to anyone with hypertension," says Dr. Duncan.

*Upper body injuries.* Walking is often a good way to stay in shape while recovering from arm, shoulder, neck and other upper-body injuries, according to Dr. Simons. "Walking may also help heal hip, knee, leg and foot injuries," she says, "but it might aggravate them as well. Before beginning a walking program to help treat lower limb conditions, consult your physician."

## Getting Started

Want to tap into all this healing potential, but you aren't quite sure of how to take those first steps? Relax—you can walk even if it's been a while since you've engaged in regular exercise.

"If you think 'exercise' means suffering, try walking," says Mark Fenton of Cohasset, Massachusetts, a five-time member of the U.S. National Racewalking Team and technical editor at *Walking* magazine. "Unlike many other fitness activities, there's nothing yucky about it. You're *already* good at it, and if you become a little more organized about it, walking can be both enjoyable and very good for you."

Here are a few tips to get you started.

**Just do it—but don't overdo it.** Think about your schedule today or tomorrow. Block out 20 to 40 minutes and take a walk. Less is okay to begin with. Walking for health should be enjoyable, not exhausting. Walk at a pace that feels comfortable— don't dawdle, but don't get yourself winded.

Fenton recommends checking your pace with the "talk test": "For noncompetitive fitness walking, you should be able to talk comfortably while walking. If you find yourself gasping for breath as you talk, you're probably pushing yourself too hard."

**Recruit a friend.** Speaking of the talk test, a great way to begin a walking program is to make a walk-date with a friend and have a conversation on the move instead of over coffee.

**Forget about the car.** Another good way to get started is to do an errand on foot instead of in your car. "If you need to carry anything," Fenton advises, "use a backpack to allow your hands and arms to swing freely at your sides. Carrying things by hand is tiring and interferes with the natural rhythm of walking."

With your hands and arms swinging freely at your sides, you can stride more comfortably for longer distances and more time without feeling winded. On your walk, appreciate the little things that are difficult to notice when driving: the warmth of the sun, architectural details, store window displays, the smiles of your neighbors.

**Listen to your body.** For the first few months, after you finish your walks, pay close attention to how you feel. Don't expect the euphoric "athletic high" that more strenuous workouts produce. There's plenty of time to experience that in the future as your walking program progresses. Instead enjoy the interesting combination of pleasant fatigue, invigoration and mood elevation that develops when formerly sedentary people start to become physically active. Assuming you didn't overdo it, your fatigue shouldn't last more than an hour or so, but your feelings of invigoration and emotional uplift should last longer.

As you continue walking and your physical condition improves, you'll feel less fatigue, more invigoration and mood elevation, and eventually an athletic high.

**Progress slowly.** Start by walking every third day for four to six weeks. Then advance to every other day for a month to six weeks. Then progress to walking four or five days for four to six weeks. Finally, move up to walking every day. It's a big mistake to progress too quickly. The body needs time to adjust to an increased level of activity. If it doesn't get the adjustment time it needs, the likelihood of injury increases.

**Chart your progress.** Don't just keep track of your walks in your head. Make a real chart, post it where you can refer to it often and record your progress weekly. Track anything that can be counted: the number of days per week you take walks, the amount of time you spend walking, the number of blocks you can walk in 45 minutes—whatever. When they're progressing the right way—slowly—people often lose track of how far they've come. Charting your progress reminds you and provides a sense of accomplishment that helps walking become a permanent part of your life.

Set modest goals and reward yourself, not with a banana split but with walking-oriented treats—a new pair of walking shoes, some new walking socks or a weekend at a country inn near inviting hiking trails.

**Check your surface.** "There are pluses and minuses for every surface," Sweetgall says. Dirt is soft, which extends shoe life and is good for shock absorption, but it's not as "springy" as harder surfaces, and if it's uneven, you might turn an ankle.

**Refine your technique.** "Many walkers can increase their walking speed and efficiency—and enjoy walking more—with a few simple changes in technique," says Suki Munsell, Ph.D., director of the Dynamic Walking Institute in Corte Madera, California. "Don't march; instead flow forward. Stand tall and roll your foot from heel to toe. It doesn't sound like much, but it makes a big difference."

Grade also affects technique. When walking uphill, Fenton advises, slow down, lean forward and put more energy into your arm swing. When walking downhill, maintain a comfortable speed, take shorter steps and plant your feet gently. "If you slap your feet down, it's hard on your knees and you may develop shin splints," he says. (Shin splints are pains that affect the front of the lower legs.)

**Vary your routine.** After walking regularly for about six months, most people can walk every day without becoming sore or unduly fatigued. Try some different walks: long walks at a moderate pace, shorter walks at a faster pace, walks on flat terrain and walks on hilly terrain. A great way to vary your routine is to leave your home neighborhood and take a walk in a park or anywhere that has beautiful scenery.

## The Sole of Walking Shoes

As fitness activities go, walking is easy on the budget, but it's well worth investing in a good pair of walking shoes. Today, walkers' feet don't have to slip into just any shoes. Walking shoes have been designed to make this sport as comfortable and enjoyable as possible.

"There are many things to look for in a walking shoe," explains Fenton, "but four are at the top of the list—fit, roll, weight and flexibility."

Fit comes first. Buy the color and style you find pleasing, but above all, make sure the shoes fit. Your arch should rest on the shoe's arch. Your heel should be held firmly but comfortably.

And there should be some space between the tips of your toes and the front of the shoe.

Many people, especially women, prefer shoes that make their feet look petite and narrow. As a result they often buy shoes that are too short and narrow. In fact, a study by the American Orthopaedic Foot and Ankle Society showed that 88 percent of women wear shoes that are too small for their feet. That's a one-way ticket to foot problems. Make sure that your toes aren't pressed up against the front of the shoe and that the sides of your shoes don't squeeze your feet.

The "roll" of the shoe will help (or hinder) your walking. The front and rear of the sole should be rounded to encourage a smooth, rolling, heel-to-toe stride. Running shoes often have flat, flared soles at the heel and toe to absorb the shock of runners' foot-strikes. Walking shoes don't need this extra shock absorption and shouldn't have it.

When it comes to weight, the rule is "the lighter, the better." *Walking* magazine's "Walking Guide" recommends shoes weighing 8 to 16 ounces.

Walking shoes should not feel stiff or restrict foot flexing. Stiff shoes cause sore feet and may contribute to muscle strains.

Here are a few more points to remember.

**Avoid pointed toes.** A square-shaped toe provides the most room and optimal comfort.

**Look for shock absorption.** The insole, midsole and outsole should feel well-cushioned but not spongy.

**Be well-padded.** The more shoe padding the better, especially on the tongue and collar and around the heel.

**Try on both shoes.** Feet can be different sizes. You may even have to buy two pairs of different sizes to fit both of your feet properly. If your feet are different sizes, call around. Some shoe stores will discount the second pair.

**Check your old shoes.** Notice where they're worn and look for extra strength in those areas.

**Check the time.** Shop for shoes in the afternoon. Feet swell a little during the day.

What if the best shoes you can buy still seem to hurt your

feet? Walking shoe manufacturers design shoes for the average foot. But with 26 bones and dozens of muscles, tendons and ligaments, there are a lot of variables—the average foot may bear little resemblance to yours. That's why many walkers' feet hurt even after they've splurged on good shoes. To soothe those sore dogs, try orthotics. Also known as arch supports, innersoles or inserts, orthotics customize mass-produced shoes to fit individual feet. Start with over-the-counter orthotics available at shoe stores, drugstores and shoe repair shops. "Ready-made orthotics are inexpensive and often effective, and they cause no harm if they don't help," says David B. Alper, D.P.M., a podiatrist in Belmont, Massachusetts.

Orthotics not only provide extra support, they also subtly reshape the feet by changing balance and the demands on some foot muscles. "This retraining takes time," Dr. Alper says. "On day one, wear your orthotics for two or three hours, then add an hour a day to allow your feet to adapt to them."

Unfortunately, not everyone finds happiness with ready-made orthotics. If your feet continue to hurt, you might want to consult a podiatrist for custom-made orthotics, suggests Dr. Alper.

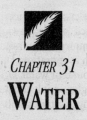

## CHAPTER 31

# WATER

*The Elixir of Life*

After oxygen, water is the second most vital component of life. People can survive about three weeks without food but only three days without water. "Life on earth evolved in water," explains Bruce Paton, M.D., professor of surgery at the University of Colorado School of Medicine in Denver and an expert on the hydration (water) needs of athletes. "Without it, there is no life."

And without *enough* water, there is no health. Most people make the mistake of taking water for granted. If you're among them, you'll change your mind once you understand the preventive and therapeutic benefits offered by this often-forgotten fluid.

*Altitude sickness.* Many people who travel quickly from lowlands to mountain elevations, especially by air, develop the headache, fatigue, limb swelling, malaise and parched feeling of altitude sickness shortly after arrival. Mountain elevations literally suck water out of lowlanders' blood, says Dr. Paton. "During your first day at altitude, fluid moves out of the blood and into the tissues," he explains. His advice: "Drink plenty of fluids on your way up and after you arrive. Drinking doesn't entirely prevent altitude sickness, but it helps minimize its discomfort."

Flying to mountain elevations exacerbates altitude sickness, not only because it's quick but also because air travel itself is dehydrating. The air in commercial aircraft is extremely dry, which boosts fluid loss through evaporation. During a two-hour flight, the body can lose one pound of water. Drink liberally before you board planes. During flights, drink nonalcoholic, noncaffeinated beverages. Take an orange or two and bottled water or juice in your carry-on baggage.

*The common cold.* The throat, explains health educator Robert K. Cooper, Ph.D., director of the Center for Health and Fitness Excellence in Bemidji, Minnesota, and author of *Health and Fitness Excellence: The Scientific Action Plan,* is covered by a layer of moist mucus that acts like flypaper. It catches many cold viruses before they can cause infection and sweeps them down into the stomach, where powerful digestive acids destroy them. Even minor dehydration can dry the mucus layer, impairing its virus-catching effectiveness.

*Diarrhea.* In reaction to this watery health problem, many people reduce their fluid intake, thinking it will help firm things up again. That's a big mistake.

Diarrhea can have many causes, explains Anne Simons, M.D., assistant clinical professor of family and community medicine at the University of California's San Francisco Medical Center and co-author of *Before You Call the Doctor.* Causes include intestinal parasites; irritable bowel syndrome; viral or bacterial infections, including food poisoning, traveler's diarrhea (*turista* or Montezuma's revenge) and salmonella and other forms of dysentery; drug side effects; and lactose intolerance, the inability of some adults to digest the milk sugar (lactose) found in dairy products and the artificial sweetener sorbitol.

The cause of everyday diarrhea is often difficult to identify. Many cases are viral, particularly in children. Sometimes combinations of foods, drugs and stress precipitate it—for example, too much pizza and coffee the night before final exams. Sometimes it's related to travel—and it doesn't have to be a full-blown case of *turista* either. Frequently when people travel, even within the United States, they react poorly to the new local water supply.

At the first sign of diarrhea, increase your fluid intake, Dr. Simons counsels. Drink eight to ten large glasses of water a day for as long as the diarrhea lasts. Often plain water is not enough, however, because water does not replace lost minerals, particularly those known as electrolytes—sodium and potassium. As a result, authorities now recommend Gatorade or other rehydration fluids that contain both of these minerals. (People with high blood pressure, heart disease, diabetes, glaucoma or a history of stroke should consult their physicians before self-treating with electrolyte-replacement beverages, because the sodium may elevate their blood pressure.) Bouillon and other clear broths are also helpful.

Gatorade is not recommended for infants and young children. Instead, give other electrolyte-rich—but less concentrated—rehydration fluids such as Pedialyte, Infalyte and Lytren. Have children sip rehydration fluids—no gulping allowed. Gulping can overstimulate the gastrointestinal tract and contribute to cramping. Flat soft drinks or dilute apple juice can also be used, but authorities say fluids like Pedialyte are preferable.

And whether the person with diarrhea is an adult or child, another rule applies—don't stop eating. People with diarrhea typically associate food with stomach distress and reduce their food intake. Like limiting drinking, this is a mistake. Reducing food consumption aggravates dehydration by denying you the water in most foods, and it impairs recovery by limiting nourishment.

Instead, change your diet to BRATT foods. BRATT is an acronym for bananas, rice, applesauce, tea and toast, all of which are binding. Bananas are also rich in potassium, so they help replenish electrolytes. But stay away from coffee, milk, fruit juices and spicy, fried and junk foods, all of which usually aggravate the problem. Also avoid alcohol, which is dehydrating. As symptoms begin to improve, gradually reintroduce other low-fat foods: crackers, cooked vegetables, skinless chicken, fish and so forth.

If diarrhea in anyone over age three does not respond to fluids and the BRATT diet within a day or two, Dr. Simons recommends trying over-the-counter Kaopectate. (The antidiarrheal fiber in applesauce is pectin. It's also the "pectate" in Kaopectate.) Adults should take four to eight tablespoons after each watery bowel movement.

For diarrhea in children under three that doesn't respond to BRATT within a day or two, Dr. Simons recommends consulting the child's physician.

*Fever.* Fever evolved for a good reason. Most disease-causing microorganisms have difficulty reproducing at temperatures much above normal body temperature. But fever also increases perspiration, which is why a fever can leave your pajamas and sheets soaking wet. All that extra perspiration can add up to dehydration, which thickens the blood, hindering recovery, and causes that out-of-it feeling because of dehydration's effects on the brain. Anyone with a fever should substantially increase water consumption.

*General illness prevention and recovery.* Your blood is 85 percent water. "Even minor dehydration thickens it, reducing circulation from the optimal level and as a result impairing the blood's ability to deliver food and oxygen to every body system and carry away wastes," says Dr. Cooper. That means that over time, chronic minor dehydration can leave your body's cells, tissues and systems somewhat undernourished and weakened. This compromises their ability to fend off disease. And once an illness develops, chronic minor dehydration may impair the blood's ability to deliver white blood cells and other components of the immune system to the affected area.

*Hangover.* Called "the moaning after" by one wit, hangovers cause headache, nausea, vomiting, thirst, mental dullness and feeling like "death warmed over." A major reason alcohol causes hangover is that it's dehydrating. This accounts for morning-after thirst and dullness and contributes to the headache and lousy-all-over feeling.

You don't have to get sloppy drunk to have a hangover the morning after. For people of average weight, the hangover-risk threshold is consumption of more than one drink per hour. If you drink at all, nurse your drinks. Alternate them with water or fruit juice to prevent alcohol-related dehydration.

And if you do imbibe to excess, drink lots of water before you go to bed. The water won't prevent a hangover entirely, but it can help minimize the misery of alcohol-induced dehydration.

If you do develop a full-blown hangover, keep drinking water until you feel human again. (For stomach distress, try adding some mint to your water. Peppermint or spearmint soothes the digestive tract.)

**Mental sharpness.** The average person's body is about 60 percent water, but this widely cited statistic actually underestimates its need for fluids. Your brain is 75 percent water. Even minor dehydration significantly impairs your concentration, memory and reaction time.

**Muscle soreness.** Physical overexertion can cause two kinds of muscle injury—the sudden sharp pain of muscle sprains or tears and a general achiness that shows up 24 to 48 hours later. That general achiness is called delayed-onset muscle soreness (DOMS). Traditionally, exercise physiologists attributed DOMS to lactic acid, a substance thought to accumulate in muscle tissue during exertion and cause soreness afterward as it dissipated. Today scientists know differently. "Lactic acid has nothing to do with DOMS," says Scott Hasson, Ed.D., associate professor of physical therapy at Texas Women's University in Houston. "It dissipates within minutes of completing exercise."

So what causes DOMS? "Microtrauma to muscle fibers," Dr. Hasson explains. "Any physical activity injures some muscle cells. But when exertion level exceeds conditioning level, enough microscopic damage occurs to cause inflammation that appears as soreness a day or two later."

Dr. Hasson's studies show that anti-inflammatory medicines—aspirin, ibuprofen or willow bark, the herbal source of pharmaceutical aspirin—help relieve DOMS. He also recommends drinking plenty of water. That's because even minor dehydration impairs the healing of damaged muscle cells.

**Muscle strength and stamina.** Even slight dehydration, too minimal to register as thirst, can reduce your strength, stamina and coordination. Not too long ago, competitive athletes did not drink during sports events because they feared abdominal cramps. Today basketball and football players start sipping water or sports drinks the moment they hit the bench. Long-distance runners grab water along the way, and bicycle racers always carry water bottles.

## Sip, Sip, Hooray!

Because dehydration causes or contributes to so many health problems, any healthy lifestyle should include drinking lots of water and other fluids. But all fluids are not created equal. Go easy on beverages containing alcohol or caffeine (coffee, tea, colas and cocoa). They act like diuretic drugs, increasing your urine production; as a result, they are dehydrating.

Don't slake your thirst with sodas, seltzer water or anything that's carbonated, warns Edward Coyle, Ph.D., director of the Human Performance Laboratory at the University of Texas at Austin. "Carbonation makes you feel fuller than you actually are," he explains, "so you may not drink as much as you should."

Of course, there's no need to avoid alcohol, caffeine and carbonated beverages altogether. You won't shrivel up and blow away from drinking a morning cup of coffee or an occasional cola, beer or glass of wine. In fact, modest consumption of alcohol, particularly red wine, appears to be one of Nature's cures for heart disease. (See Ornish Therapy on page 368.) And caffeine is often considered a natural therapy for chest congestion and pain relief. Just don't use these beverages to the exclusion of good old $H_2O$. Drink water, juices and noncaffeinated teas regularly. And when you drink alcohol or anything caffeinated or carbonated, do what restaurants do—serve yourself water on the side.

How much water should a person drink each day? Considerably more than you may be drinking now. The average American takes in about 3½ cups of water daily from food and produces about a ½ cup as a by-product of metabolism, a total nonbeverage intake of approximately 4 cups a day. Meanwhile, average daily water loss amounts to 6 cups through elimination functions, 2 cups through routine, invisible perspiration (independent of sweating caused by exercise) and 2 cups through breathing, because every exhalation contains water vapor—a total of about 10 cups.

"Even without exercising, which is a necessity for good health, the average American is looking at a six-cup-a-day water deficit," Dr. Cooper says, "and moderate exercise can sweat off another cup or two." That's why nutritionists generally recommend drinking six to eight cups of water a day.

Most people find it nearly impossible to guzzle that much water every day. "Gulping is not the way to go," Dr. Cooper says, "Instead of drinking whole glasses of water all at once, it's easier to take sips frequently throughout the day."

Keep a glass or small bottle of water or juice within arm's reach at work, by your TV, in your car or wherever you spend time. To keep your beverage of choice either hot or cold while you sip, invest in an insulated cup. They're available at most kitchen and variety stores for less than $10.

## Thirst Is Worst

When should fluids be replaced? *Before* you feel thirsty.

"By the time you become conscious of thirst, you're already significantly dehydrated, and your concentration, coordination, memory, reaction time and athletic stamina are already suffering," explains Nancy Clark, R.D., director of nutrition services at SportsMedicine Brookline in Massachusetts and a fellow of the American College of Sports Medicine. "In addition, drinking in response to thirst replaces only about half of lost fluid."

In addition to sipping water throughout the day, Clark recommends drinking one to two cups about 15 minutes before even moderate exercise like walking or gardening, taking water breaks during workouts and downing a few more cups after you've finished your workout. The hotter the weather, the more important adequate hydration becomes. Take a water bottle with you during warm-weather walks and take drink breaks frequently.

And don't ignore fluid needs during cold weather. "People don't drip sweat during winter workouts," Dr. Paton says, "but they're still losing water and should drink frequently."

Independent of exercise, individual fluid needs vary. Children need more water than adults. Comparing body mass to skin surface, children have more skin surface than adults, resulting in greater water loss through perspiration. Men need more water than women of the same height, weight and build because men have a larger proportion of muscle tissue, and muscles are sponges for water.

Diet also affects fluid needs. Fresh fruits and vegetables are largely water. Oranges, grapes and melons are about 85 percent water. Apples are about 80 percent water. Even "dry" fruits like bananas are 75 percent water. Some foods, however, are actually dehydrating. Foods high in protein (meat, eggs and cheeses) increase blood levels of chemicals called ketones, which are dehydrating.

To gauge your own hydration level accurately, Clark recommends paying close attention to urination. "If you don't urinate several times a day," she warns, "you're not drinking enough." Urine color is also important. It should be pale yellow. If it looks as bright or dark as it does in the morning (after a night of dehydrating sleep), start drinking water immediately.

## Troubled Waters

Unfortunately, when many Americans turn on their faucets, what flows from the tap is more than just Nature's cure for dehydration. In the words of singer/satirist Tom Lehrer, it just might be "hot and cold running sludge."

During the last 25 years, the quality of the nation's drinking water has gone right down the drain. The U.S. water supply is free of serious bacterial contamination, notably cholera, a waterborne biblical plague that is still very much with us. Within the last few years major cholera outbreaks have sickened thousands and killed several hundred in South America. But freedom from cholera does not make the nation's drinking water pure.

# Sports Drinks versus Water

Few people outside physiology laboratories knew what electrolytes were until the late 1960s, when Gatorade commercials began proclaiming, "We've got 'em and plain water doesn't."

Electrolytes are minerals, primarily sodium and potassium. In the body, they become electrically charged. Electrolytes are involved in muscle contraction, nerve impulse conduction, blood chemistry and maintenance of normal heart rhythm.

Do you need to be concerned about electrolytes? For most people who engage in regular, moderate exercise, the answer is no. "Casual, noncompetitive exercisers whose workouts don't exceed two hours can usually replace lost electrolytes simply by eating and drinking at meals," explains Nancy Clark, R.D., director of nutrition services at SportsMedicine Brookline in Massachusetts and a fellow of the American College of Sports Medicine. "They don't need sports drinks."

But strenuous, sustained athletic activity can deplete electrolytes, impairing performance and triggering muscle cramps. In addition, sports drinks contain carbohydrate, the body's main fuel. As they rehydrate the body, they also provide an energy boost.

Several studies have shown that sports drinks have some advantages over plain water. They're absorbed faster, provide more complete rehydration and even enhance performance a bit. But since most of these studies have been conducted by scientists supported by Gatorade, many nutritionists and exercise physiologists look askance at the results.

Investigators from the General Accounting Office (GAO)—the investigative arm of Congress—have discovered "serious health risks," including waterborne diseases and contamination with pesticides, heavy metals and cancer-causing chemicals (carcinogens), in many water supplies around the country.

A GAO survey in the late 1980s showed that 28 percent of community water systems reported violating at least one water

"Commercial hype," sniffs Bruce Paton, M.D., professor of surgery at the University of Colorado in Denver and an expert on athletic hydration. Dr. Paton contends that plain water works just fine even for strenuous, extended workouts if you also munch a few pretzels (carbohydrate plus sodium in the salt) or a banana (carbohydrate plus potassium).

To increase the speed of water absorption, Robert K. Cooper, Ph.D., director of the Center for Health and Fitness Excellence in Bemidji, Minnesota, and author of *Health and Fitness Excellence: The Scientific Action Plan,* recommends drinking it chilled. Cool water passes through the stomach faster than warm or hot water, and contrary to popular mythology, it doesn't cause cramping.

Then there's the issue of the sodium in sports drinks. Sodium may be an electrolyte, but most Americans consume too much. The recommended daily intake is 500 milligrams. The typical American consumes 3,000 to 7,000 milligrams. Many nutritionists question the wisdom of guzzling down more sodium in the name of better rehydration because dietary sodium can raise blood pressure and increase risk of heart attack and stroke. If your blood pressure is high, consult your physician before using sports drinks.

But even skeptical Dr. Paton concedes one advantage to sports drinks—convenience. He prefers to eat a light lunch during all-day cross-country ski excursions, and sports drinks offer a convenient way to obtain some carbohydrate without chewing it. If you steer clear of big lunches during your workouts, a sports drink might be a good way to go—except for the "lite" brands. They're low in carbohydrate.

purity standard set by the Environmental Protection Agency (EPA). A 1993 report by the National Resources Defense Counsel, an environmental organization in Washington, D.C., alleged 250,000 violations of the Safe Drinking Water Act in just two years (1991 and 1992) affecting 43 percent of the nation's water systems serving 120 million Americans. A 1993 EPA report said that more than 800 of the nation's water systems, serving 30 million Americans, had excessive levels of lead, a highly toxic mineral that can cause learning disabilities and even mental retardation in children.

The EPA requires public water systems to conduct purity tests regularly, keep careful records of them, release test records to the public and inform consumers of any problems. But GAO investigators have discovered "ample evidence" that water system employees have falsified test data and failed to report problems they have discovered. Ironically, given pollution in and around the nation's industrial cities, the dirtiest drinking water is in rural areas, home to 25 million Americans, where wells are often contaminated with fertilizers and pesticides. Meanwhile, the EPA's water-purity enforcement program has been chronically underfunded for years, and the GAO calls its enforcement efforts spotty at best.

The nation's water quality crisis has been simmering for years: Contamination caused 485 disease outbreaks affecting 110,000 Americans from 1971 to 1985, according to the Centers for Disease Control and Prevention in Atlanta.

It's no wonder then that in recent years, millions of Americans have either fitted their faucets with home water filters or abandoned municipal drinking water altogether in favor of bottled water. But according to GAO investigators, the sales tactics of the burgeoning "pure water" industry are sometimes dirtier than tapwater. Some marketers of bottled water and home filters have used scandalously deceptive tactics to scare consumers into spending small fortunes for water no purer than the $H_2O$ that flows from their taps. In fact, some bottled and filtered waters are more contaminated than tapwater.

## Let the Buyer Beware

Since 1985, annual sales of home water filters have jumped 49 percent, to almost $2 billion. The most popular water treatment units—activated charcoal filters—remove chlorine and many organic compounds but may not remove some microorganisms, heavy metals (including lead) and other contaminants routinely removed by well-maintained municipal water systems. In addition, the charcoal filter units must be changed regularly, otherwise they can release hazardously high concentrations of pollutants back into the water.

The water-filter industry is also poorly regulated. No federal agency tests or approves home filters, and only three states—Wisconsin, Iowa and California—require manufacturers to submit test results to prove that their units perform as advertised. The industry trade association has developed voluntary standards but does not enforce them, and only 54 of the estimated 600 manufacturers meet them. Only 43 manufacturers have submitted their units for testing by the National Sanitation Foundation (NSF), an independent, nonprofit food-equipment inspection company.

Finally, according to the GAO, some water-filter marketers have lied about the ability of their units to remove contaminants, rigged in-home tests to show pollution that did not actually exist and used "scare tactics" about poor tapwater quality to sell their products. Attorneys-general in Wisconsin, California and New York have prosecuted filter makers for deceptive sales practices, and the Federal Trade Commission successfully prosecuted one distributor whose filter released a suspected carcinogen. More than 350,000 of these filters were sold.

What about bottled waters? In the last decade, annual sales have quadrupled, to almost two billion gallons. A typical family that drinks and cooks with bottled water can spend several hundred dollars a year—but they may not be getting what they pay for.

In 1990, Perrier recalled millions of gallons of its upscale water because of contamination with benzene, a potent carcinogen. The voluntary recall combined with the company's pronouncements about its commitment to quality averted a public relations disaster. But according to a GAO investigation, contrary to Perrier's press releases, company testers did not discover the contamination and did not immediately announce the recall. The benzene was discovered accidentally by employees at a North Carolina water-testing laboratory who were using the supposedly super-pure water to calibrate their testing equipment. When the scandal broke, Perrier records showed benzene contamination for eight months before the North Carolina lab discovered it.

More recently, University of Delaware researchers analyzed 37 brands of bottled water. Twenty-four violated at least one of 31 U.S. drinking water standards.

As a result of the Perrier incident, the Food and Drug Administration (FDA) launched a national survey of bottled water safety. But according to GAO investigators, the FDA tested only 10 percent of the nation's bottled waters for only 9 of 31 regulated contaminants. Nonetheless, this survey and the FDA's ongoing bottled-water monitoring program turned up dozens of "violations requiring immediate correction."

The FDA requires bottlers to test their waters, but unlike municipal water systems, bottlers are essentially unaccountable. The FDA does not require bottlers to use certified laboratories or keep test records, so the agency has no way of knowing if required purity tests are even performed.

## Finding a Safe Supply

What's a nervous consumer to do? Don't stop drinking water. Instead take a few precautions. Here's what experts, including the Western Water Foundation in Sacramento, California, a nonprofit organization that educates consumers about water issues, recommend.

**Cook with cold water only.** Lead leaches more readily into hot water than cold. Start your soups, stews and other water-containing dishes with cold water. The few extra minutes you save by starting them with hot water may be giving you a dose of toxic metals from your plumbing.

**Be patient.** Let your cold water run for 30 seconds before using it for drinking or cooking. Water that sits in household piping—especially overnight—may pick up contaminants. Thirty seconds of flushing eliminates this water and allows you to draw from the main line outside your home.

Consider calling a plumbing inspector. Lead solder is no longer used in household plumbing, but it used to be. Old plumbing may contain the toxic metal.

Call your local water department. The EPA requires municipal water suppliers to inform consumers of regular test results, point out any problems and advise consumers what the supplier is doing to correct them. The phone number should be on your bill.

Call your county or state water agency. If your local water supplier gives you the runaround, you can appeal to these agencies. Check the government pages of your phone book.

Contact the EPA. The EPA operates a toll-free Safe Drinking Water Hotline. Check the Federal Government pages of your phone book. The EPA Hotline can answer questions about federal water regulations and send you free booklets: "Is Your Drinking Water Safe?" describes how the government monitors drinking water safety. "Citizen Monitoring: Recommendations to Public Water System Users" describes common water pollutants and suggests steps for investigating and correcting any suspected problems. "Lead and Your Drinking Water" answers questions about this waterborne neurological hazard and what consumers can do about it.

Do some checking before you buy a home water filter. Buy a filter certified by the NSF. The NSF charges manufacturers to analyze filter performance and certifies tested models with a label listing the contaminants the filter actually removes. Look for an NSF label or contact NSF at 3475 Plymouth Road, Ann Arbor, MI 48105 for a list of certified filters. Once you select a home filter, have the water it produces independently tested.

Do some checking before you buy bottled water. To join the trade group—the International Bottled Water Association (IBWA)—bottlers must have their water tested by NSF. Avoid waters marketed by companies outside the IBWA. To find out if a particular brand is a member, contact the IBWA at 113 North Henry Street, Alexandria, VA 22314. Once you select a brand, have it independently tested.

Have your water tested. It doesn't matter what kind of

water you drink, you can't be sure it's pure until you've had it independently tested. For referrals to water-testing laboratories around the country, contact the American Council of Independent Laboratories, 1629 K Street, N.W., Suite 400, Washington, D.C. 20006. One member, the National Testing Laboratory (NTL) in Cleveland, tests water for 93 pollutants, including microorganisms, pesticides, PCBs, industrial chemicals, lead and other heavy metals.

You receive sampling test tubes packed in a Styrofoam box. Fill them with water and return the box to NTL. You receive the test results with an explanation and, if necessary, suggestions for eliminating any contaminants. Cost: about $150. This may sound high, but a year of bottled water or many brands of home filters cost more.

Once you know how pure or impure your water is, you can make an informed decision about what to drink. Contact the National Testing Laboratory at 6555 Wilson Mills Road, Cleveland, OH 44143.

## CHAPTER 32

# WEIGHT TRAINING

*Putting Muscle to Work for Health*

**M**ention "pumping iron," and most people think of Arnold Schwarzenegger or some other macho body-builder with rock-hard biceps as big as the average person's thighs. But strength training is no longer just for gym rats who aspire to be Mr. Universe. It's for men and women of *all* ages who are looking for a way to boost their health. There's one gym in Boston where the weight-lifters are every bit as serious as Olympic hopefuls. But these iron pumpers' average age is 90, and since news of their remarkable muscle development hit the media in 1990, they've been turning more heads than Arnold himself.

The nonagenarian weight-lifters all live at the Hebrew Rehabilitation Center for Aged (HRCA) in Boston. For more than 50 years, none had been physically active, until gerontologist Maria Fiatarone, M.D., assistant professor of medicine at Harvard Medical School, began wondering if muscle development had an upper age limit. She recruited ten HRCA residents, ages 85 to 96, and measured the strength of their quadriceps leg muscles. The average participant's "quad" could lift 16 pounds. Dr. Fiatarone then placed the ten on a modest weight-training program designed to challenge them but not overtax their elderly quads.

"After eight weeks," she explains, "their lifting ability almost tripled, to 42 pounds. Their quadriceps size increased 10 percent, and their walking speed also increased significantly. The study proved that you can increase strength and muscle size at any age. The physical deterioration we have traditionally associated with aging actually has nothing to do with years. It's entirely due to lack of use."

One of Dr. Fiatarone's elderly weight-lifters was Sara Chiller, age 85. "I worked all my life in an office and never exercised," she says. "As I got older, I had problems with my hip. I broke it twice and now have a stainless steel pin and a limp. I joined the study because I wanted to improve my walking. And I did. Thanks to the weight-lifting, I walk more easily now, and I'm less afraid of falling."

In 1994, Dr. Fiatarone released the results of a repeat study involving ten times as many HRCA residents—100 instead of 10. Their average age was 87, and one-third were in their nineties. For several weeks, they strengthened their leg muscles using weight-lifting resistance machines similar to those found in health clubs. Compared with their abilities before they began pumping iron, the individuals participating in the study increased their walking speed an average of 12 percent and their stair-climbing ability 28 percent. The weight-lifters also reported mood elevation. Happier and stronger, they became more involved in HRCA group activities, thus increasing feelings of companionship, which also contribute to heath and well-being.

Dr. Fiatarone is not the only researcher to show that the elderly benefit from strength training. Robert Marcus, M.D., professor of medicine and endocrinology at Stanford University, placed 27 women ages 65 to 87 on a modest weight-training program that focused on their leg muscles. After a year, their leg muscle mass increased 20 percent and their leg strength doubled.

## How Strength Benefits the Body

A generation ago, only young men lifted weights—largely to impress young women who wouldn't be caught dead curling a dumbbell. Today men and women of all ages are curling, pressing and pumping up because it's an integral part of a well-rounded exercise program.

"Strength training," says Robert K. Cooper, Ph.D., director of the Center for Health and Fitness Excellence in Bemidji, Minnesota, and author of *Health and Fitness Excellence: The Scientific Action Plan,* "does more than increase the size of the major muscle groups. It confers real health benefits as well." Here are some of the conditions that medical research has shown can benefit from strength training.

*Arthritis.* At the U.S. Department of Agriculture's Human Nutrition Research Center on Aging at Tufts University in Boston, Ronenn Roubenoff, M.D., assistant professor of medicine, has obtained promising results in a pilot study of weight training for people with rheumatoid arthritis, the most severe form of joint disease. Dr. Roubenoff suggests that weight training increases joint mobility and reduces pain because stronger muscles function as shock absorbers for the joints near them.

*Depression.* In one study at the University of Rochester Medical Center in New York, 40 women with serious depression began either running or strength training (four weekly half-hour sessions on a universal weight machine). After eight weeks, a nonexercising group showed no change in depression, but both exercising groups showed significantly more upbeat mood and greater self-esteem. Like aerobics and other less rigorous exercise programs (walking, gardening or yoga), strength training releases endorphins, the body's feel-good chemicals.

The elderly participants in Dr. Fiatarone's study all reported mood elevation from their weight-lifting. The phenomenon, which many exercisers compare to a drug-induced "high," is a key reason that people continue to exercise. "The high that exercise produces," Dr. Cooper says, "is a positive addiction, something you crave that's good for you."

*Diabetes.* Muscle cells are big consumers of glucose, the blood sugar that people with diabetes have trouble using. As muscle mass increases, glucose leaves the bloodstream to nourish the muscles, which prevents the buildup of glucose responsible for diabetic complications. Weight training does not free people who have Type I, or insulin-dependent, diabetes from their injections, but it can help them (and those with Type II, or non-insulin-dependent, diabetes as well) maintain tighter blood sugar control.

*Gastrointestinal diseases.* As visible muscles grow stronger, some invisible ones do too—specifically the muscles whose wavelike contractions push food through the gastrointestinal (GI) tract. Studies by exercise physiologist Bernard Hurley, Ph.D., associate professor of kinesiology at the University of Maryland in College Park, show that after several months on a weight-training program, sedentary men cut their GI transit time in half. Transit time measures how long it takes for food to pass through the digestive system. A slow transit time is associated with increased risk of hemorrhoids, diverticulitis (inflammation of tiny pouches that develop in the colon) and colon cancer. Reducing transit time helps prevent these conditions.

*Heart disease.* Like other forms of exercise, strength training reduces blood pressure, conditions the heart and reduces cholesterol—by 4 percent, according to an analysis by University of Northern Colorado researchers who reviewed the results of 11 studies. In addition to decreasing total cholesterol, weight training also changes the ratio of low-density lipoprotein, or LDL ("bad") cholesterol to high-density lipoprotein, or HDL ("good") cholesterol. It decreases LDL by 13 percent according to the Colorado researchers, while boosting HDL by 5 percent.

*Muscle weakness.* Strength training produces noticeable results more quickly than more popular cardiovascular conditioning programs. With a few workouts a week, most people feel stronger within a month, and those who are new to strength training often double their strength in two to three months.

Dr. Fiatarone's elderly weight-lifters almost tripled their strength in eight weeks. If you have trouble opening jars or lifting grocery bags, a modest strength-training program can make life easier and more enjoyable.

*Osteoporosis.* Bone-thinning osteoporosis can lead to fractures, especially hip fractures, a major medical problem for the elderly. One way to maintain strong, healthy bones is to get plenty of calcium. Certain kinds of exercise, including strength training, also help keep bones healthy. In addition, weight training helps prevent fractures by strengthening the leg muscles, contributing to improved balance and decreasing the likelihood of falls, the cause of most fractures in the elderly.

*Overweight.* Without weight training, after about age 30 youthful muscle loses its tone, giving us that middle-aged, flabby look. From age 20 to 70, Americans uninvolved in strength-building programs typically lose almost one-third of their muscle cells from lack of use. Much of that tissue is replaced by fat. Muscle is much more metabolically active than fat; it burns calories instead of simply storing them.

As the body's proportion of muscle tissue declines and its fat increases, basal metabolic rate (BMR), the rate at which the body burns calories while at rest, slows by about 2 percent per decade. As BMR slows, you burn fewer calories per hour and store more as fat, a phenomenon that leads to middle-age spread. Weight training helps preserve calorie-burning muscle tissue. Less muscle turns to flab, and your BMR stays high, meaning less weight gain.

## Getting Started

To add strength training to your exercise program, you don't have to spend a fortune or join a fancy health club. Dumbbells, also known as free weights, are inexpensive and sold at most sporting goods stores. Start with two- or three-pound weights and as you grow stronger, move up to five- to seven-pound weights. You can try weights that wrap around your ankles or wrists or simply use weighty household objects: cans of beans, a hammer or a few hardcover books.

Most people can start a weight-training program on their own. Check with your physician first, however, if you're a sedentary man over 40 or a sedentary woman over 50 or if you have any chronic medical condition or significant risk factors for one.

Here are some weight-training exercises you can try on your own. For a more complete program, consult a trainer at your local gym or Y.

*Curl.* This targets the biceps, located in the upper arm. Stand with your arms at your sides and your palms facing forward. Grasp a weight with each hand and bend your elbows, holding your upper arms vertical. Keeping your elbows at your sides, bring the weights up to your shoulder, then let them back down slowly. Start with one set of five to ten repetitions ("reps"). Over time, work up to three sets.

*Upright row.* This exercise develops the muscles of the neck, shoulders and upper back. Hold a weight in each hand with the palms facing inward and the weights against your upper thighs. Raise the weights by bending your elbows and pointing them outward until the weights are even with your chin and about ten inches apart. Let them back down using the reverse motion. Start with one set of five to ten reps. Over time, work up to three sets.

*Seated press.* Sit in a chair with your feet flat on the floor and a weight in each hand. Raise the weights to shoulder height, then extend your arms directly over your head. Lower the weights to shoulder level, then lower them back to the starting position. Start with one set of five to ten reps. Over time, work up to three sets.

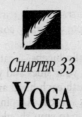

## CHAPTER 33

# YOGA

## Stretch the Body, Mind and Spirit

**W**hen she was in her thirties, Mary Pullig Schatz, M.D., a Nashville pathologist on the staff of the Centennial Medical Center, endured terrible chronic back pain.

"I was miserable," recalls Dr. Pullig Schatz, who is also a member of the American College of Sports Medicine. "I had constant pain that took all the fun out of my life."

Dr. Pullig Schatz tried: pain relievers, bed rest, chiropractic, physical therapy—you name it. Then a friend suggested she try yoga. She was skeptical. Yoga conjured up images of emaciated men in loincloths and turbans contorting themselves into pretzels for no apparent reason. But she felt she had nothing to lose. "I viewed yoga as my last resort before back surgery, which I really didn't want," she recalls.

At her first yoga class, Dr. Pullig Schatz thought she might have accidentally wandered into an aerobic dance studio. Students in leotards or sweat suits were distributed around a large open room, unrolling exercise mats. But unlike aerobics, jazzercise or any of today's other dance-for-fitness programs, yoga involves neither loud music nor cheerleader-style choreography. Instead the room stays quiet and participants spend a good deal of time remaining relatively still as the teacher leads them in a

60- to 90-minute series of stretches that resemble the warm-up exercises athletes do before events. But on closer inspection, yoga differs tremendously from athletic warm-ups.

*Yoga is slower.* Students might take as long as a minute to ease into stretched postures and then hold them for up to several minutes before changing positions.

*Yoga is gentler.* The old locker-room adage "no pain, no gain" has no place in this mind/body workout that comes from ancient India. If participants feel the least bit uncomfortable attempting any movement, they signal the teacher, who works with them individually to modify the pose so they can perform it comfortably. If that's not possible, they don't do it.

*Yoga involves the whole body.* Most exercise programs concentrate on the large muscle groups: the arms, legs and abdominals. The typical yoga class works these muscles but also spends time flexing the fingers and toes and rolling the eyes, wrists and ankles, thus exercising muscle groups most other fitness programs ignore.

*Yoga is surprising.* It works up a sweat, but it's not aerobically strenuous. After class, participants usually feel more relaxed than tired. People of any age can practice it, and unlike most exercise programs, so can those with serious physical limitations, such as heart disease, multiple sclerosis and severe arthritis. (People with serious conditions, however, should check with their doctors first.)

*Yoga is meditative.* While stretching into the various postures—some as simple as standing up straight, others as challenging as headstands—participants breathe slowly and deeply and enjoy the relaxation and mind-clearing benefits of meditation.

Yoga was certainly different from anything Dr. Pullig Schatz had tried for her back. Its results were different as well. Almost immediately, her back began to feel less painful and more flexible. As she continued to practice, her back pain disappeared.

"Yoga was amazingly therapeutic for me," says Dr. Pullig Schatz. "I can honestly say that it changed my life. Now I practice yoga every day. My husband does it when his back hurts.

And my stepson has used it to control the knee pain he developed playing basketball." Dr. Pullig Schatz also used yoga as the basis for her book, *Back Care Basics*.

## Doctors Take a Stand

Dr. Pullig Schatz is not the only physician to discover the healing power of yoga. About 15 years ago, William E. Connor, M.D., professor of medicine and clinical nutrition at the Oregon Health Sciences University in Portland, developed chronic hip pain. "My daughter practiced yoga and encouraged me to try it," recalls Dr. Connor. "I was very skeptical, but she insisted, so I figured I'd humor her for a while. At first I couldn't even do the poses she showed me. But after a while, they came more easily—and my hip improved. Now I don't have hip pain anymore, except when I don't do yoga for a few days."

A year after Dr. Connor began practicing yoga regularly, his wife had to have surgery after a skiing accident. "She couldn't take pain relievers because of a stomach problem, so I encouraged her to try yoga," says Dr. Connor. "It helped her considerably. Now we do it together."

Dr. Connor particularly enjoys the fact that yoga is completely portable. "All you need is about ten square feet of floor space," he says. "You don't need any special clothing or equipment or a gym. It's as easy to do in a hotel room as it is at home. I practice ten minutes a day and take an hour-long class once a week. Yoga has improved my body, mind and spirit. No wonder it's been around for thousands of years."

Another physician who uses yoga therapeutically is Dean Ornish, M.D., president of the Preventive Medicine Research Institute in Sausalito, California, whose revolutionary natural treatment for heart disease is the subject of Ornish Therapy on page 368.

Yoga is generally practiced by healthy people who want a gentle, relaxing form of exercise that develops flexibility and strength. But as Dr. Pullig Schatz, Dr. Connor and Dr. Ornish attest, yoga has become increasingly popular for those with chronic medical conditions. Lorna Bell, R.N., co-author of *Gentle Yoga* and former director of the YMCA Health and Fitness Program in Cedar Rapids, Iowa, developed a yoga class specifically for people with disabilities, particularly arthritis, multiple sclerosis, stroke and paraplegia. Participants have reported significant physical benefits and general improvement in their quality of life.

"Yoga has helped me considerably," says John Jenney, a retired salesman who was diagnosed with multiple sclerosis in 1977. "My balance definitely improved."

## Science Documents Yoga's Benefits

Testimonials like those above may be moving, but most scientists dismiss them as merely "anecdotal evidence"—curiosities that may or may not hold up under rigorous experimental scrutiny.

But yoga has also been subjected to rigorous medical research. Its benefits have been demonstrated over and over again in more than 100 scientific studies. Most have been conducted in India, yoga's birthplace, where it is a major pillar of India's traditional healing therapy, Ayurvedic medicine. Studies showing the many benefits of yoga have also been conducted in the United States and Europe and published in leading Western scientific journals. Here is a sampling of recent findings.

*Arthritis.* Gentle stretching exercises that move sore joints through their full range of motion are a key to managing arthritis. Dr. Connor says yoga stretches and postures encourage range-of-motion movements without unduly stressing arthritic joints.

*Asthma.* Many studies have shown that yoga helps people with asthma reduce the amount of medication they take and gain control over their breathing by relaxing the respiratory system. In 1992, at the annual meeting of the American Academy of Allergy and Immunology in Orlando, Florida, Pudupakkam K. Vedanthan, M.D., an allergist in Fort Collins, Colorado, described a study he conducted. Dr. Vedanthan divided 17 people with asthma, ages 19 to 52, into two groups. Both groups received standard medical care, but one also took part in a yoga class three times a week for 12 weeks. Afterward, the yoga group reported decreased use of asthma medication, fewer bronchial spasms, less anxiety about their condition, improved physical condition and less likelihood of experiencing exercise-induced asthma symptoms.

Several other studies have produced similar results. A 1993 Indian study of 46 people with chronic asthma showed that yoga's benefits—decreased medication needs, improved lung function and ability to exercise—endured one year after the yoga class ceased. A 1991 study showed similar improvement in 46 children with asthma. And a 1990 British experiment showed that yoga eases breathing in people with asthma and reduces the likelihood of asthma attacks.

**Bad moods and low energy levels.** In a 1993 study, British researchers tested three different relaxation techniques—chair sitting, visualization and 30 minutes of yoga—on 71 people ranging in age from 21 to 76. Yoga produced the greatest increase in feelings of alertness, mental and physical energy and enthusiasm for life. "Yoga," the researchers concluded, "is simple to learn and can be practiced even by the elderly. It had a markedly invigorating effect and increased positive mood."

**Diabetes.** People with diabetes who are not dependent on insulin injections may still have trouble maintaining normal blood sugar (glucose) levels. A 1993 Indian experiment enrolled 149 people with Type II, or non-insulin-dependent, diabetes in a yoga class lasting 40 days and then assessed any effects on their condition. Yoga helped normalize their blood glucose levels, reducing their need for medication.

**Mental retardation.** In a 1989 study, scientists at the Yoga Research Foundation in Bangalore, India, divided 90 mentally retarded children into two groups. Both received standard education and medical care, but in addition, one group practiced yoga for five hours a week for one school year. The yoga group showed "highly significant improvement" in IQ and social skills.

(continued on page 520)

# A Yoga Sampler

Most yoga sessions involve 15 to 30 poses. Here are 7 that almost anyone can do. The directions come from two longtime teachers of Iyengar yoga, Donna Farhi, a frequent contributor to *Yoga Journal* who teaches yoga workshops around the world, and Patricia Walden, star of the Yoga for Beginners video, who teaches in Somerville, Massachusetts.

***Mountain Pose.*** The basis for all standing poses, Mountain Pose teaches correct posture, which is a boon to health and well-being even when you're not practicing yoga. Stand with your feet together, your big toes touching, your heels slightly apart and your arms hanging at your sides. (If you feel unstable with your feet together, separate them slightly.) Distribute your weight evenly between your feet and between the ball and heel of each foot. Your kneecaps should face forward. Focus on your pelvis. Balance it atop your legs, neither tucking the tailbone (which pushes the pelvis forward) nor overarching the back (which pushes it back). Feel your body rise upward from your feet. Stretch your inner legs up from the inner heels to the groin. Relax your diaphragm and extend your spine upward from the pelvis. Open your chest. Breathe deeply and slowly from your diaphragm. Drop your shoulders and relax your face and eyes. Your shoulders, hips and heels should be in a line. Hold the pose for up to one minute.

***Jumping to the Wide-Leg Standing Pose.*** Jumping is both a pose and an elegant transition from Mountain Pose to the other standing poses. Do it on a nonslip surface. If you have ankle, knee, hip or back problems or if you are pregnant, however, step instead of jumping. To jump, begin in Mountain Pose, then inhale and bend your knees slightly. Also raise your arms to shoulder height and bend them at the elbow so that your middle fingers touch in front of your lower neck. Then jump your feet outward as you extend your arms straight out. There's no need to jump high. The jump should be silent and graceful.

You should end up with your feet parallel, pointing forward, three to four feet apart and in line with your wrists. To return to Mountain Pose, follow this sequence in reverse.

***Triangle Pose.*** Begin in Mountain Pose, then jump to the Wide-Leg Standing Pose. Pivot on your heels, turning your left foot in 60 degrees and your right foot out 90 degrees. Place a prop block or a pile of books behind your right ankle. Distribute your weight evenly between your feet and the ball and heel of each foot. Spread and lengthen your toes. Do not overextend your knees. Use your front thigh muscles to draw your kneecaps upward.

Inhale, then as you exhale, bend from the hips and extend your torso over your right leg. Place your right hand down on the block. (If you can reach it comfortably, place your hand on the floor.) Raise your left arm over your head, palm forward. On an exhalation, turn your head and look up at your left hand. Feel the floor beneath your feet and relax into lengthening your spine, legs and arms. If your neck begins to ache, look forward.

Hold the pose for up to 30 seconds on each side. Afterward, return to the Wide-Leg Standing Pose and then jump to Mountain Pose.

***Side Stretch Pose.*** Begin in Mountain Pose, then jump your feet wider apart than you would for Triangle Pose, so your ankles and wrists are in line. Turn your left foot in and your right foot out. Bend your front (right) leg so that your thigh and lower leg form a right angle at the knee. Your right knee should be directly above your right ankle. Keep your left leg strong and planted as you bend your right knee. Bending from the hips, extend your torso over your right thigh. Place your right hand on a block (or the floor). Press your feet into the floor and extend your left arm overhead, palm forward. Feel your spine stretch up through the fingertips of your left hand.

On an exhalation, gently turn your neck and look up at the ceiling. Hold the pose for up to one minute on each side. Afterward, return to the Wide-Leg Standing Pose and then jump to Mountain Pose.

***Proud Warrior Pose.*** Begin in Mountain Pose, then jump to Wide-Leg Standing Pose, with your feet under your wrists. Imagine a line from the top of your head down through the center of your torso to your tailbone. Maintain an awareness of this line as you turn your

*(continued)*

## A Yoga Sampler—*Continued*

left foot in and your right foot out. On an exhalation, bend your right knee to form a right angle, with your knee directly over your right ankle. On your next exhalation, turn your head and look at your right hand. Press your feet into the floor and feel your spine lengthen. Afterward, return to the Wide-Leg Standing Pose and then jump to Mountain Pose.

***Standing Forward Bend Number One.*** Begin in Mountain Pose, standing two to three feet behind a chair with your feet parallel and hip-width apart. Place your hands on your hips and on an exhalation, bend forward from the hips. Bend your arms, clasping your elbows. Place your forearms on top of the back of the chair and rest your forehead on your arms. Relax your spine. Hold the pose for up to one minute. Afterward, return to Mountain Pose. (If you're pregnant, don't do this pose; it could strain your back.)

***Standing Forward Bend Number Two.*** Begin in Mountain Pose, standing with your back about one foot away from a wall. Place your palms on the wall and rest your buttocks against the wall. Move your feet about hip-width apart, keeping them parallel. Lengthen and spread your toes. Inhale, placing your hands on your hips. On an exhalation, bend forward from the hips. As you bend forward, bend your arms and clasp your elbows. Relax your spine, releasing your head and neck. Extend your arms beneath your head. Hold for up to one minute. Afterward, return to Mountain Pose. (If you're pregnant, don't do this pose; it could strain your back.

***Pain.*** A 1991 report published in the *International Journal of Psychosomatics* urges physicians to recommend yoga for the management of chronic pain. Effective nondrug approaches to pain control include relaxation training, deep breathing and gentle exercise, all of which are combined in yoga.

***Stress.*** "Deep breathing and moderate exercise are two fundamentals of many stress management programs," Dr. Pullig

Schatz says. "Yoga includes both. Most people who practice regularly usually say it helps them control everyday stresses, tensions and anxieties."

Yoga also helps improve the overall level of physical conditioning. In a 1993 study, Indian researchers recruited 40 physical education teachers who were in excellent shape but had never done yoga. They measured the teachers' blood pressure, lung function, heart and respiratory rates and hand steadiness before and after three months of yoga training. Despite the teachers' admirable initial physical condition, yoga conferred many benefits: improved lung function, reduced blood pressure, decreased heart and respiratory rates and improved hand steadiness.

A 1992 Indian study tested yoga's effects on hand grip strength and reaction times to visual and auditory cues. Twenty-seven college students were tested before and after 12 weeks of yoga training. The class significantly increased their grip strength and improved their reaction times. Faster reaction times suggest that yoga might improve highway safety.

"Exercise advocates generally tout aerobic exercise for cardiovascular fitness," Dr. Connor says. "Cardiovascular fitness is certainly worth developing, but aerobic exercise isn't everything. The body also needs workouts that build flexibility, and it's hard to top yoga for flexibility."

Finally, yoga offers mental and spiritual benefits, Dr. Connor says. "They're hard to measure, but most people who practice regularly report mental invigoration and feelings of greater well-being. I don't consider yoga a religion. But many people say that like meditation, it has deepened their appreciation for the spiritual side of life."

Of course, yoga is no cure-all. Dr. Conner and Dr. Pullig Schatz say that people with asthma, arthritis, diabetes, back problems and other medical conditions should not throw away their medications or abandon their physicians in favor of yoga classes. "But in addition to regular medical care, yoga can be quite beneficial for many chronic illnesses," Dr. Connor says.

# Yoga, American-Style

To many Americans, the 4,000-year-old art of yoga is still an exotic import from India, a workout for spiritual seekers who have gurus. But during the century since Swami Vivekananda was first applauded for his yoga performance at the 1893 Chicago World's Fair, yoga's combination of gentle postures, stretches and deep breathing has become as American as several other Indian imports, such as ginger and cinnamon.

The word yoga comes from the Sanskrit for "yoke," as in the joining of two oxen in a disciplined union. To appreciate what yoga is, it helps to understand what it is not. It's not a religion, although it developed from Hinduism. It's not calisthenics, although it works up a sweat and tones and strengthens the muscles and joints as well as—or better than—most forms of exercise. And it's not meditation, although its slow pace, deep breathing and focus on the moment open a door to meditative relaxation. Longtime practitioners describe yoga as a physical path to uniting the mind, body and spirit.

There are six major types of yoga, but only two have gained a foothold in the West—hatha yoga and tantra yoga. Hatha is by far the more popular. It's what people mean when they say "yoga"—the stretches and postures Indian yoga masters call asanas. Hatha means "forceful," which is ironic because a hallmark of American yoga is its gentleness. But hatha yoga's roots penetrate deep into the same spiritual soil that nurtured the martial arts in China, the energy that uses physical determination to achieve spiritual goals.

Today there are several schools of hatha yoga. The most popular is Iyengar yoga, developed by B. K. S. Iyengar, who modified the classic hatha poses for the comfort of Western practitioners.

Tantra yoga is a meditative form of self-transcendence through elaborate rituals, including ritual sexuality, the focus of its practice in the West. But genuine tantra involves a great deal more than sex; many Indian schools of tantra yoga recommend celibacy.

Hatha yoga dates back to the eleventh century, when Gorakshanatha distilled several thousand years of yogic practices into the forerunners of the asanas practiced today, focusing on posture and breath control (pranayama). Hatha yoga was meant for what Hindus call kali-yuga, a time when few people can devote themselves entirely to spiritual pursuits yet still crave some activity that unites the mind, body and spirit.

## How to Learn the Moves

The best way to learn yoga, Dr. Pullig Schatz says, is to enroll in a class taught by a well-trained teacher you like. "There are many different styles of yoga," she says, "but Iyengar yoga instructors are rigorously trained, not only in the postures themselves but also in adapting them to beginners and to those with disabilities, chronic illnesses or other special needs."

Yoga classes abound around the United States, in every metropolitan area and in many out-of-the-way places as well. Ask friends, inquire at your local gym or aerobic studio or look in the Yellow Pages under Yoga.

If you're traveling or can't get to a yoga class, you can turn on the TV and do yoga with Lilias, whose early-morning program is nationally syndicated on PBS. "She's very good," Dr. Connor says. Or try *Yoga for Beginners*, an engaging 75-minute video produced by *Yoga Journal*, a monthly magazine devoted to yoga and a leading resource in the field.

Dr. Connor says yoga is "generally safe" but says some postures aren't for everyone. "Depending on a person's disease or disability, certain poses might cause problems," he says. "Headstands can be a problem for people with glaucoma. And certain stretches might need to be modified for people with back, knee or other musculoskeletal problems. But one of yoga's attractions is that, unlike so many other forms of exercise, good teachers can usually adapt the postures to the special needs of people with chronic medical conditions. Yoga is usually a good form of exercise for people with health problems."

Before enrolling in a yoga class (or starting any exercise program), people over 60 or those with disabilities or chronic medical conditions should consult their physicians. In addition, anyone with a medical problem who decides to pursue yoga should confer with the teacher before enrolling to discuss modifying or abstaining from any problematic postures.

## For Best Results

Once you've found a teacher and learned some postures, here are some tips to enhance your practice. These come from Iyengar yoga teachers Hart Lazer of Winnipeg, Canada, and Donald Moyer of Berkeley, California.

**Be a regular.** Devote at least one session a week to yoga. The ideal would be one session a day at the same time six days a week, with the seventh a rest day.

**Pick your space.** Practice in a clean, quiet, flat space, out of direct sunlight.

**Think empty.** Don't eat for two hours before practicing.

**Feel good.** Practice only when you're in reasonably good health. Don't practice when you feel ill, especially if you have a fever.

**Go easy on yourself.** Learn to distinguish between stretching sensations, which are beneficial, and pain, which is not. If you feel any sharp pain, stop what you are doing and try to modify the pose. If pain persists, stop doing the posture until you consult a yoga teacher.

**Honor your cycles.** During menstruation, women should not perform inverted postures—headstands or shoulder stands. And consult a yoga teacher about practicing while pregnant. Abdominal postures are not recommended, and others will need to be modified as pregnancy progresses.

**Don't forget to warm up.** Begin yoga sessions with several nondemanding warm-up postures.

**Stay focused.** While practicing, keep your mind on the pose, your breathing and your emotional responses to your practice of yoga.

**Flow into postures.** "In each pose," Iyengar quips, "there should be repose." Don't bounce into postures or force yourself into them. Allow them to develop gradually. Beginners who cannot perform the postures unassisted should use props: a chair, blocks or books and rolled-up towels or blankets.

# BIBLIOGRAPHY NOTE

Space limitations preclude listing the 148 books, 244 medical journal articles and 257 other resources used to prepare *Nature's Cures*. To obtain the complete bibliography, send a check or money order for $4 (for reproduction, postage and handling), payable to: Self-Care Associates, P.O. Box 460066, San Francisco, CA 94146-0066. Please allow three weeks for delivery.

# RESOURCES

*Nature's Cures* emphasizes self-care, but some natural therapies may require professional practitioners. This list of resources can help you find them. In addition, each year the *Holistic Health Directory* publishes a comprehensive national guide that lists the names, addresses, phone numbers and specialties of more than 7,000 practitioners throughout the United States. For more information, write to the Holistic Health Directory, 42 Pleasant St., Watertown, MA 02172.

## Acupuncture

**Books**

*Acupressure's Potent Points: A Guide to Self-Care for Common Ailments* by Michael Reed Gach (New York: Bantam Books, 1990). The best book on acupressure. Gach, founder and director of the Acupressure Institute of America in Berkeley, California, provides clear, concise, step-by-step directions for using about 75 points to treat 40 common conditions, including allergies, anxiety, arthritis, asthma, back pain, constipation, headaches, insomnia, motion sickness and sinus problems.

*Between Heaven and Earth: A Guide to Chinese Medicine* by Harriet Beinfield and Efrem Korngold (New York: Ballantine Books, 1991). The best in-depth introduction to Chinese medical philosophy. More than any other guide, it explains Chinese medicine in terms Western readers can comprehend.

*Beyond Yin and Yang: How Acupuncture Really Works* by George A. Ulett (St. Louis, Mo.: Warren H. Green, 1992). A fascinating though technical treatise by one of the few American scientists who has seriously researched acupuncture.

*Bioenergetic Medicine East and West: Acupuncture and Homeopathy* by Clark A. Manning and Louis J. Vanrenen (Berkeley, Calif.: North Atlantic Books, 1988). This engaging book makes the case that both Chinese medicine and homeopathy work because of their subtle but powerful neuroelectrical effects.

*Feet First: A Guide to Foot Reflexology* by Laura Norman and Thomas Cowan (New York: Fireside/Simon & Schuster, 1988). This is a good reference. Norman also conducts training programs around the country. (For information, contact Laura Norman and Associates Reflexology Center, 41 Park Ave. #8-A, New York, NY 10016.)

*The Web That Has No Weaver: Understanding Chinese Medicine* by Ted Kaptchuk (New York: Congdon and Weed, 1983). This was the first book to explain Chinese medicine to a Western audience. Though somewhat less accessible than *Between Heaven and Earth*, it's still excellent.

## Organizations

The Acupressure Institute of America
1533 Shattuck Ave.
Berkeley, CA 94709
The institute, founded by Michael Reed Gach, offers several acupuncture training programs.

American Academy of Medical Acupuncture (AAMA)
5820 Wilshire Blvd., Suite 500
Los Angeles, CA 90036
Open to M.D.'s and D.O.'s who practice acupuncture, the AAMA sponsors a certification program that requires 200 hours of training and two years' experience. For referrals to AAMA members in your area, contact the AAMA.

* * * *

National Commission for the Certification of Acupuncturists (NCCA)
1424 16th St. NW
Washington, DC 20036
More than 3,000 acupuncturists have been certified around the United States. Contact the organization for referrals to certified practitioners in your state.

# Aromatherapy

**Books**

   *The Aromatherapy Book* by Jeanne Rose (Berkeley, Calif.: North Atlantic Books, 1992). A quirky, personal, often delightful guide by one of the nation's best-known herbalists.

   *The Aromatherapy Workbook* by Marcel Lavabre (Rochester, Vt.: Healing Arts Press, 1990). An excellent brief introduction.

   *The Complete Book of Essential Oils and Aromatherapy* by Valerie Ann Worwood (San Rafael, Calif.: New World Library, 1991). The most comprehensive guide to home medical aromatherapy.

**Products**

   More than 100 essential oils, plus a large variety of aromatic soaps, candles, bath and massage oils and hair- and skin-care products. For a free catalog, contact:
Aroma-Vera, Inc.
5901 Rodeo Rd.
Los Angeles, CA 90016-4312

   Approximately 75 essential oils; specializes in creating natural perfumes. For a free catalog, contact:
Santa Fe Fragrance
P.O. Box 282
Santa Fe, NM 87504

Approximately 60 essential oils. For a free catalog, contact:
Windrose Aromatics
12629 N. Tatum Blvd., Suite 611
Phoenix, AZ 85032

# Biofeedback

## Organization
Association for Applied Psychophysiology and Biofeedback
10200 West 44th Ave., Suite 304
Wheat Ridge, CO 80033
This international organization has more than 2,000 members
who teach and do research in biofeedback. It also operates the
Biofeedback Certification Institute of America, which grants credentials to biofeedback therapists. Write for a list of certified
biofeedback therapists.

## Products
Home biofeedback equipment—the GSR-2—with an instruction booklet and several programs that combine the device
with visualization audiotapes for specific personal goals: improving athletic performance, overcoming dental phobia, flying
relaxed, enhancing immune function, relieving insomnia, overcoming chemical dependency, controlling pain, managing stress,
taking tests and speaking in public with greater confidence, and
losing weight. For information, contact:
Thought Technology
2180 Belgrave Ave.
Montreal, Quebec H4A-2L8, Canada

# Cognitive Therapy

## Book
*The Feeling Good Handbook* by David D. Burns (New York:
Plume/Penguin Books, 1989). A pioneering book about cognitive therapy.

**Program**
Depression/Awareness, Recognition and Treatment (D/ART)
National Institute of Mental Health
Rockville, MD 20857
1-800-421-4211
This program provides free information on depression. If you are in crisis or know someone who is, D/ART does not offer counseling but can refer you to a crisis center near you.

# Companionship

**Book**
    *We Can Work It Out: Making Sense of Marital Conflict* by Howard Markham and Clifford Notarius (New York: Putnam, 1993). Thought-provoking first-aid for couples who feel stuck in a fight style they dislike.

**Organizations**
American Self-Help Clearinghouse (ASHC)
St. Clares–Riverside Medical Center
Denville, NJ 07834
This organization focuses primarily on self-help groups in New Jersey. People from other states are usually referred to their own state or regional self-help clearinghouses—which currently number about 35—or to the national organization that deals with their concern, which can often refer them to a group in their area. The best way to find a support group or launch one is to buy a copy of Edward Madara's *Self-Help Sourcebook,* which describes groups around the country that deal with more than 600 concerns. It also lists every state and regional self-help clearinghouse in the United States and Canada. For information, contact the ASHC.

Prevention and Relationship Enhancement Program (PREP)
1780 S. Bellaire St., Suite 621
Denver, CO 80222
Write for information about weekend workshops.

# Complementary Cancer Care

## Book

*Choices in Healing: Integrating the Best of the Conventional and Complementary Approaches to Cancer* by Michael Lerner (Cambridge, Mass.: MIT Press, 1994). A comprehensive look at complementary cancer care around the world.

## Programs

Besides the two listed below, hundreds of cancer support groups meet regularly around the country. For referrals, contact the American Cancer Society or other cancer organizations in your area or ask your oncologist for a referral to a social worker knowledgeable about community cancer resources.

Commonweal Cancer Help Program
P.O. Box 316
Bolinas, CA 94924
Founded by Michael Lerner, this organization sponsors six week-long Cancer Help Programs a year. About ten people with cancer attend each session, typically more women than men. Participants have every type of cancer, but the most frequent diagnosis is breast cancer. Participants may bring a spouse or significant other, but most come by themselves.

The Wellness Community (TWC)
2716 Ocean Park Blvd., Suite 1040
Santa Monica, CA 90405
TWC facilities currently operate in seven states: California, Maryland, Massachusetts, Missouri, Ohio, Pennsylvania and Tennessee.

# Dreams

## Books

*Exploring the World of Lucid Dreaming* by Stephen La Berge and Howard Rheingold (New York: Ballantine Books,

1990). An elaboration on LaBerge's earlier book, *Lucid Dreaming*, with exercises to increase the likelihood of having lucid dreams.

*The Healing Power of Dreams* by Patricia Garfield (New York: Fireside/Simon & Schuster, 1992). An intimate look at using dreams to point to diagnoses and recovery from illness and trauma.

*Lucid Dreaming* by Stephen LaBerge (New York: Ballantine Books, 1985). An introduction to conscious dreaming.

*The Sleepwatchers* by William Dement (Stanford, Calif.: Stanford Alumni Association, 1992). A fascinating, amusing tour through sleep research by a leading authority (Stanford Alumni Association, Bowman Alumni House, Stanford, CA 94305-4005).

*What Your Dreams Can Teach You* by Alex Lukeman (St. Paul, Minn.: Llewellyn Publications, 1990). A guide to exploring what your unique dreams mean for you. P.O. Box 64383-475, St. Paul, MN 55164-0383.

**Magazine**
*Dream Network*
1337 Powerhouse Lane, Suite 32
Moab, UT 84532
A magazine devoted to dreams as tools for personal growth, change and healing.

**Organization**
The Lucidity Institute
2555 Park Blvd., Suite 2
Palo Alto, CA 94306
The institute, founded by Stephen LaBerge, Ph.D., markets DreamLink, NovaDreamer and DreamLight, devices for inducing lucid dreams. Income from the sale of these products finances continuing investigations of lucid dreaming. The institute also publishes a quarterly newsletter, *NightLight,* and sponsors workshops and a home study course on lucid dreaming. Free catalog.

## Elimination Diets

**Books**

*In Bad Taste: The MSG Syndrome* by George Schwartz (Santa Fe, N.M.: HealthPress, 1988).

*The Complete Guide to Food Allergy and Intolerance* by Jonathan Brostoff and Linda Gamlin (New York: Crown, 1989).

*The Multiple Sclerosis Diet Book: A Low-Fat Diet for the Treatment of MS* by Roy. L. Swank and Barbara B. Dugan (New York: Doubleday, 1987).

**Organizations**

Food Allergy Network
4744 Holly Ave.
Fairfax, VA 22030
The network's purpose is to provide educational material, coping strategies and emotional support. Write for free information.

## The Healing Foods

**Books**

*Food—Your Miracle Medicine* by Jean Carper (New York: HarperCollins, 1993).

*The Healing Foods* by Patricia Hausman and Judith Benn Hurley (Emmaus, Pa.: Rodale Press, 1989).

## Healing Humor

**Book**

*The Healing Power of Humor* by Allen Klein (Los Angeles: Jeremy Tarcher, 1989).

**Newspaper**

*Funny Times: A Monthly Humor Review*
3108 Scarborough Rd.
Cleveland Heights, OH 44118
This newspaper scours the print media for cartoons, jokes and humorous stories.

**Organizations**
American Association of Therapeutic Humor
222 South Merimac #303
St. Louis, MO 63105
A professional organization of nurses, psychologists, clergy and social workers who use humor in their work. Write for free information.

Big Apple Circus Clown Care Unit
35 W. 35th St.
New York, NY 10011
This group works in hospitals, cheering children with "clown rounds."

Carolina Health and Humor Association/Ruth Hamilton
5223 Revere Rd.
Durham, NC 27713
This group is responsible for the Laugh Mobile for cancer patients at the Duke University Medical Center.

Comedy Carts/Leslie Gibson
430 Park Place Blvd.
Clearwater, FL 34619-3926
Members of this group tour hospitals with carts that supply all types of humorous materials—books, videos, games and gags—for patients.

The Humor Project
110 Spring St.
Saratoga Springs, NY 12866-3397
Founded by Joel Goodman, Ed.D., the project sponsors an annual conference in Saratoga Springs on "The Positive Power of Humor and Creativity." Speakers have included Jay Leno, Steve Allen and Bernie Siegel, M.D. The project publishes a "jest-selling" quarterly magazine, Laughing Matters, and Humo–Resources, an extensive catalog of materials both silly and serious about using humor for fun and profit. It also provides "fun-

ding" for innovative efforts to incorporate humor into the serious business of life.

# Healthy Habits

## Books

*How to Become Naturally Thin by Eating More* by Jean Antonello (New York: Avon Books, 1989). Antonello argues persuasively that fear is the key obstacle to major life changes.

*The No-Nag, No-Guilt, Do-It-Your-Own-Way Guide to Quitting Smoking* by Tom Ferguson (New York: Ballantine 1988). This is the best book on quitting. Dr. Ferguson, an ex-smoker himself, was asked by the American Cancer Society to offer suggestions for improving the organization's smoking cessation program. He asked 200 smokers what information would help them quit and then compiled it in a book that thoroughly lives up to its title.

## Organization

American Self-Help Clearinghouse (ASHC)
Saint Clares–Riverside Medical Center
Denville, NJ, 07834
If there's a self-help group that deals with your bad habit, the ASHC can put you in touch with it. If not, the ASHC can help you launch one in your area. Their database includes thousands of groups around the country.

# Herbal Healing

## Books

*The Healing Herbs* by Michael Castleman (Emmaus, Pa.: Rodale Press, 1991). A comprehensive guide to using medicinal herbs confidently, effectively and safely.

*Herbal Medicine* by Rudolf Fritz Weiss (London, England: Beaconsfield Publishers, 1988). Herbal medicine is much more mainstream in Germany than it is in the United States, and Dr. Weiss is a leading German physician who specializes in herbal therapy. This is a medical text for those who want technical information.

*Natural Health, Natural Healing* by Andrew Weil (New York: Houghton Mifflin, 1990). Has an excellent introduction to herbal medicine.

## Magazine

*HerbalGram*
American Botanical Council
P.O. Box 201660
Austin, TX 78720
The best source for recent new herbal medicine research.

## Products

A selection of 350 herbs and spices. For a free catalog, contact:
Nature's Herbs
1010 46th St.
Emeryville, CA 94608

More than 200 herbs. For a free catalog, contact:
The Herb and Spice Collection
P.O. Box 118
Norway, IA 52318

# Homeopathy

## Books

*Discovering Homeopathy: Your Introduction to the Science and Art of Homeopathic Medicine* by Dana Ullman (Berkeley, Calif: North Atlantic Books, 1991).

*Everybody's Guide to Homeopathic Medicines* by Stephen Cummings and Dana Ullman (Los Angeles: Jeremy Tarcher, 1991).

*Homeopathy at Home: Natural Remedies for Everyday Ailments and Minor Injuries* by M. B. Panos and Jane Heimlich (Los Angeles: Jeremy Tarcher, 1980).

**Organization**
National Center for Homeopathy
801 North Fairfax #306
Alexandria, VA 22314
Promotes homeopathy, sponsors a training program and study groups around the country and publishes a monthly magazine, *Homeopathy Today.*

**Products**
A large selection of homeopathic books, medicines and other resources. For a free catalog, contact:
Homeopathic Educational Services
2124 Kittredge St.
Berkeley CA 94704

# Heat and Cold Therapies

**Book**
*Fodor's Healthy Escapes* by Bernard Burt (New York: Fodor, 1993). This book from the well-known travel publisher describes 250 health spas around North America. Available from bookstores.

# Low-Fat Eating

**Books**
*Choose to Lose: A Food Lover's Guide to Permanent Weight Loss* by Ron Goor and Nancy Goor (Boston: Houghton Mifflin, 1995). An excellent guide to low-fat eating that limits total fat to less than 20 percent of calories. With 73 recipes.

*Eat More, Weigh Less: Dr. Dean Ornish's Life Choice Program for Losing Weight Safely While Eating Abundantly* by Dean Ornish (New York: HarperCollins, 1993). An excellent guide to ultra-low-fat eating. With 250 recipes by famous chefs. All recipes derive less than 10 percent of calories from fat.

*Eater's Choice: A Food Lover's Guide to Lower Cholesterol* by Ron Goor and Nancy Goor. A fine introduction to lower-fat eating that focuses on limiting saturated fat to less than 10 percent of calories. With more than 300 delicious recipes for soups, chicken, turkey, fish, seafood, vegetables, pizza, pastas, breads, salads, sandwiches and desserts.

# Massage

**Book and Videos**

*Accepting Your Power to Heal: The Personal Practice of Therapeutic Touch* by Dolores Krieger (Santa Fe, N.M.: Bear, 1993).

"Massage Your Mate." This 92-minute, color VHS cassette has a misleading title, because it's not just for spouses. It's recommended by the American Massage Therapy Association. Rebecca Klinger, a licensed massage therapist in New York, is your guide through this excellent introduction to Swedish and shiatsu techniques (V.I.E.W. Video, 34 East 23rd St., New York, NY 10010).

"Massage for Health." Shari Belafonte Harper (Harry Belafonte's daughter) is part of the ensemble cast in this 70-minute, color VHS cassette that also introduces viewers to a relaxing combination of Swedish and shiatsu massages. Includes a 40-page booklet (Healing Arts, 321 Hampton Dr., Suite 203, Venice, CA 90291).

**Organizations**

American Massage Therapy Association (AMTA)
820 Davis St., Suite 1000
Evanston, IL 60201
The association provides referrals to certified massage therapists and certified massage schools in your area.

Associated Professional Massage Therapists and Bodyworkers (APMTB)
1746 Cold Blvd. Suite 225
Golden, CO 80401
This group works to promote professional massage and bodywork.

# Meditation

**Book and Audiotapes**

*Full Catastrophe Living: Using the Wisdom of Your Body and Mind to Face Stress, Pain and Illness* by Jon Kabat-Zinn (New York: Delta, 1990). An exhaustive discussion of meditation, with instruction in mantra and breath meditation, mindfulness, body scan, autogenic training and progressive muscle relaxation.

Harvard cardiologist Herbert Benson, M.D., has developed a series of audiocassettes that teach the relaxation response and mindfulness, body scan, autogenic training and progressive muscle relaxation. For a free catalog, contact:

Mind/Body Medical Institute
Deaconess Hospital
185 Pilgrim Rd., Boston, MA 02215

Jon Kabat-Zinn, Ph.D., has also produced a series of audiotapes covering meditation and body scan. For information, contact:

Stress Reduction Tapes
P.O. Box 547
Lexington, MA 02173

# Mind/Body Healing

**Newsletter**

*Mental Medicine Update*
Institute for the Study of Human Knowledge
P.O. Box 176, Los Altos, CA 94023
Edited by David Sobel, M.D., and Robert Ornstein, Ph.D., this is a lively, scientifically referenced quarterly newsletter of mind/body healing.

# Music Therapy

**Book**

*Healthy Pleasures* by Robert Ornstein and David Sobel (Reading, Mass.: Addison-Wesley, 1989).

**Organizations**

American Association for Music Therapy
P.O. Box 80012
King of Prussia, PA 1948-0012
The association provides information about music therapy and referrals to training programs and therapists.

The Bonny Foundation
2020 Simmons St.
Salina, KS 67104
Helen Bonny founded this organization to promote her program of guided imagery and music. Write for information.

Hearing Education and Awareness for Rockers (H.E.A.R.)
P.O. Box 460847
San Francisco, CA 94146
This group educates young people about the hazards of noise, particularly loud rock music.

National Association for Music Therapy
8455 Colesville Rd., Suite 930
Silver Spring, MD 20910
The association provides information about music therapy and referrals to training programs and therapists.

**Products**

Original sedative music by Steven Halpern. A newsletter, *Brainwaves, Relaxation, and Music,* is also available. For a free catalog, contact:
Sound Rx
P.O. Box 2644
San Anselmo, CA 94979

Original sedative music by Marcey Hamm. For a free catalog, contact:
Music by Marcey
Box 831210
Richardson, TX 75083

# Sleep

**Book**

*No More Sleepless Nights* by Peter Hauri and Shirley Linde (New York: Wiley & Sons, 1991). The best self-care guide to overcoming insomnia.

**Organization**

American Sleep Disorders Association (ASDA)
1610 14th St., NW
Rochester, MN 55901
The ASDA refers to the more than 125 accredited sleep centers in the United States.

# Tai Chi and Chi Gong

**Book and Video**

*Ride the Tiger to the Mountain: Tai Chi for Health* by Martin and Emily Lee and JoAn Johnstone (Reading, Mass: Addison-Wesley, 1991). A poetic introduction to tai chi, with directions for performing a form.

"Tai Chi for Health" with Terry Dunn. A two-hour color video that teaches one tai chi form. (Healing Arts Publishing, 321 Hampton Dr., Venice, CA 90291).

For other books and videos about tai chi, chi gong and the martial arts, contact:
Wayfarer Publications
P.O. Box 26156
Los Angeles, CA 90026

# Vegetarianism

**Books**

*Food for Life* by Neal Barnard (New York: Crown, 1993).
*Green Groceries: A Mail Order Guide to Organic Foods* by Jeanne Heifetz (New York: HarperPerennial, 1992).

*The Juicing Book* by Stephen Blauer (Garden City, N.Y.: Avery, 1989).

For other books about vegetarianism, many of which are hard to find in bookstores, contact:
The Mail Order Catalog
P.O. Box 180
Summerton, TN 38483

**Magazines**
*Organic Gardening*
33 East Minor St.
Emmaus, PA 18098
Published by Rodale Press, *Organic Gardening* is a respected source of information on growing foods organically.

*Vegetarian Journal*
P.O. Box 1463
Baltimore, MD 21203
Published by the Vegetarian Resource Group, this is a national guide to vegetarian restaurants and other information.

*Vegetarian Times*
P.O. Box 570
Oak Park, IL 60303
1-800-435-9610
The best all-around guide, this monthly magazine emphasizes the health advantages of vegetarianism, and each issue contains many good recipes.

# Vitamins and Minerals

**Books**
*The Doctor's Vitamin and Mineral Encyclopedia* by Sheldon Saul Hendler (New York: Fireside/Simon & Schuster, 1990). Written by an authority with a firm grasp of the scientific literature, this book is fully referenced and discusses prudent dose ranges for preventive and optimal health purposes. It contains

comprehensive discussions of possible toxicity and interactions with drugs and other nutrients.

*Prevention's Food and Nutrition* by the editors of *Prevention* magazine (Emmaus, Pa.: Rodale Press, 1993). More than just a supplement guide, this book is a nutritional encyclopedia.

*The Real Vitamin and Mineral Book* by Shari Lieberman and Nancy Bruning (Garden City, N.Y.: Avery, 1990). With many of the same features as *The Doctor's Vitamin and Mineral Encyclopedia*, this book is authoritative and comprehensive.

# Vision Therapy

**Organizations**
Cambridge Institute for Better Vision
65 Wenham Rd.
Topsfield, MA 01983
The institute sponsors weekend vision-improvement workshops around the country and markets a do-it-yourself home study course that includes a manual, three audiocassettes and some vision therapy activity items. Executive director Martin Sussman is co-author (with Ernest Loewenstein and Howard Sann) of *Total Health at the Computer* (Barrytown, N.Y.: Station Hill Press, 1993).

Optometric Extension Program
2912 South Daimler St.
Santa Ana, CA 92705
The program promotes behavioral optometry and vision therapy and publishes many brochures, books and training materials related to vision therapy for both behavioral optometrists and the public, particularly educators.

Vision WorkOut
911 West Moana Lane
Reno, NV 89509
This is a video-based home program of eye exercises and relaxation techniques for a wide range of eye problems.

# Visualization, Guided Imagery and Self-Hypnosis

## Book and Audiotapes

*Total Visualization: Using All Five Senses* by William Fezler (Englewood Cliffs, N.J.: Prentice-Hall, 1992). An excellent introduction to visualization, with descriptions of 35 different scenes, including a farm, a mountain cabin, a mansion, a jungle, a picnic and a hayloft.

In addition to basic relaxation tapes, psychiatrist Emmett Miller, M.D., a pioneer in visualization cassettes, offers tapes for specific health and behavior problems, among them "Smoke No More," "The Sleep Tape," "Imagine Yourself Slim," "Letting Go of Stress," "Free Yourself from Fear," "Successful Surgery and Recovery," "Images for Optimal Health" and "Positive Images for People with Cancer." Contact:
Source Cassette Learning Systems
P.O. Box W
Stanford, CA 94305

Martin Rossman, M.D., and pain specialist David Bressler, Ph.D., offer a six-tape series on illness recovery and health enhancement ("Healing Yourself"), and many visualization tapes for specific health and behavior problems, including "Mind-Controlled Anesthesia for Pain," "A Restful Sleep," "Listening to Symptoms," "Chest Pain, Anxiety and Heartbreak" and "Forgiveness in Healing." Contact:
The Image Store
P.O. Box 2070
Mill Valley, CA 94942

## Organizations

Society for Clinical and Experimental Hypnosis
6728 Old McLean Village Dr.
McLean, VA 22101

American Society of Clinical Hypnosis
2200 East Devon Ave., Suite 291
Des Plaines, IL 60018

Both of these professional organizations represent physicians, dentists, psychologists and social workers who use and investigate hypnosis. Contact either one for referrals to qualified hypnotherapists in your area. Include a stamped, self-addressed envelope.

# Walking

**Organizations**
American Hiking Society (AHS)
P.O. Box 21060
Washington, DC 20041
The AHS boasts more than 300,000 members in more than 100 affiliated hiking clubs. $25 annual membership includes the quarterly magazine, *American Hiker*.

American Volkssport Association (AVA)
Phoenix Square, Suite 203
1001 Pat Booker Rd.
Universal City, TX 78148
Volks is German for "folks." This organization of more than 600 local clubs sponsors noncompetitive, family-oriented events in walking, bicycling, swimming and cross-country skiing.

Creative Walking, Inc.
P.O. Box 50296
Clayton, MO 63105
Rob Sweetgall is the founder and president of this organization that trains more than 35,000 educators and corporate and health-care managers a year to support walking programs in schools, corporations, and health care facilities. Write for information on Sweetgall's 96-page book, *Walking Off Weight*, or a free catalog of other publications.

Pedestrian Federation of America (PFA)
1818 R St. NW
Washington, DC 20009

An offshoot of the Bicycle Federation of America, the PFA organizes walking events and acts as an advocate for pedestrian safety.

# Weight Training

**Video**

"Keys to Weight Training for Men and Women." This 80-minute video uses ordinary people of all ages as models for the strength-training program. The exercises were developed in consultation with biomechanics specialist Gary Moran, Ph.D., a fellow of the American College of Sports Medicine. The program host is Bill Pearl, a professional weight-training coach. A 20-page booklet and training log are included (KTWT Productions, 2040 Polk St., San Francisco, CA 94109).

# Yoga

**Books and Videos**

*Back Care Basics* by Mary Pullig Schatz (Berkeley, Calif.: Rodmell Press, 1992). You don't have to have a bad back to benefit from this clear, basic introduction to yoga.

*Gentle Yoga: For People with Arthritis, Stroke Damage, Multiple Sclerosis, in Wheelchairs, or Anyone Who Needs a Guide to Gentle Exercise* by Lorna Bell and Eudora Seyfer (Berkeley, Calif.: Celestial Arts, 1987).

*Light on Yoga*, rev. ed., by B. K. S. Iyengar (New York: Schocken Books, 1979). Iyengar's adaptations of the classic postures were instrumental in popularizing yoga in the United States. Includes 600 photos.

"Yoga for Beginners." Produced by *Yoga Journal*, this 75-minute, color video stars Patricia Walden, who teaches at the B. K. S. Iyengar Yoga Center in Somerville, Massachusetts. Comes with a 52-page instruction booklet (Healing Arts Publishing, 321 Hampton Dr., Suite 203, Venice, CA 90921). *Yoga Journal* and Healing Arts have also collaborated on three other videos: "Yoga for Relaxation," "Yoga for Flexibility" and "Yoga for Strength."

**Magazine**
*Yoga Journal*
2054 University Ave.
Berkeley, CA 94704
The most comprehensive yoga resource, this magazine lists classes and workshops around the country.

# INDEX

Note: <u>Underscored</u> page references indicate boxed text.

# ABOUT THE AUTHOR

Michael Castleman has been called "one of the nation's leading health and medical writers" (*Portland Oregonian*). He is the author of seven previous consumer medical guides, including *The Healing Herbs* (Rodale Press, 1991). In addition, he writes frequently for many national magazines and teaches health and medical writing as an adjunct professor in the Graduate School of Journalism at the University of California at Berkeley. He lives in San Francisco with his wife, who is a family physician, and their two children.